D1433687

Core Topics in Obstetric Anaesthesia

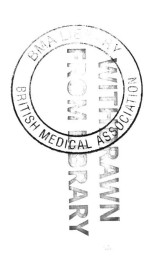

Core Topics in Obstetric Anaesthesia

Edited by

Kirsty MacLennan
Consultant Obstetric Anaesthetist, St Mary's Hospital, Central Manchester University Hospitals NHS Trust, Manchester, UK

Kate O'Brien
Consultant Obstetric Anaesthetist, St Mary's Hospital, Central Manchester University Hospitals NHS Trust, Manchester, UK

W. Ross Macnab
Consultant Obstetric Anaesthetist, St Mary's Hospital, Central Manchester University Hospitals NHS Trust, Manchester, UK

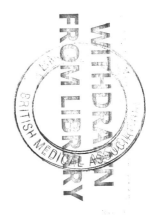

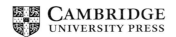

CAMBRIDGE
UNIVERSITY PRESS

CAMBRIDGE
UNIVERSITY PRESS

University Printing House, Cambridge CB2 8BS, United Kingdom

Cambridge University Press is part of the University of Cambridge.

It furthers the University's mission by disseminating knowledge in the pursuit of education, learning and research at the highest international levels of excellence.

www.cambridge.org
Information on this title: www.cambridge.org/9781107028494

© Cambridge University Press 2015

First published 2015

Printed in the United Kingdom by TJ International Ltd. Padstow Cornwall

A catalogue record for this publication is available from the British Library

Library of Congress Cataloguing in Publication data
Core topics in obstetric anaesthesia / edited by Kirsty MacLennan, Consultant Obstetric Anaesthetist, St Mary's Hospital, Central Manchester, University Hospitals NHS Trust, Manchester, UK, Katherine O'Brien, Consultant Obstetric Anaesthetist, St Mary's Hospital, Central Manchester, University Hospitals NHS Trust, Manchester, UK, William MacNab, Consultant Obstetric Anaesthetist, St Mary's Hospital, Central Manchester, University Hospitals NHS Trust, Manchester, UK.
   pages   cm
ISBN 978-1-107-02849-4 (hardback)
1. Anesthesia in obstetrics.   I. MacLennan, Kirsty.   II. O'Brien, Katherine, 1962–   III. MacNab, William, 1969–
RG732.C68   2015
617.9′682–dc23

2015021141

ISBN 978-1-107-02849-4 Hardback

....

Contents

Contents

Contributors

Cathy Armstrong
Consultant Anaesthetist, Manchester Royal
Infirmary, Manchester, UK

Dougal Atkinson
Consultant in Anaesthesia and Critical Care, Central
Manchester University Hospitals, Manchester, UK

Jacqueline E. A. K. Bamfo
Subspeciality Trainee in Maternal Fetal Medicine, Fetal
Medicine Unit, St Mary's Hospital, Manchester, UK

Kailash Bhatia
Consultant Anaesthetist, Department of Anaesthesia,
Central Manchester University Hospitals NHS
Foundation Trust, Manchester, UK

Sophie Bishop
Consultant Anaesthetist, University Hospital of South
Manchester, Wythenshawe, UK

Karen Butler
Consultant Anaesthetist, Anaesthetic Department,
Blackburn Hospital, Blackburn, UK

Craig Carroll
Consultant Neuroanaesthetist, Salford Royal Hospital
NHS Foundation Trust, Salford, UK

K. Chan
Consultant Obstetrician, Department of Obstetrics
and Fetal Medicine Unit, St Mary's Hospital,
Manchester, UK

Desiree M. A. Choi
Consultant Obstetric Anaesthetist, Nuffield
Department of Anaesthetics, John Radcliffe Hospital,
Oxford, UK

Ross Clark
Consultant Obstetric Anaesthetist, Central
Manchester University Hospitals NHS Foundation
Trust, Manchester, UK

Ian Clegg
Consultant Anaesthetist, East Lancashire Hospitals
NHS Trust, UK

Malachy Columb
Consultant in Anaesthesia and Intensive Care
Medicine, University Hospital of South Manchester,
Wythenshawe, UK

John R. Dick
Consultant Anaesthetist, University College London
Hospital, London, UK

Tomaz Garcez
Consultant Clinical Immunologist, Central
Manchester University Hospitals NHS Foundation
Trust, Manchester, UK

Khaled Girgirah
Specialty Trainee in Anaesthesia, North West
Deanery, Central Manchester Children's Hospital,
Manchester, UK

Kate Grady
Consultant Anaesthetist, University Hospital of South
Manchester, Manchester, UK

Nigel J. N. Harper
Consultant Anaesthetist, Department of Anaesthesia,
Central Manchester University Hospitals NHS
Foundation Trust, Manchester, UK

Alex Heazell
Senior Clinical Lecturer and Honorary Consultant in
Obstetrics, St Mary's Hospital, Manchester, UK

Andrew Heck
Specialty Trainee in Anaesthesia, North West
Deanery, Department of Anaesthesia, St Mary's
Hospital, Manchester, UK

Tim Holzmann
North Western Deanery, Manchester, UK

Allison C. L. Howells
Consultant Anaesthetist, Central Manchester University Hospitals NHS Foundation Trust, Manchester, UK

Lorna A. Howie
Specialist Trainee in Anaesthesia, North West Deanery, St Mary's Hospital, Manchester, UK

Emma Ingram
Academic Health Science Centre, Manchester, UK

Suraj Jayasundera
Specialty Trainee in Anaesthesia, North West Deanery, Royal Manchester Children's Hospital, Manchester, UK

Tracey Johnston
Consultant Obstetrician, Birmingham Women's NHS Foundation Trust, Birmingham, UK

Edward D. Johnstone
Senior Clinical Lecturer, St Mary's Hospital and Central Manchester University Hospitals NHS Foundation Trust, Manchester, UK

Christopher Kelly
Specialty Trainee, in Anaesthesia, North West Deanery, University Hospital of South Manchester, Wythenshawe, UK

M. Kingston
Consultant Physician in Genitourinang Medicine, Manchester Royal Infirmary, Manchester, UK

Gareth Kitchen
Specialty Trainee in Anaesthesis, North Western Deanery, Manchester, UK

Pavan Kochhar
Consultant Obstetric Anaesthetist, St Mary's Hospital, Manchester, UK

Jessica Longbottom
Specialty Trainee in Anaesthesia, North West Deanery, Manchester, UK

Kirsty MacLennan
Consultant Obstetric Anaesthetist, St Mary's Hospital, Manchester, UK

Anita Macnab
Consultant Cardiologist, University Hospital of South Manchester, Manchester, UK

W. Ross Macnab
Consultant Obstetric Anaesthetist, St Mary's Hospital, Manchester, UK

Simon Maguire
Consultant Anaesthetist, South Manchester University Hospital Trust, Manchester, UK

Dan Mallaber
Consultant Anaesthetist, Central Manchester University Hospitals NHS Foundation Trust, Manchester, UK

Suna Monaghan
Consultant Anaesthetist, Central Manchester University Hospitals NHS Foundation Trust, Manchester, UK

Jenny Myers
Senior Clinical Lecturer, Maternal and Fetal Health Research Centre, St Mary's Hospital, Manchester, UK

M. Nirmalan
Professor of Medical Education and Honorary Consultant in Anaesthesia, Manchester Royal Infirmary, Manchester, UK

N. J. Nirmalan
Senior Lecturer, Programme Leader, Biomedical Sciences, University of Salford, Manchester, UK

Kate O'Brien
Consultant Obstetric Anaesthetist, St Mary's Hospital, Manchester, UK

Matthew D. Phillips
Manchester Royal Infirmary, Manchester, UK

Catherine Robinson
Consultant Anaesthetist, Manchester Royal Infirmary, Manchester, UK

Kim G. Soulsby
Specialist Registrar in Anaesthesia, Oxford University Hospitals, Oxford, UK

Clare Tower
Consultant in Obstetrics and Maternal
and Fetal Medicine, Central Manchester University
Hospitals NHS Foundation Trust, Manchester, UK

Lawrence C. Tsen
Associate Professor, Harvard Medical School,
Department of Anesthesiology, Perioperative and
Pain Medicine, Brigham and Women's Hospital,
Boston, MA

Akbar Vohra
Consultant Anaesthetist Central Manchester
University Hospitals NHS Foundation Trust,
Manchester, UK

Richard Wadsworth
Consultant Anaesthetist, Department of Anaesthesia,
Central Manchester University Hospitals NHS
Foundation Trust, Manchester, UK

Carolynn Wai
Specialty Trainee in Anaesthesia, North West
Deanery, Manchester, UK

Sarah Wheatly
Consultant Anaesthetist, University Hospital of South
Manchester, Manchester, UK

Gordon Yuill
Consultant Anaesthetist, Department of Anaesthesia,
Stepping Hill Hospital, Stockport, UK

Preye Zuokumor
Consultant Anaesthetist, Central Manchester
University Hospitals NHS Foundation Trust,
Manchester, UK

Preface

Navigating through the minefields of obstetric anaesthesia is becoming more and more challenging. Obstetric anaesthetists are encountering a much broader range of pathologies owing to the ever increasing morbidity affecting women of childbearing age. This book aims to provide healthcare professionals caring for parturients with a wealth of up-to-date information on a broad range of aspects affecting obstetric care.

The book is divided into six sections. Section 1 addresses the basic sciences, including expected physiological and pharmacological alterations associated with pregnancy, and epidemiology. Section 2, entitled obstetric aspects, includes maternal critical care, antenatal assessment and a chapter authored by an obstetrician, dedicated to obstetrics for the anaesthetist.

Section 3 covers all aspects of provision of anaesthesia, including incidental anaesthesia (for those parturients requiring non-obstetric surgery whilst pregnant), regional and non-regional analgesia for labour, regional and general anaesthesia for operative delivery and anaesthesia for specific obstetric indications. Section 4 is divided into easily navigable chapters that cover the common conditions encountered during pregnancy, ranging from obesity and pre-eclampsia to allergy, sepsis and HIV. Dedicated chapters for individual systems detail commonly encountered conditions, how these conditions can be affected by pregnancy and suggested peripartum management plans.

Section 5 focuses on postpartum complications and maternal collapse. Section 6 changes the direction away from clinical practice and addresses ethics and consent, clinical governance and multidisciplinary training for members of the delivery suite.

By combining obstetric and anaesthetic authorship on many chapters, we aspire to give the reader a well-founded knowledge base with which to approach situations on the delivery suite. This book is a must have for current, easily accessible opinion, making it valuable for anaesthetic trainees sitting examinations, occasional dabblers in obstetric anaesthesia and full-time obstetric anaesthetic consultants alike. Most up-to-date literature and initiatives, including National Audit Project 5, Cochrane reviews, guidelines and enhanced recovery after surgery are discussed.

We hope that this addition to the core topic range will assist healthcare professionals in the rapidly changing complex field of obstetric anaesthesia.

**Kirsty MacLennan, Kate O'Brien and
W. Ross Macnab**

Chapter

1

Physiology of pregnancy

N. J. Nirmalan and M. Nirmalan

Introduction

Maternal physiology undergoes complex changes during pregnancy in order to enable the female reproductive system to nurture and adapt to the fetus and placenta. The changes are predominantly either secondary to hormonal responses to female sex hormones or physical adaptations to increasing fetal size. The definition and detailed understanding of the normal physiological changes occurring in the antepartum, intrapartum and postpartum periods of pregnancy are crucial to recognize pathophysiological deviations as a result of disease and anaesthesia. Even though the changes are in fact quite widespread, this chapter will focus on some of the key physiological systems that are of direct relevance to the anaesthetist's management of a pregnant woman during the peripartum period.

Haematological system

Antepartum period

Pregnancy and the neonatal period result in significant changes in the haematological system with an associated increased risk for the development of complications, such as anaemia, thromboembolism and consumptive coagulopathies. Most haematological parameters are progressively altered during pregnancy and are reflected in laboratory investigations. Blood and plasma volumes increase, resulting in an adaptive hypervolaemia. An increase of 30–45% in the blood volume occurs, with changes starting at 6–8 weeks and peaking at 28–34 weeks, approximately 1.5 L higher than the prepregnant state. The increased blood volume is accompanied by increases in red cell mass secondary to increased erythropoiesis stimulated by high circulating levels of renal erythropoietin (Epo). The changes in erythropoiesis begin by week 10 and progressively accelerate through the second and

third trimesters and are accompanied by erythroid hyperplasia of the bone marrow and an increase in the reticulocyte counts. While the early increases in erythropoietin may be due to the decreased oxygen-carrying capacity, in the last two trimesters, the increase is thought to be induced by progesterone, prolactin and human placental lactogen. Pregnancy-induced physiological changes are also responsible for a rise in red blood cell 2,3 diphosphoglycerate (2,3-DPG) levels leading to a gradual rightward shift of the maternal oxygen–haemoglobin dissociation curve, with improved oxygen transfer from mother to fetus. Red cell parameters like the mean corpuscular volume (MCV) and mean corpuscular haemoglobin concentration (MCHC) remain relatively stable in the absence of iron deficiency anaemia.

Circulating oestrogen and progesterone act directly on the kidney, inducing the release of renin with activation of the aldosterone–renin–angiotensin mechanism resulting in Na^+ retention and an associated increase in total body water. The resultant increase in plasma volume (~45%) is relatively greater than accompanying increases in red cell mass (~33%). The consequent haemodilution causes decreases in haematocrit (33–39% at term) and haemoglobin concentrations (~150 g/L prepregnancy to ~120 g/L in the third trimester) leading to physiological anaemia of pregnancy. White cell counts can increase by ~8% from the second month of pregnancy, predominantly due to an oestrogen-induced neutrophilia. While T- and B-lymphocyte counts do not change, their function is suppressed leading to increased susceptibility to infections. Platelet levels generally remain within the normal range during pregnancy. There is some evidence of increased production and increased consumption. Gestational thrombocytopenia is a physiological condition that occurs in a small number of parturients.

Core Topics in Obstetric Anaesthesia, ed. Kirsty MacLennan, Kate O'Brien and W. Ross Mcnab.
Published by Cambridge University Press. © Cambridge University Press 2015.

Hypervolaemia and the ensuing haemodilution can cause significant changes in other plasma components as well (plasma proteins, electrolytes, lipids, enzymes, serum iron etc.). Total plasma protein is reduced by 10–14%, particularly during the first trimester. Despite an absolute increase in serum albumin concentrations, the relative decrease due to haemodilution results in decreased oncotic pressure, contributing to oedema, which is further aggravated by increased venous hydrostatic pressure in the third trimester. The albumin-to-globulin ratio decreases due to absolute and relative increases in globulin concentrations. Increases in fibrinogen levels of 50–80% are reported in pregnancy, which, together with elevations in serum globulins, cause progressive elevations in the erythrocyte sedimentation rate (ESR) in pregnancy. A combination of hypervolaemia and effects of alterations in the respiratory system (low CO_2 levels) result in a decrease of serum electrolyte levels with reduced plasma osmolarity. Increases in serum lipids (40–60% at term), particularly cholesterol and phospholipids, occur due to increased fetal and placental demands. With poor iron supplementation, serum iron and ferritin levels decrease. Reduction of serum ferritin – a more precise indicator of reticuloendothelial iron stores – peaks in the second trimester in parallel with the rapid expansion in maternal red blood cell mass. An increase in serum alkaline phosphatase is a common finding and is usually attributed to increased placental production.

Pregnancy induces a hypercoagulable state with an increased risk of thrombosis and coagulopathies due to an intrinsic activation of the coagulation system in the uteroplacental circulation. The majority of the coagulation factors are elevated, particularly Factors I, VII, VIII, X, XII, prekallikrein and the von Willebrand factor (vWF). Activated partial thromboplastin time (APTT) and prothrombin time (PT) decrease after mid pregnancy, while the bleeding time remains normal. The overall effect on the coagulation system during pregnancy is an increase in thrombin generation due to increased activity of procoagulant proteins and suppression of the fibrinolytic system. The resultant hypercoagulable state facilitates and stabilizes clot formation. Haematological changes occurring in pregnancy are summarized in Table 1.1 below.

The physiological changes in the haematological and haemostatic system during pregnancy are essential to meet the demands of the fetus and protect against intrapartum blood loss. An understanding

Table 1.1 The most significant haematological changes in pregnancy

Physiological anaemia
Neutrophilia
Mild thrombocytopenia
Increased procoagulant factors
Diminished fibrinolysis

of the normal physiological process is vital, given the influence of these changing parameters on the interpretation of laboratory investigations and the increased susceptibility to thromboembolism and coagulopathies. The haematological changes revert to prepregnancy status at 2 weeks post partum.

Intrapartum and postpartum phases

Maternal adaptions in the haematological system during the intrapartum phase of the pregnancy are primarily aligned to coping with and minimizing the impact of significant blood loss associated with the delivery of the fetus. The efficacy of this adaptation is reflected in the ability to withstand losses of up to 1000 mL of blood (~500 mL in a normal vaginal delivery; up to ~ 1000 mL for a caesarian section or normal twin delivery) with minimal resultant effects on the blood and pulse pressures estimated to be around half the extra blood volume acquired antepartum.

A stress-induced increase in erythropoiesis coupled with muscular exertion and dehydration result in haemoconcentration and mild increases in haemoglobin levels in the peripartum period. The stress response also contributes to neutrophilia and increased WBC counts that could confound or mask the diagnosis of infection. Some authors have documented a physiological increase in white cell counts of up to 30 000 mm^3 in the postpartum period.

An enhancement of the hypercoagulable state of pregnancy and activation of the clotting cascades and platelets ensures a more stringent control on the blood losses in the peripartum phase. In order to minimize blood losses from the endometrial placental separation site, fibrinolytic activity decreases during partus, promoting clot formation. Placental and decidual tissue factor, a membrane bound protein that initiates coagulation, increases during labour, as does Factor VIII complex and Factor V. Prothrombin time decreases, particularly in the final stages of labour.

The reduction of fibrinolytic inhibitor levels following placental detachment results in normal fibrinolytic activity 48 h after the delivery. By week 6 post partum, the haemostatic system returns to the prepregnant state. These changes in the pro- and anticoagulation systems account for the marked increase in the risks of venous thrombosis in women during this period.

The cardiovascular system

Physiological changes in pregnancy

The increased metabolic demands of the mother and fetus during pregnancy result in a range of physiologically significant, but reversible adaptive changes in the maternal cardiovascular system. In most instances, the increased demands on the maternal cardiovascular system are met adequately by the ensuing physiological adaptations. If, however, there is underlying maternal cardiovascular compromise due to disease, or the normal physiological haemodynamic changes fail to occur, the adverse effects on the uteroplacental circulation could result in fetal and maternal disease.

Most cardiovascular and haemodynamic changes are initiated in the early stages of pregnancy due to high circulatory levels of the vasoactive reproductive hormones oestrogen, progesterone and prostaglandins (PGE1 and PGE2). The resulting vasodilation and reduction in systemic and pulmonary vascular resistance (~20%) cause a fall in systolic and diastolic blood pressures triggering reflex increases in the stroke volume (~25–30%) and heart rate (~10–20), and increases in cardiac output by approximately 30–50% of the prepregnancy states. Changes in heart rate and stroke volume are detected as early as 5 weeks and 8 weeks, respectively. Stroke volume peaks around 16–24 weeks and decreases in the last trimester to reach prepregnancy values by term. The increased cardiac outputs are facilitated by physiological hypertrophy and dilatation of the left ventricles and, together with increases in total blood volume, plasma volume and red cell mass, aid in increasing the capacity of the maternal cardiovascular system to effectively respond to the increased demands imposed by the fetal and uteroplacental circulations. A further increase in cardiac output may occur during labour in response to the sympathetic and catecholamine drives.

Maternal blood volume increase starts as early as 6 weeks' gestation and progressively rises through pregnancy peaking at 30% at 28–32 weeks of gestation. Increases in the total volume are consequent to increases in plasma volumes and red blood cell volumes. While changes in the blood volume during pregnancy are mediated primarily by hormonal effects, vasoactive mediators like nitric oxide are largely responsible for the vasodilatation that is commonly seen within the maternal circulation. This combination of increased circulating volume and vasodilatation will result in an increase in stroke volume and cardiac output. While much of the increased cardiac output is redistributed in the uteroplacental circuit, organs like the mammary glands, skin, uterus and kidneys also have increased perfusion. Uterine blood flow increases from ~50 mL/min at 10 weeks' gestation to 500–600 mL/min at term. The elasticity of the uterine spiral arteries is severely compromised, resulting in permanent dilatation and unresponsiveness to circulating vasopressor agents and the autonomic nervous system. The resulting pooling of uterine blood aids in the maintenance of the uteroplacental blood circulation.

Arterial and venous blood pressures during pregnancy do not show increases, despite the significant perturbations in blood volume and cardiac output. Inferior vena caval compression, particularly post 20 weeks of gestation, may result in decreases in cardiac output and placental perfusion and cause maternal hypotension. Positional changes in blood pressure are more evident in diastolic pressures, with average decreases of 10–15 mmHg, while systolic blood pressures remain constant. Consequent to these changes the pulse pressure increases in the third trimester.

Some of the physiological changes in pregnancy may also be reflected in an electrocardiogram (ECG) and need to be defined in order to be differentiated

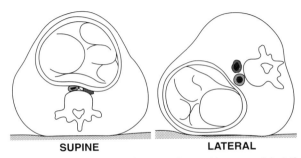

Figure 1.1 The relationship between the gravid uterus and the IVC in the supine and lateral positions. For the colour version, please refer to the plate section.

SUPINE   LATERAL

3

Table 1.2 Summary of key cardiovascular changes in pregnancy

Parameter	Change
Stroke volume	+30%
Heart rate	+15–20%
SVR	−5% (approximately)
SBP	−10 mmHg
DBP	−15–20 mmHg
MAP	−15–20 mmHg
Oxygen consumption	+20%
Cardiac output	+50–70% (increase is more dramatic in late pregnancy)

from pathological changes. Diaphragmatic elevation due to increased uterine size causes a deviation of the position of the heart to the left. A 15° left axis deviation may be seen with Q waves in leads III and AVF. Unspecific ST changes and inverted T waves in lead III may also occur.

Intrapartum period

The stress-induced release of catecholamines and an increased sympathetic drive during labour and delivery of the fetus result in significant haemodynamic and cardiovascular perturbations. A significant increase occurs in cardiac output as a result of the additional circulatory load secondary to each uterine contraction (approximately 300–500 mL). Cardiac output rises progressively throughout labour, peaking immediately after delivery. Rises in systolic and diastolic blood pressure occur during the contractions. Heart rate changes in the intrapartum period are variable, although SVR remains constant. Arrhythmias may occur in subjects with pre-existing cardiac diseases and occasionally in subjects with no previous cardiac disease in response to these changes. These arrhythmias include sinus tachycardia/bradycardia, supraventricular tachycardia and premature ventricular/atrial and nodal contractions.

Postpartum period

While blood loss during delivery can be significant (up to 10% (500 mL) with vaginal deliveries and 15–30% with caesarean sections), the compensatory increase in stroke volume and therefore cardiac output seen in early pregnancy could last for up to 2 hours after delivery of the fetus. The cardiac output continues to decline by a further 30% over 2 weeks, reaching prepregnant values by 6–12 weeks in most cases.

The respiratory system

Antepartum period

The increased demands of pregnancy require an associated expansion in the efficacy of tissue oxygenation, and maternal alterations during pregnancy are designed to accommodate this. A 30–50% increase in the minute ventilation is achieved through a series of hormonal and biochemical changes, ensuring enhanced oxygen availability and more efficient carbon dioxide removal. In addition to hormonal effects, several mechanical factors influence respiratory function.

The progressive enlargement of the gravid uterus causes progressive cranial displacement and alterations in the movement of the diaphragm. The increased intra-abdominal pressures lead to a flaring of the lower thorax and an increase in the thoracic circumference by ~ 6 cm. The hormonal and biochemical effects on respiration may occur through either central effects on the respiratory centre or via direct local effects in the respiratory smooth muscles. Increasing levels of serum progesterone, a known respiratory stimulant, are primarily responsible for these changes, aided by high circulating levels of oestradiol and prostaglandins. The mechanism of action is postulated to be a progesterone-induced enhanced sensitivity to CO_2 (up to 60% by 20 weeks), a lowering of the carbon dioxide thresholds in the respiratory centre and a consequent increase in minute ventilation. The consequent reduction in maternal $PaCO_2$ facilitates a greater carbon dioxide pressure gradient ($PaCO_2$) between the maternal and fetal circulations resulting in a more efficient transfer via the placental circulation. In addition, progesterone-induced relaxation of the bronchial and tracheal smooth musculature results in decreased airway resistance and increased respiratory air volumes in pregnancy, often causing symptoms attributed to asthma to lessen in pregnancy. The increased respiratory rate and increased minute ventilation result in a fall in $PaCO_2$ (to ~ 4.1 kPa, 31 mmHg) by the end of the first trimester. A small increase in PaO_2 (to ~ 14 kPa, 105 mmHg) is also observed during the third trimester. Nearer to term however, the inability of increases in cardiac output to fully compensate for the increased oxygen demand results in a small reduction in PaO_2 to less than 13.5 kPa (101 mmHg). The changes in PaO_2 alluded to above, however, are too small to have any important consequences on maternal or fetal physiology. O_2 consumption and CO_2 production increase by 60% of prepregnant values at term.

Changes in respiratory volume become apparent at around 20 weeks' gestation and progress throughout the pregnancy. A 30–40% increase in tidal volume (Vt) is accompanied by an increased inspiratory reserve volume (IRV) and decreases in expiratory reserve volume (ERV, 20–30%), residual volume (RV, ~20%) and functional residual capacity (FRC, 20%). The decrease in FRC as a result of decreases in ERV and RV could make parturients more prone to respiratory collapse in the supine position. The vital capacity (VC), forced expiratory volume in 1 second (FEV1) and the FEV1/VC ratios remain unchanged during pregnancy. An increase in the physiological dead space up to a volume of ~60 mL may occur. The reduction in FRC by approximately 20% and an increase in minute ventilation by 30–50% have major implications for changes to alveolar gas compositions (anaesthetic agents as well as PaO_2) in response to changes in alveolar ventilation. This includes a faster rise in the concentration of anaesthetic agents during induction of anaesthesia and a faster fall in PaO_2 in response to upper airway obstruction or central respiratory depression.

Airflow is mainly determined by bronchial smooth muscle tone and the degree of congestion in the bronchial capillaries, particularly in the smaller airways.

Table 1.3 Changes in lung function tests during the late stages (third trimester) of pregnancy

Respiratory rate	Unchanged
FEV1	Unchanged
PEFR	Unchanged
Minute volume/ventilation	Increased by 30–50%
Tidal volume	Increased by 30–50%
FVC	Unchanged
FEV1/FVC	Unchanged
Maximum mid-expiratory flow rate (forced expiratory flow rate 25–75)	Unchanged
Functional residual volume	Decreased by 18%

The net effect on airway resistance is probably determined by the balance between factors enhancing bronchoconstriction (e.g. PFG2a, decreased RV and decreased $PaCO_2$) and those enhancing bronchodilatation (PGE$_2$ and progesterone). In the small airways (< 1 mm), airway closure in pregnancy occurs above the FRC nearer term with a higher tendency for closure in the supine position. This may result in an alteration in PaO_2 due to ventilation–perfusion (V/Q) mismatch in the lung bases.

Diffusing capacity, a measure of the ease with which gas transfers across the pulmonary membrane, may show an increase in early pregnancy, although the changes are not deemed to be clinically significant.

Changes in the intrapartum and postpartum periods

The specific changes during these phases will largely be dependent on the effect of pain, anxiety, airway congestion and posture on alveolar ventilation, airflow resistance and arterial $PaCO_2$ levels along the lines described above. As the size of the gravid uterus gets smaller, the FRC and minute ventilation are returned to prepregnant values over the first few weeks after delivery.

Acid–base regulation in pregnancy

Pregnancy induces a state of respiratory alkalosis and a left shift of the oxyhaemoglobin dissociation curve. The respiratory alkalosis drives CO_2 transfer from the fetus to the mother by increasing the arterial CO_2 pressure gradient between the maternal and fetal circulations. Increased renal excretion of bicarbonate metabolically compensates for the respiratory alkalosis, with maternal pH levels at the higher end of normal values (pH 7.4–7.45). Changes are stable throughout pregnancy until the onset of labour. Maternal hyperventilation associated with labour results in an acute left shift of the oxyhaemoglobin dissociation curve. The resultant increase in the affinity of maternal haemoglobin for oxygen compromises oxygen delivery to the fetus. In addition, prolonged, painful labour results in increases in the basic metabolic rates and oxygen demand, which cannot be compensated by further increases in cardiac output. Effective administration of regional anaesthesia could prevent further exacerbations in BMR and hyperventilation and serve to minimize potentially detrimental effects on the fetus.

Oxygen–haemoglobin dissociation curve in pregnancy

The oxygen dissociation curve demonstrates the equilibrium between the partial pressure of oxygen in the blood (PaO_2) and the saturation of haemoglobin with oxygen. The sigmoid nature of the curve dictates that once the plateau stage has been reached, large changes in oxygen partial pressures are required to make relatively small differences in percentage haemoglobin saturation (SaO_2). The left/right shift in the position of the curve is determined by the affinity of haemoglobin for oxygen, with a shift to the right implying lowered affinity, and vice versa. The affinity is expressed by the P_{50} values, i.e. the oxygen tension at 50% haemoglobin saturation. The normal adult P_{50} (at pH 7.4, 37 °C) is 26 mmHg (3.4 kPa). Throughout pregnancy there is a gradual rightward shift of the curve due to a progressive increase in P_{50}. At term, the P_{50} is approximately 30 mmHg, resulting in decreased haemoglobin affinity and therefore increased oxygen transfer to the fetus. These changes are mediated by increases in 2,3-DPG levels seen throughout pregnancy. The median concentration of red cell 2,3-DPG in the first trimester of pregnancy is approximately 16.1 μmol/gHb and this may increase to a level of approximately 17.0 μmol/gHb by the end of the third trimester. Red cell 2,3-DPG levels decrease rapidly during the postpartum period. These changes in 2,3-DPG levels and the consequent reduction in oxygen affinity may partially compensate for the physiological anaemia seen during pregnancy.

The gastrointestinal system

Anatomical and physiological alterations in the maternal gastrointestinal and hepatic systems during pregnancy are essential to support the increased nutritional demands of the fetus. The changes are primarily due to either mechanical changes imposed by the growing fetus and/or hormonal effects of progesterone and oestrogen. Appetite and food consumption are increased during pregnancy, although variations can occur in the food types desired, with avoidance of certain items and cravings for others. Although the basis for these changes is unclear, a combination of hormonal changes (oestrogens and progesterone), insulin/glucagon levels and alterations in taste etc. are postulated to have a role to play.

A combination of increased abdominal pressure due to the growing fetus and a progesterone-induced decrease in the lower oesophageal sphincter tone result in gastro-oesophageal reflux in as many as 80% of term parturients. Most of the clinical changes occur in the third trimester at about 36 weeks. The flattening of the hemidiaphragm could result in the reduction of the normally acute gastro-oesophageal angle, thereby contributing to the reflux. The alterations in lower oesophageal sphincter tone are also primarily responsible for heartburn in pregnancy. Although a progesterone-induced decreased gastric tone can result in delayed gastric emptying and increased gastric volumes during pregnancy, the effects are more significant during labour. The effects may be exaggerated due to the administration of opiate analgesics and general anaesthetics, thereby increasing the risk of vomiting and aspiration pneumonia on induction of general anaesthesia. Preventive measures include administration of H_2 blockers, neutralization of gastric contents and rapid sequence induction with cricoid pressure.

Similarly, a progesterone-induced decrease in smooth muscle tone and motility can also occur in pregnancy, prolonging intestinal transit times, particularly during late pregnancy. Histological changes in the intestinal villi show villus hypertrophy and increased absorptive capacity to cope with corresponding increases in demand. Together with the increased absorptive surface, decreased motility allows for increased absorption of fluids and nutrients, including amino acids, glucose, sodium chloride and water. Iron absorption in the duodenum increases twofold by the third trimester. Calcium absorption is enhanced primarily due to increased levels of 1,25-dihydroxy-vitamin D. All pregnancy-associated changes to the gastrointestinal system are thought to revert to normal by 48 hours post partum.

The hepatic system

Pregnancy-associated changes in the hepatic system are primarily related to the effects of oestrogens on liver metabolism. The enlarging uterus displaces the liver superiorly, posteriorly and anteriorly. Small but significant increases in the plasma concentrations of all liver enzymes, including gamma-GT, ALT, AST and LDH are demonstrable in pregnancy. In most patients, however, these changes do not imply liver dysfunction and are clinically insignificant. These small increases in liver enzymes and the presence of some of the clinical signs – usually attributed to liver disease, such as spider naevi and palmar erythema, in otherwise normal pregnancies may render the diagnosis of liver disease more challenging in pregnant women. The placenta is a rich source of alkaline phosphatase and consequently plasma concentrations of alkaline phosphatase may be increased almost threefold in the late stages of pregnancy. Pregnant women also have a slightly greater tendency to develop gall stones due to a progesterone-induced reduction in cholecystokinin release and a reduced contractile response of the gall bladder, resulting in biliary stasis. Plasma cholinesterase levels may be almost 25% lower in the third trimester due to reduced hepatic synthesis and, theoretically, this reduction may prolong the duration of action of succinylcholine. Even though these differences are not clinically important in the majority of women who receive suxamethonium, a small group of women with increased succinylcholine sensitivity (who are heterozygote for an abnormal cholinesterase gene) may show prolonged neuromuscular block following the administration of suxamethonium during pregnancy.

Renal system

As a result of an increase in blood volume, stroke volume and cardiac renal blood flow, and renal plasma flow and glomerular filtration rate are increased in pregnancy. In fact, renal plasma flow and GFR may be 40–65% greater in a pregnant woman at term when compared to her prepregnant values. This is reflected by an increased clearance of urea, creatinine, urate and excretion of bicarbonate, resulting in a corresponding reduction in the plasma levels of these solutes. Through increased activity of the renin–angiotensin–aldosterone axis and the effects of circulating progesterone, increased free water retention is seen and this leads to a reduction in plasma osmolality. It has been shown that plasma osmolality starts to decline soon after conception and reaches a value almost 10 mosmol/kg lower than preconception values by the 10th week of pregnancy, changing very little after this. Glycosuria can be observed in 40% of parturients secondary to increased filtration (due to raised GFR) and the filtered load of glucose exceeding the tubular maximum for glucose.

Urinary tract infections are also more common in pregnant patients due to urinary stasis from progesterone-mediated ureteric smooth muscle relaxation and the direct effects of the gravid uterus on the bladder. Finally the changes in the ECF volume and GFR may alter the volume of distribution and

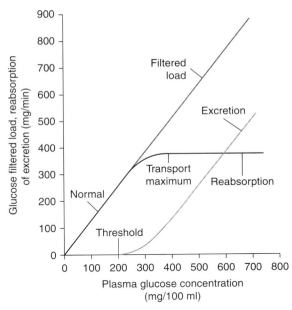

Figure 1.2 Relationship between filtered/reabsorbed glucose levels and the inability of the renal tubules to indefinitely reabsorb all the filtered glucose due to saturation of the relevant transport systems. When the filtered load exceeds the tubular transport systems, glucose will appear in the urine – renal glycosuria.

clearance of some drugs that are of considerable importance to anaesthetists. For example, although some studies show conflicting results, it is generally seen that the plasma concentrations of anticonvulsant drugs may be decreased considerably in the third trimester of pregnancy. A combination of factors including changes to protein binding, increased GFR and expansion of plasma volume may account for these observed changes in the pharmacokinetics of some of the common drugs used in clinical practice

Endocrine system

Pregnancy is frequently associated with increased insulin production and increased insulin resistance. These changes are brought about largely through the effects of human placental lactogen (HPL), which is also known as the human chorionic somatomammotropin (HCS). HCS is a polypeptide placental hormone that is secreted by the syncytiotrophoblast of the developing embryo. Structurally and functionally HCS mimics the effects of human growth hormone and modifies the metabolic state of the mother during pregnancy. The changes brought about by the actions of HCS facilitate the constant and uninterrupted supply of glucose and other energy substrates to the

Table 1.4 Changes in GFR in pregnancy

Normal adult female	106 to 132 mL/min
Trimester one	131 to 166 mL/min
Trimester two	135 to 170 mL/min
Trimester three	117 to 182 mL/min

growing fetus. HPL has anti-insulin properties and consequently relative hyperglycaemia and impaired glucose tolerance is common in pregnancy. Approximately 6% of pregnancies are complicated by maternal diabetes mellitus (80% of which are gestational). Maternal hyperglycaemia can result in fetal hyperglycaemia, which is usually accompanied by fetal hyperinsulinism. This results in large fetal sizes (macrosomia), which may have considerable implications for delivery and hypoglycaemia during the immediate peripartum periods. In addition to the above, pregnancy is also associated with an increase in the production of prolactin, parathyroid hormone and the adrenal cortical hormones, such as cortisol and aldosterone.

Key points

1. The complex changes in maternal physiology are predominantly secondary to hormonal responses to female sex hormones or physical adaptations to increasing fetal size.
2. Significant changes in the haematological system increase the risk for development of anaemia, thromboembolism and consumptive coagulopathies.
3. Cardiovascular adaptations occur early, with an increase in stroke volume and heart rate and a reduction in SVR, PVR and blood pressure.
4. The respiratory system undergoes significant changes to improve efficacy of tissue oxygenation.
5. Acid–base regulation changes alter normal non-pregnant parameters.
6. Gastrointestinal, hepatic, endocrine and renal physiology undergoes significant alterations to support the development of the fetus.

Further reading

Bassell, G. M. and Marx, G. F. (1981). Physiological changes of normal pregnancy and parturition: In E. V. Cosmi (ed.), *Obstetrical Anaesthesia and Perinatology*. New York: Appleton Century-Crofts.

Blackburn, S. T. (2007). *Maternal and Fetal Neonatal Physiology: A Clinical Perspective*, 3rd edn. Philadelphia, PA: Elsevier Saunders.

Cunningham, F. G., Leveno, K., Bloom, S. *et al.* (2005). *Williams Obstetrics*, 22nd edn. New York: McGraw-Hill.

Duffy, T. P. (2004). Haematological aspects of pregnancy. In Burrows, G. N., Duffy, T. P. and Copel, J. A. (eds.), *Medical Complications During Pregnancy*, 6th edn. Philadelphia, PA: Saunders.

Hellgren, M. (2003). Haemostasis during normal pregnancy and puerperium. *Semin. Thromb. Hemost.*, **29**, 125.

McAuliffe, F., Kametas, N., Costello, J. *et al.* (2004). Respiratory function in singleton and twin pregnancy. *BJOG*, **108**, 980.

Monga, M. (2004). Maternal cardiovascular and renal adaptations to pregnancy. In Creasy, R. K., Resnik, R. and Iams, J. D. (eds.), *Maternal-Fetal Medicine: Principles and Practice*, 5th edn. Philadelphia, PA: Saunders.

Pritchard, J. A. (1965). Changes in blood volume during pregnancy and delivery. *Anaetheioslogy*, **26**, 393.

Van Thiel, D.H. and Shade, R. R. (1996). Pregnancy: Its physiologic course, nutrient cost and effects on gastrointestinal function. In Rustgi, V. K. and Cooper, J. N. (eds.), *Gastrointestinal and Hepatic Complications in Pregnancy*. New York: John Wiley & Sons, Inc.

Wise, R. A., Polito, A. J. and Krishnan, V. (2006). Respiratory physiologic changes. *Immun. Allergy Clin. North Am.* **26**, 1.

Placental physiology

Carolynn Wai and W. Ross Macnab

Introduction

The placenta is an organ that connects a developing fetus to the uterine wall for exchange of oxygen, nutrients, antibodies and hormones between the mother and fetus. It is required for the removal of waste products. The development of the placenta is essential for normal fetal growth, development, and the maintenance of a healthy pregnancy.

Embryological development

The placenta begins to develop upon implantation of a blastocyst into the maternal endometrium, leading to rapid proliferation and differentiation of trophoblasts. This leads to the formation of two layers: the cytotrophoblast and syncytiotrophoblast. As the blastocyst implants in the uterine lining, vacuoles and lacunae form within the syncytiotrophoblast. This network of lacunae eventually become the intervillous spaces. The cytotrophoblast erodes deeper into the endometrial tissues leading to formation of chorionic villi, which will cover the entire surface of the chorionic sac. Transformation of the narrow spiral arteries into wide uteroplacental arteries also takes place, due to invasion of cytotrophoblasts into the vascular smooth muscle and endothelial cells. The maternal endometrium undergoes various changes, known collectively as the decidual reaction, forming the decidua, which is shed at delivery.

Anatomical structure

The placenta is discoid in shape with a diameter of 15 to 25 cm. A full-term placenta is approximately 2–3 cm thick and weighs about 500–600 g. The growth of the placenta roughly parallels that of the expanding uterus and covers approximately 15 to 30% of the internal surface of the uterus. It consists of two components: a fetal and a maternal portion.

The fetal component of the placenta is formed by the wall of the chorion (chorionic plate). The villi that arise from it project into the intervillous spaces which contain maternal blood. The maternal component of the placenta, on the other hand, is formed by the decidua basalis, which is the endometrium, deep into the fetal component of the placenta. The two components are held together by the cytotrophoblastic shell. Wedge-shaped areas of decidual tissues, known as placental septa, form as the villi invade the decidua, leading to grooves when viewed from the maternal side of the placenta. Cotyledons are easily recognizable bulging areas that are covered by a thin layer of decidua basalis. These areas of irregular convexities within the fetal part of the placenta result from the formation of the placental septa. These septa contain two or more stem villi and their branches. Anastomoses are formed between the dilated spiral arteries from the decidua and endometrial veins. These anastomoses result in the formation of sinusoids which drain into the lacunar network, establishing the uteroplacental circulation (see Figures 2.1 and 2.2).

Placental circulation

The placenta receives the highest blood flow of any fetal organ (40% of fetal cardiac output). The maternal and fetal circulations are separated by a placental membrane consisting of fetal tissue.

Maternal placental circulation

Maternal blood fills the intervillous space through 80 to 100 spiral arteries in the decidua. Remodelling of these arteries causes them to be wider and less convoluted, and this in turn increases maternal blood flow to the placenta. This pulsatile flow of blood bathes the fetal villi with oxygenated blood. The pressure from the arteries forces the blood deep

Core Topics in Obstetric Anaesthesia, ed. Kirsty MacLennan, Kate O'Brien and W. Ross Mcnab.
Published by Cambridge University Press. © Cambridge University Press 2015.

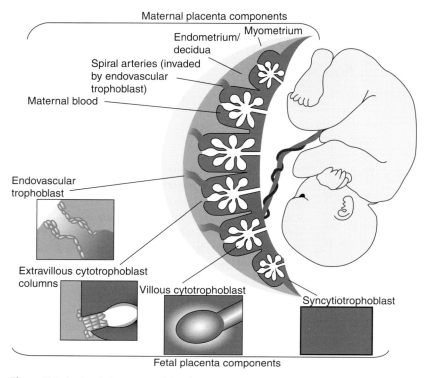

Figure 2.1 Anatomical structure of the placenta.

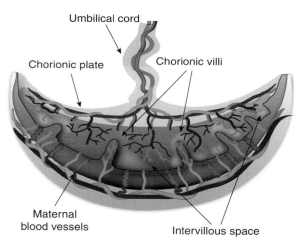

Figure 2.2 Structure of the placenta. For the colour version, please refer to the plate section.

spaces of a mature placenta. It is replenished about three to four times a minute and is affected by uterine contractions.

Placental membrane

This membrane separates the maternal and fetal blood. In the first four months of pregnancy, it consists of four layers: the endothelial lining of the fetal vessels, the connective tissue of the villus, the cytotrophoblast layer and the syncytiotrophoblast layer. This gradually thins out to permit closer contact between the fetal endothelium and the syncytial membrane, allowing greater exchange of compounds between mother and fetus. Although also called a 'barrier', this is a misnomer, as many substances pass through freely.

Fetal placental circulation

Deoxygenated fetal blood leaves the fetus through umbilical arteries to the placenta. The umbilical arteries then branch radially, forming the chorionic arteries at the junction of the umbilical cord and the placenta; these arteries further branch into cotyledon

into the intervillous spaces to allow gas and metabolic exchange. As the pressure decreases, the deoxygenated maternal blood re-enters the circulation through the endometrial veins. There is a total of approximately 150 mL of blood within the intervillous

10

arteries. Within the villi, the vessels form an extensive arterio–capillary–venous system, bringing the fetal blood extremely close to the maternal blood. There is no intermingling of fetal and maternal blood; however, small gaps exist within the placental membrane, leading to small amounts of fetal blood entering the maternal circulation.

Oxygenated fetal blood passes into thin-walled veins that map the placental arteries back to the site of attachment of the umbilical cord. Here, they merge to form the umbilical vein, which supplies oxygenated blood to the fetus.

Placental transfer

The efficient exchange of compounds between maternal and fetal circulation occurs at the syncytiotrophoblast layer and utilises several mechanisms:

1. Passive transport:
   a. Simple diffusion
   b. Osmosis
   c. Facilitated diffusion
2. Active transport:
   a. Carrier-mediated active transport
   b. Ion channels
3. Vesicular transport:
   a. Endocytosis
   b. Exocytosis

Functions

The placenta has three main functions: metabolism, exchange of metabolic and gaseous products between maternal and fetal circulations, and the production of hormones.

Metabolism

The placenta has the ability to synthesize glycogen, protein, cholesterol and fatty acids, which serve as a source of nutrients and energy for the developing fetus. Glycogen is synthesized and stored as an energy reserve for the fetus.

The high demand for cholesterol by the fetus is initially supplied by maternal cholesterol, but as gestation progresses, the placenta synthesizes cholesterol from fatty acid stores. Placental cholesterol is an important precursor for placental production of steroid hormones, such as progesterone and oestrogen.

Lactate is produced as a waste product of metabolism by the placenta and has to be removed via the maternal circulation.

Exchange of metabolic and gaseous products

Gaseous transfer

The placental membrane is highly permeable to oxygen and carbon dioxide, which cross the placenta rapidly by simple diffusion. Therefore, the rate-limiting step for exchange is the blood flow. Fetal haemoglobin has a higher affinity for oxygen and a lower affinity for carbon dioxide in comparison to maternal haemoglobin. This therefore favours oxygen uptake by the fetus and carbon dioxide excretion to the mother.

Glucose and carbohydrates

The fetus relies on glucose as the primary substrate for its oxidative metabolism. The placenta is unable to produce sufficient amounts of glucose until later in gestation and therefore relies on transfer of glucose from the maternal circulation. This is achieved via protein-mediated facilitated diffusion. A few glucose transporters (GLUTs) have been identified in the human placenta, with GLUT1 being the most abundant subtype.

Proteins and amino acids

Amino acids are essential for protein synthesis by the fetus. The maternal transfer of amino acids occurs via the microvillous and basal membranes of the syncytiotrophoblast, utilizing an active transport mechanism.

Lipids and fatty acids

Fatty acids are essential components for fetal development. Many lipids are bound to plasma proteins, which can be released by lipoprotein lipase found on the maternal surface of the placenta. Free fatty acids and glycerol cross the placental membrane via simple diffusion, as well as facilitated diffusion via fatty-acid binding proteins. They are re-esterified when they reach the cytoplasm of the placental trophoblast.

Immunoglobulins and antibodies

The fetus is unable to produce antibodies until well after birth, and placental transfer of maternal antibodies confers passive immunity to the fetus. Immunoglobulin

G is the predominant means of fetal immunity and is transported via pinocytosis.

Water and electrolytes

These compounds are freely exchanged between maternal and fetal circulations. The basal membrane of the placenta contains a Na^+-K^+ pump but net movement of Na^+ and Cl^- is by simple diffusion. This maintains similar concentrations of these ions between maternal and fetal circulations. Water passes freely by osmosis, whilst Ca^{2+} utilizes an active transport mechanism, which is still poorly understood. Fetal ionized Ca^{2+} levels are higher compared to maternal levels and are regulated by parathyroid hormone-related peptides (PTHrP).

Drugs

Most drugs and metabolites cross the placental membrane by simple diffusion, but a few may utilize any of the transport mechanisms described above. This is dependent on the drug's molecular weight, degree of ionization, lipid solubility, protein binding and the blood flow.

Hormone production

The placenta has no innervation and therefore relies on secretion of humoral agents to communicate between maternal and fetal circulations. These substances can act locally within the placenta or the uterus (autocrine and paracrine regulations). The two main groups of hormones produced by the placenta are peptide and steroid hormones.

1. Peptide hormones are mainly produced by the trophoblast cells of the chorionic villi. The main ones are:
   a. Human chorionic gonadotrophin (hCG)
   b. Human placental lactogen (hPL)
   c. Insulin-like growth factors (IGFs)
   d. Corticotropin-releasing hormone (CRH)

2. Steroid hormones are derived from a common precursor, cholesterol. They are lipophilic molecules which readily cross the cell membranes:
   a. Progesterone
   b. Oestrogen
   c. Glucocorticoids

3. Others
   a. Growth factors, including vascular endothelial growth factors and placental growth factors
   b. Cytokines, chemokines, eicosanoids.

Key points

1. Placental development begins at the point of blastocyst implantation into maternal endometrium.
2. Two layers are formed, the cytotrophoblast and the syncytiotrophoblast, that develop into the chorionic villi and intervillous spaces, respectively.
3. Placental function includes exchange of metabolic and gaseous products, metabolism and hormone production.

Further reading

Baker, P. and Kenny, L. (eds.) (2011). *Obstetrics by Ten Teachers, 19th edn.* Boca Raton, FL: CRC press.

Moore, K., Persaud, T. and Torchia, M. (eds.) (2012). *The Developing Human, 9th edn.* Philadelphia, PA: Saunders.

Roberts, V. and Myatt, L. (2014). Placental development and physiology, *UpToDate* http://www.uptodate.com/contents/placental-development-and-physiology (accessed April 2015).

Langman, J. and Sadler, T. (2012). *Langman's Medical Embryology, 12th edn.* Philadelphia, PA: Lippincott Williams & Wilkins.

Gude, N. M., Roberts, C. T., Kalionis, B. and King, R. G. (2004). Growth and function of the normal human placenta. *Thromb. Res.*, **114**, 397–407.

Chapter 3

Pharmacology relevant to pregnancy

Christopher Kelly and Malachy Columb

There are specific issues with regard to therapeutics and pharmacology in the expectant mother and during the postpartum period. There are general changes in the pharmacokinetics and pharmacodynamics, considerations relating to the placenta, potential effects on the fetus and impacts on breastfeeding.

Pharmacokinetics

Bioavailability

The absorption of a drug is the method by which it moves into the body and into the circulating blood, and is characterized as the bioavailability. This can be via a wide range of routes, those used most commonly by the anaesthetist are intravenous (IV), inhalational, epidural, intrathecal, oral, intramuscular (IM), sublingual, intranasal, rectal and transdermal. Despite the enhanced cardiac output in pregnancy, the absorption of drugs is minimally affected, but pregnancy-induced emesis may reduce the bioavailability of orally administered drugs. The increased minute ventilation associated with pregnancy can speed the onset and offset of inhalational agents.

Volume of distribution (V_D)

The distribution of a drug throughout the body is dependent on various factors: physicochemical characteristics of the drug (molecular size, lipid solubility, ionization and protein binding), regional blood flow and any cellular transport mechanisms. The volume of distribution (V_D) can be greatly affected by pregnancy. Increases in circulating blood volume and total body water provide a larger V_D for most drugs. Pregnancy alters the plasma protein profile, potentially changing binding characteristics and the fraction of free drug available for action. Increased cardiac output will speed the distribution of drugs.

Placental transfer

The fetus is also, in effect, an additional compartment into which drugs may distribute. The factors affecting the extent to which drugs cross the placenta into fetal circulation are similar to those for any phospholipid membrane bilayer. Placental transfer will be facilitated for more lipid-soluble drugs, compared to hydrophilic polar or ionized molecules. Likewise, the greater the proportion that is free drug or in the unbound state, the faster it will equilibrate. The extents to which the drug is ionized and protein bound may be different in mother and fetus because of the reduced pH in the fetus, and this may impact on the effective concentration gradients. This situation may change or be exacerbated by labour, during which maternal and fetal acidoses may develop.

Metabolism

Metabolism of drugs is largely unaffected by normal pregnancy. It is possible that the pathological state of HELLP (Haemolysis, Elevated Liver enzymes, Low Platelets) syndrome may impair liver function and thus the metabolism of drugs. A special situation is the relative reduction in the levels of circulating plasma cholinesterases as a result of the increased plasma volume in pregnancy. This can lead to prolonged duration of action of drugs metabolized by these enzymes e.g. *suxamethonium*. Elimination of most drugs is increased during pregnancy. Glomerular filtration rate is increased by 50%, peaking at the end of the first trimester, leading to greater plasma clearance. Pre-eclampsia is a potential exception to this, with associated reduction in renal function.

Core Topics in Obstetric Anaesthesia, ed. Kirsty MacLennan, Kate O'Brien and W. Ross Mcnab.
Published by Cambridge University Press. © Cambridge University Press 2015.

Pharmacodynamics

In general, pharmacodynamics are relatively unaffected by pregnancy. An important exception is the reduction in minimum alveolar concentration (MAC) of inhaled anaesthetic agents that is required for anaesthesia in pregnancy with a resulting increase in the relative potencies of these agents. Likewise the potencies of local anaesthetics are increased in pregnancy and the altered coagulation of the pregnant state may affect the efficacies of anticoagulants.

Local anaesthetics

A local anaesthetic is an agent that produces temporary blockade of neuronal transmission when applied to a nerve axon. The amide local anaesthetics *bupivacaine* and *ropivacaine* are commonly used for analgesia in obstetric patients in the UK.

At rest, the interior of a nerve is negatively charged due to the greater concentration of sodium ions in the extracellular space relative to the intracellular. The propagation of an action potential is dependent on opening of sodium channels in the cell membrane, allowing net influx and depolarization of the cell. Local anaesthetics prevent this sequence of events by first diffusing into the cell in an unionized state, then, having been ionized in the more acidic cytoplasm, binding the cytosolic aspect of the sodium channel. This prevents sodium influx and depolarization and hence propagation of the action potential.

The physiochemical properties of local anaesthetics affect their behaviour clinically. As with all anaesthetic agents, potency is related to lipid solubility. The more lipid soluble drugs are more potent. Unlike general anaesthetics, there appears to be a ceiling effect; above an oil:water partition coefficient of four there is no further increase in potency. *Bupivacaine* is more lipid soluble than *lidocaine* and concentrations of 0.25%wt/vol compared to 1% wt/vol will produce anaesthesia.

Greater protein binding of the drug will lead to a longer duration of action. The longer the aliphatic chain on the compound the greater the protein binding will be. Both *bupivacaine* and *ropivacaine* are extensively (95% and 94%, respectively) bound to both albumin and α_1-acid glycoprotein hence the relatively long duration of action. Lidocaine is only 64% bound and consequently has a shorter duration of action.

The pK_a of the agent impacts the time to onset of action of the drug because it determines the ratio of the ionized to the unionized lipid-soluble fraction at any given pH. A large fraction of lipid-soluble unionized drug will facilitate diffusion of the anaesthetic into the axon where it will take effect. In practice, the lower the pK_a of these basic compounds, the greater the unionized fraction at physiological pH and the faster the onset of action. *Lidocaine*, for example, has a pK_a of 7.9 so is 33% unionized at pH 7.4, whereas *bupivacaine*, with a pK_a of 8.1, is only 15% unionized at the same pH.

Local anaesthetic agents become toxic once they reach sufficient plasma concentrations. Although guidance is given for maximum safe doses, there are a variety of factors in determining toxicity. The vascularity and presence of fat, which fixes local anaesthetic, at the injection site will influence eventual plasma concentration. There is also evidence to suggest that the rate of change of the plasma concentration will impact toxicity as well as peak concentration. So, as well as mass of the drug, its concentration and speed of administration will be relevant.

As blood concentrations increase, central nervous system (CNS) symptoms will develop. Initially there is a period of excitation (due to inhibition of inhibitory fibres) followed by generalized depression and eventually respiratory arrest. Cardiovascular effects will follow the onset of CNS features, but vary from agent to agent. Bupivacaine is said to be maximally cardiotoxic causing re-entrant tachyarrhythmias and eventually ventricular fibrillation and cardiac arrest. The situation is then worsened as the patient becomes more acidotic, reducing protein binding and increasing free drug. Resuscitation attempts can be prolonged and *intralipid* is recommended to reduce free drug concentrations. The ratio of concentrations required for CNS to cardiovascular toxicities is considered to be a safety margin. This is lower for *bupivacaine* than all the other agents in use.

Because of these safety concerns, the pure *S*-enantiomer of *bupivacaine*, *levobupivacaine*, has been developed with a more favourable side effect profile. Likewise, *ropivacaine* is a pure *S*-enantiomer, which is also less cardiotoxic and less potent than bupivacaine.

Systemic analgesia

A variety of systemic analgesics are in common use today. Generally they are cheap, easy to administer and have few contraindications. They can be of great value when epidural analgesia is refused or contraindicated.

Parenteral opioids have a long history of use and are still popular today.

Pethidine

Since 1950 in the UK it has been legal for midwives to administer *pethidine* to labouring women and so it is the most commonly administered analgesic. It is a synthetic opioid and phenylpiperidine derivative, and is usually given at a dose of 1 mg/kg IM by midwives. There is some evidence to suggest that the reduction in pain scores is greater when administered by the IV route with no associated increases in negative outcomes. The efficacy of *pethidine* has been questioned by a National Childbirth Trust (NCT) survey showing that women more often find it unhelpful than helpful. This is likely due to side effects of the drug on the mother. CNS effects include sedation, confusion and dysphoria. *Pethidine* is metabolized by the liver to inactive *pethidinic acid* and *norpethidine* which has half the activity of *pethidine*. *Norpethidine (N-desmethyl pethidine)* may accumulate in renal failure and has been linked to grand mal epilepsy. For this reason it is relatively contraindicated in patients with raised blood pressure or other potential for seizures, such as eclampsia.

Pethidine reduces gastric motility and will lead to increased aspiration risk should general anaesthesia be required. It is common practice to co-administer ranitidine and metoclopramide in an attempt to offset this effect. Like other opioids there is the potential to cause nausea and vomiting, although *phenothiazine* antiemetics should be avoided specifically with *pethidine* because of the increased sedation and antagonism of the analgesia that may ensue. There is a dose-dependent respiratory depression with all opiates. The dosage should be titrated to effect and respiratory rate. This can be particularly problematic if the patient is also using *Entonox*. *Pethidine* has not been shown to have any effect on uterine contractility.

The fetus and neonate can also be affected by the administration of opiates. *Pethidine* is nearly 30 times more lipid soluble than *morphine* and as a result will equilibrate across the placenta within minutes. Here the half life is around 20 hours, as compared to 3 hours in the mother. Fortunately this does not appear to be detrimental to the neonate, although some authors argue that the maternal respiratory alkalosis associated with pain will facilitate ion trapping of *pethidine* base within the relatively acidic fetal circulation. Cardiorespiratory effects have been noted. Heart rate variability may be reduced and some studies have shown reduced S_pO_2 values in mother and baby while sleeping, but none of these findings have been associated with adverse long-term outcomes.

Morphine

Morphine is a naturally occurring phenanthrene derivative. It is typically given as a bolus of 2–5 mg IV or 5–10 mg IM. It shares many of the systemic effects of *pethidine*, but is cleared more quickly, with duration of action of 3–4 hours. There is deemed to be less potential for accumulation of active metabolites than with *pethidine* and a reduced concern for convulsions. This drug can only be prescribed by doctors, so does not allow midwives the autonomy afforded with *pethidine*.

Diamorphine

Diamorphine is a diacetylated morphine derivative; it is a prodrug with 1.5 to 2.0 times the potency of *morphine*. The NCT survey found that mothers and midwives rated it more useful than *pethidine*. It is more lipid soluble than morphine and as a result would be expected to have a faster onset of action. This drug is not available for clinical use in the US. It is associated with the same sedation, respiratory depression and nausea that come with all opiates.

Patient-controlled analgesia (PCA)

There has been great enthusiasm for PCA in labour. Many different agents have been administered in this way because of the potential benefits to patients, fetus and staff:

- Increased patient satisfaction
- Lower total dose of drug delivered
- Less respiratory depression
- Less nausea and vomiting
- Increased patient autonomy and less intensive for carers
- Few contraindications.

Remifentanil is an ultra short-acting pure μ-opioid agonist that is rapidly metabolized by non-specific plasma esterases. With a half life of only 3–7 minutes, independent of hepatic or renal function, it would appear to be ideal for rapidly fluctuating pain in labour. Recently this has been used to good effect in patients refusing epidural analgesia or where it is contraindicated. Mothers must be taught to coordinate the timing of the bolus dose to cover their contraction. Monitoring of S_pO_2 and one to one nursing care is advised, although any respiratory depression is likely to be short lived and *naloxone* is rarely required. The initial bolus is often set at 0.25 μg/kg of lean body weight, with a three minute lockout. This can then be titrated to effect.

Ketamine

Ketamine is a phencyclidine derivative presented as a mixture of two enantiomers and at low doses can have potent analgesic effects. It has a reasonably short duration of action of around 10 minutes but may accumulate with repeated doses. It may be helpful during the second stage of labour, but use is limited by the potential for psychomotor effects and at higher doses increased uterine tone. Interest has been renewed in this agent with the advent of the pure *S*-enantiomer, which may have fewer side effects.

Inhalational analgesia

A wide range of inhalational anaesthetic agents have been used over more than 150 years. During this time they have been shown to be effective and safe. Some of the oldest anaesthetics such as *ether* and *chloroform* gave way to *trichloroethylene* and *methoxyflurane*, subsequently the more recent agents such as *isoflurane*, *sevoflurane* and *desflurane* have also been used. Despite this, the most commonly used agent by far is a 50:50 *nitrous oxide* in *oxygen* mix known as *Entonox*.

Nitrous oxide has a low blood:gas partition coefficient of 0.47, leading to rapid onset and offset of action. Although quick, the peak effect does not come on immediately and mothers must be taught the timing to begin inspiring the mixture 20–30 seconds before the peak pain sets in. Incorrect timing can lead to the unfortunate situation of poor analgesia then disproportionate sedation following the contraction. It is thought to act at the μ-opioid receptor and can transiently give analgesia of similar potency to *morphine*.

The Medical Research Council, in conducting studies with different ratios of *nitrous oxide* to *oxygen*, concluded that the 50:50 mix was safest. Although higher proportions of *nitrous oxide* would be more efficacious, there is increased risk that patients would become unduly sedated. Less than 0.5% of mothers will become excessively drowsy with *Entonox* alone, but this figure would rise if other respiratory depressants are co-administered. Whether or not any significant desaturation occurs with the use of *Entonox*, it is estimated that 25 million administrations occur in the USA annually without obvious problems.

Drugs affecting the uterus

Drugs reducing uterine tone

Tocolysis is indicated to prevent preterm labour and to aid intrauterine resuscitation of the fetus. Due to the pressure in the uterus there is no blood flow to the fetus during contractions. Because of this, once a decision has been made to proceed to operative delivery, attempts are often made to improve blood flow. A variety of agents are in use to reduce uterine tone, none of these have been studied extensively and a degree of controversy exists over their use.

β-adrenoceptor agonists such as *salbutamol* and terbutaline (*ritrodrine* is no longer available as it has been discontinued) will bind $β_2$ receptors in the myometrium. There is subsequent activation of adenylyl cyclase with increasing concentrations of the secondary messenger 3′-5′-cyclic adenosine monophosphate (cAMP). The increased concentrations reduce free ionized calcium, which is required for the interaction of myofilaments, hence the smooth muscle of the uterus relaxes. These agents can be given orally or by infusion and can cause tremor, restlessness and tachycardia. Rarely pulmonary oedema is seen, but this is thought to be an indirect mechanism partially due to fluid overload.

The calcium channel dihydropyridine blocker *nifedipine* blocks voltage-gated calcium channels, which then limits the release of calcium into the sarcoplasmic reticulum and prevents muscle contraction. None of the other calcium channel blockers are used for this purpose.

Atosiban is the only *oxytocin* antagonist available. It has similar effect to the outmoded *ritrodrine*, but has a more favourable side effect profile. The usual rise in intracellular calcium that is prompted by secondary messenger systems is blocked by *atosiban*. An advantage of this agent is that it can be used in conjunction with other tocolytics with potentially synergistic effect.

Glyceryl trinitrate (GTN) acts as a nitrate donor and increases concentrations of *nitric oxide* in the smooth muscle of the uterus. *Nitric oxide* is normally responsible for regulating blood flow within the uterus. The lipophilic molecule easily crosses cell membranes, where it activates guanylyl cyclase. This enzyme increases intracellular concentrations of cyclic guanosine monophosphate (cGMP) and thus activates protein kinases, protein phosphorylation and causes smooth muscle relaxation. The drug can be given sublingually or intravenously and can lead to the familiar side effects of headache, hypotension and reflex tachycardia. Pulmonary oedema has been reported with its use, potentially due to changes in vascular permeability.

Magnesium sulfate has a wide range of clinical applications, several of which are relevant to the obstetric anaesthetist. *Magnesium* is the fourth most common cation in the body and is involved in a variety of body systems. Its effects as a tocolytic arise from the physiological antagonism of *calcium*. This is mediated via two separate mechanisms: high intracellular concentrations of magnesium prevent influx of calcium in a non-competitive way and there appears to be competitive inhibition of calcium binding at the sarcoplasmic reticulum.

The *volatile anaesthetic agents* all cause dose-dependent reductions in uterine tone.

Drugs that stimulate the uterus

Oxytocin is the first-line drug for prophylaxis and treatment of uterine atony. Endogenous *oxytocin* is produced in the supraoptic nucleus of the hypothalamus and stored in the neurohypophysis or posterior pituitary gland. It is normally responsible for controlling lactation and acts at receptors in the uterine myometrium. In early pregnancy there are few of these receptors and so the response to *oxytocin* is greatly reduced when compared to that at term. The exogenous drug was historically derived from animal extracts and had significant quantities *of antidiuretic hormone (ADH)* in the mixture. This is far less of a problem with newer synthetic agents such as *syntocinon*, but there is still potential for the problem because the nine amino-acid polypeptide *oxytocin* differs from *ADH* by only two amino acids. It is therefore possible that small quantities of *ADH* are present. This is part of the rationale for the administration of *syntocinon* in normal saline to prevent excessive doses.

Syntocinon will increase the frequency and force of contractions via its action on the oxytocin receptors in the myometrium. It also causes clinically significant reductions in systemic vascular resistance at therapeutic doses, resulting in hypotension and tachycardia. These side effects can be reduced by ensuring that

large doses (>5 units) are not given and that the drug is not given quickly. Many authors suggest giving the dose as an infusion over several minutes to reduce haemodynamic instability and to allow compensatory responses. It follows that patients with a fixed cardiac output state, such as those with aortic stenosis or pulmonary hypertension would be particularly susceptible to the deleterious effects of reduced afterload. The effects of the drug, however, are only short lived and have a half life of approximately 10 minutes, potentially adding further weight to the argument for infusion rather than bolus injection of the drug.

The ergot alkaloids are second-line agents used in the treatment of uterine atony, a class of chemicals produced by a common fungus. *Ergometrine* is the most commonly used agent today and has activity at α-adrenergic, dopaminergic and serotoninergic (5-HT$_3$) receptors. In addition to causing uterine tetany, it causes generalized vasoconstriction, hypertension, bronchospasm and nausea. The drug should therefore be used only with caution in patients with pre-existing hypertension, pre-eclampsia, pulmonary hypertension or asthma. It is generally not given IV because the IM route is preferred as onsets of action are comparable and there is some potential to reduce some of the side effects. Interestingly the combination of *syntocinon* (5 units) and *ergometrine* (500 μg) known as *syntometrine* seems to reduce the side effect profile further and is said to be safer in patients with asthma when given IM.

Should first- and second-line treatments fail in treating uterine atony, *prostaglandins (PG) E* and *F* may be useful. Endogenous *PG* concentrations increase during labour and are responsible for uterine contraction after placental separation; however, this system may be deficient in some women. The effects of *PG* are twofold; they directly increase the concentration of free intracellular calcium and potentiate the effect of the oxytotics. *15-Methyl PG F$_{2\alpha}$ (carboprost, Hemabate)* is now the agent of choice, given at a dose of 250 μg IM and has been given directly to the myometrium. Doses can be repeated not more than every 15 minutes to a maximum dose of 2 mg. Common side effects are fever, flushing, diarrhoea, nausea and vomiting. *Carboprost* may also cause bronchospasm, ventilation–perfusion inequality and shunt leading to hypoxaemia. For this reason it is relatively contraindicated in asthmatics. *PG E$_2$* is an alternative option for those with asthma as it causes bronchodilatation and in some studies has caused increases in PaO$_2$.

Anaesthetic agents and pregnancy

Anaesthesia may be necessary during the course of the pregnancy and there are special considerations to consider. As for any patient a safe anaesthetic must be provided for the mother but minimizing the potential for teratogenesis and maximizing fetal viability are additional challenges. This can be aided in part by timing of surgery, but choice of agents is paramount.

Induction agents

Thiopentone is the sulfur analogue of *pentobarbitone*. It is used for induction of anaesthesia and treatment of status epilepticus. Animal studies in rats and mice have not demonstrated any adverse effects at anaesthetic doses and indeed this agent has a long history of use in pregnant women without any evidence of teratogenicity. There is a theoretical risk with barbiturates at very high doses when used to control seizure activity in that it has been suggested that dysmorphism in children of mothers with epilepsy may not be entirely due to complications of convulsions.

There is evidence from animal models that *thiopentone* causes a significant (20%–35%) reduction in uterine blood flow. This is transient and of unknown significance to viability of the pregnancy, but it has been postulated that this could be associated with reduced birthweight and increased risk of miscarriage.

Propofol has animal data to support its use in that it is not known to be teratogenic and has not been shown to affect oocyte maturation. It has been used in many pregnant women both for anaesthesia and sedation in intensive care without obvious problems. The manufacturer data sheets, however, do not recommend use during pregnancy. Similar studies to those performed with *thiopentone* have been performed in sheep and despite maternal hypotension on induction, uterine blood flow remained stable. This provides a theoretical advantage to the use of *propofol*.

Ketamine is perhaps less well studied than some other agents and less experience has been amassed. There is no evidence to suggest that it is teratogenic in doses used clinically for anaesthesia. Again knowledge of response to this drug comes from studies in sheep. During the third trimester ketamine causes hypertension and increases uterine blood flow, but earlier in pregnancy it causes profound uterine hypertonus. This almost certainly has negative implications for fetal blood flow.

Etomidate is not recommended for use in expectant mothers. Although no evidence exists for teratogenicity it is accepted that cortisol levels are suppressed with its use. This may have consequences for glucose homeostasis in the unborn child.

Benzodiazepines (BDZ) do have some evidence to suggest teratogenicity. Retrospective studies showed an association between *BDZ* use in the first trimester and cleft lip or palate, although this finding is not universal. Indeed, prospective investigations have not repeated the finding and many experts do not consider these to be teratogenic. Most authors agree that the risk posed by single-dose short-acting agents is of negligible risk. Large doses of *BDZ* immediately prior to delivery can have lasting impact on the neonate. Hypotonus, respiratory depression and hypoxia have all been reported, so it is advised to avoid these agents if possible. When required, personnel trained in neonatal resuscitation should be present at delivery.

Opioids have been investigated thoroughly in animal models. Early concerns that these agents may cause growth and developmental problems have been put down to study design and the consequent effects of opiates such as respiratory depression and reduced nutritional intake. These issues have been circumvented by improved study design and even large sustained doses of opiate such as 500 µg/kg/day *fentanyl* and 8 mg/kg/day *alfentanil* through pregnancy have shown no teratogenic effects whatsoever. Observational studies in mothers on *methadone* programmes have not found congenital anomalies, but systematic study is lacking in this area. It is highly unlikely that standard dosing of opioid analgesia for surgery is of any risk to the fetus.

Muscle relaxants

There are obvious difficulties when testing for the teratogenicity of muscle relaxants. The agents are not usually given in clinically relevant doses alone and there is always potential for hypoxia and hypercarbia, both of which are known to have deleterious effects on the fetus. Observational studies have not demonstrated any problems with the use of non-depolarizing agents. Cultured rat embryo studies have shown dose-dependent growth retardation and morphological changes, but only at concentrations 30 times clinical levels. These bulky polar molecules do not readily cross the placenta where typically concentrations are one-tenth the levels found in maternal blood. It is widely accepted they are safe to use, particularly if they facilitate ventilation and oxygenation where the balance of risk certainly favours them.

Volatile anaesthetics

As with agents discussed so far, much of the evidence we have on volatile agents comes from animal models and observational studies in human populations. Similar problems arise from experiments with inhaled anaesthetics as with muscle relaxants, namely distinguishing between genuine teratogenicity and consequences of hypoxia, hypercarbia, hypothermia and nutritional issues. Attempts have been made to see if either prolonged low-dose or intermittent, but frequent, high-dose exposures have deleterious effects.

Chronic exposure to sub-anaesthetic concentrations of *halothane* in pregnant rats caused growth restriction, but no other abnormalities. Although repeated and prolonged exposures of mice to clinically relevant concentrations of *halothane* (4 MAC hours per day) caused skeletal abnormalities, it is not clear if this link is causal. Indeed in other studies in rats where temperature, feeding and sleep patterns were preserved *halothane, isoflurane* and *enflurane* showed no teratogenicity. Most authors agree that *isoflurane* is safe to use in pregnancy as no studies have shown conclusive effects. Since *halothane* has a theoretical impact on pregnancy it is suggested that it is not given to expectant mothers.

There is a paucity of information on agents more commonly used in anaesthetic practice today. *Sevoflurane* and *desflurane* have been animal tested by manufacturers in unpublished work. Their suggestion is that pregnancies were only negatively impacted by concentrations associated with maternal mortality. It is widely accepted that these agents are safe to use in pregnancy.

Nitrous oxide has been shown to have teratogenic effects in animal models when administered in concentrations greater than 50% for prolonged periods. It was initially hypothesized that the inhibition of the methionine synthase-tetrahydrofolate reductase system was causing impaired DNA synthesis and hence abnormalities. This was shown to be incorrect because the effect could not be blocked by *folinic acid* supplementation, which should correct this effect. Perhaps surprisingly the effect is corrected by the co-administration of volatile anaesthetics. The precise mechanism by which this happens has not been confirmed. Observational studies in humans during the 1960s and 1970s suggested that members of the healthcare professions in theatre environments were more prone to spontaneous abortion and congenital malformations. This was, at the time, attributed to chronic exposure to sub-anaesthetic doses of the volatile agents. The study design was criticized and felt to be impacted by reporting bias. Subsequent studies have failed to find such a link and prospective trials have reported female anaesthetists to have similar rates of reproductive success as other female physicians.

Antiemetics

Nausea and vomiting unfortunately affect many mothers and hyperemesis gravidarum is a potential cause of serious morbidity for mother and fetus. As a consequence, the arsenal of drugs usually employed perioperatively to combat nausea and vomiting has been used extensively in pregnant women.

Prochlorperazine has been assessed in a large prospective clinical study and not found to have negative sequelae. Despite this, manufacturers advise caution following case reports of jaundice in late-term mothers taking large doses of this antiemetic. It can be considered safe.

Metoclopramide is a popular agent when treating pregnancy-related nausea. As well as many years of experience of the drug in this population, animal studies have not demonstrated teratogenic effects. There is, however, controversy in the literature as to how effective an antiemetic it is.

Cyclizine has no evidence to suggest that it causes problems during pregnancy. Manufacturers do advise caution because a related piperazine-derived antihistamine has caused teratogenicity in high doses in rats.

The *serotonin (5-HT$_3$) antagonists*, such as *ondansetron*, have not been found to be teratogenic in animal studies. Since these agents have been in general use for less time than other agents, there are fewer data from human studies. For this reason caution is advised, particularly in the first trimester.

NSAIDs

The non-steroidal anti-inflammatory drugs (NSAIDs) have a long history of use perioperatively in pregnancy in spite of some evidence from animal models that they may be harmful at very high concentrations. The Collaborative Low-dose *Aspirin* Study in Pregnancy (CLASP) study followed the children of mothers through early childhood and found no increased congenital or behavioural abnormalities from the background rate.

A possible exception in this class is *ketorolac*, where the product literature provided by the manufacturer described studies in which rats given the drug had offspring with high rates of vascular malformations. Aside from this specific case NSAIDs are thought to be safe in early pregnancy. In later pregnancy (after 32 weeks gestation) these agents may have a range of unfavourable impacts on the unborn child. By inhibiting cyclo-oxygenase enzymes the NSAIDs alter the synthesis of prostaglandins, impacting the circulatory system. Indeed these drugs can cause premature closure of the fetal ductus arteriosus, with resulting pulmonary hypertension and if severe enough, tricuspid incompetence. Paradoxically they may also cause delayed closure of the ductus arteriosus after birth, which can be refractory to standard medical treatments. The manufacturers also express caution with regard to the consequences of platelet dysfunction with intracranial and gastrointestinal haemorrhage and perforation. There are possible links with renal failure and necrotizing enterocolitis.

Acetaminophen

There is no known teratogenic effect with *acetaminophen (paracetamol)* and it has been used extensively in pregnancy without cause for concern. Pregnancy does not seem to alter the kinetics or dynamics of this useful drug. It does not appear to cause any lasting changes to the expression of prostaglandins.

Catecholamines and the vasoactive drugs

Should surgery be required, it is desirable to keep maternal haemodynamics as stable as possible. There are additional considerations when manipulating the blood pressure of the pregnant patient, paramount in this is the maintenance of blood flow to the uterus and placenta. Blood flow is dependent on the arterial to venous pressure gradient and vascular resistance of the uterus. Pregnancy reduces the sensitivity to vasopressors, but this reduction in sensitivity is not consistent, nor is it the same for all vascular beds to all agents. It was argued in the past that *ephedrine* was the agent of choice in treating maternal hypotension relating to regional or general anaesthesia. The justification for this was that the β-adrenergic effects of the drug would increase cardiac output. This

increased output would offset the increase in uterine vascular resistance and maintain or correct reductions in uterine blood flow. This was supported by some early work demonstrating favourable umbilical cord pH values with the use of *ephedrine*. Equally, it was noted that stressed women, due to pain or anxiety, with elevated blood pressure in response to endogenous *norepinephrine* had reduced uterine blood flow.

More recently some carefully designed studies have demonstrated value in using the α-adrenoceptor agonist *phenylephrine* by infusion to maintain normotension. Previous fears that this would cause disproportionate constriction of the uterine vessels compared to systemic vasculature have not materialized. Research has not confirmed that umbilical cord pH and fetal outcomes are improved with phenylephrine delivered this way and it has become standard practice in many centres to combat hypotension associated with intrathecal block. Both of these agents have an established history of use in the pregnant woman without any observed teratogenic effect. Equally they have been studied extensively in animal models of uteroplacental blood flow without any risk of congenital malformation. As is often the case, the risk of hypoperfusion of the placenta with ensuing hypoxaemia and acidosis is a far greater risk to the fetus than the theoretical potential these drugs may have for teratogenicity.

Antihypertensive agents

It may become necessary to pharmacologically reduce blood pressure in the pregnant patient mother, particularly in the event of craniofacial surgery in response to conditions raising intracranial pressure.

Labetalol has combined α- and β-adrenoceptor blocking effects, α-blockade is specific to α_1 receptors but β-blockade is non-specific. The ratios of the relative activities at these two receptors vary, depending on the route of administration from 1:7 for intravenous to 1:3 for oral. IV administration has been shown to lower blood pressure in hypertensive, pregnant rats. This reduction in blood pressure is not accompanied by reduction in uterine blood flow, presumably because of α-mediated vasodilatation. It is for this reason it has become so popular for use in hypertensive pregnant women and those with pre-eclampsia.

Esmolol is a cardioselective ultra-short-acting β_1-blocker that undergoes rapid ester hydrolysis in the plasma. It is a highly lipophilic agent that crosses the placenta readily and is responsible for a degree of β-blockade in the fetal heart with resultant bradycardia. This, coupled with the tendency to significantly reduce uterine blood flow, can cause fetal metabolic disturbance. For these reasons this otherwise useful agent should be avoided in pregnancy.

Hydralazine is a direct-acting vasodilator. The precise mechanism of action is not clear, but is thought to involve activation of guanylyl cyclase increasing concentrations of cGMP and resultant reduction in intracellular calcium. This relaxes smooth muscle and causes vasodilatation. It is effective in lowering blood pressure and seems to have favourable characteristics for uterine blood flow in animal models. Some argue it should be used with caution in situations of raised intracranial pressure or cerebral irritation as it markedly increases cerebral blood flow. It is a useful agent for women with pre-eclampsia, particularly where β-blockers are contra-indicated, such as in asthma.

GTN reduces smooth-muscle tone and reduces blood pressure by mechanisms discussed previously. Animal models of uterine blood flow do not demonstrate significant reductions, even when maternal blood pressure has fallen. Furthermore, prolonged infusion has not been shown to cause metabolic disturbance in the sheep fetus.

Sodium *nitroprusside* is becoming increasingly rare as a choice for treatment of hypertension. The production of cyanide as a by-product of metabolism has been of concern in all patient groups, but this may be even more so when the fetus will also be exposed. There are case reports of it being used successfully in pregnancy during neurosurgery, but it appears to have negative effects on uterine blood flow. Its use cannot be routinely recommended.

Dihydropyridine calcium-channel blockers such as *nifedipine* and *nimodipine* have been used to treat hypertension in pregnancy. They are often used in neurosurgical conditions because their benefits go beyond those of blood pressure control. They are particularly useful in the treatment of cerebral artery vasospasm. There have, however, been animal studies in sheep that have demonstrated fetal hypoxaemia and acidosis in response to infusions of these drugs. These unwanted effects can persist even after the drug is discontinued. For this reason most authors now agree that calcium-channel blockers should not be used routinely unless the secondary benefits on brain vasculature are required.

Magnesium sulfate has a wide range of interesting uses for the anaesthetist including an antiadrenergic effect by inhibiting the release of catecholamines. It slows cardiac conduction and reduces force of contraction while reducing afterload. In normotensive and hypertensive animals it can increase uterine blood flow by 10%. Although it poorly crosses the blood–brain barrier it interferes with the release of all neurotransmitters and accordingly has antiseizure activity. This combination of features explains why it has been shown to be so useful in the management of pre-eclampsia. Infants born to mothers given *magnesium* sulfate show reduced rates of cystic periventricular leucomalacia and cerebral palsy. Magnesium is presumed to have neuroprotective effects by blocking *N*-methyl, *D*-aspartate (NMDA) receptors and acting as a calcium antagonist and reducing calcium influx into cells. Other proposed mechanisms include protection against free radicals, vasodilatation, increased vascular stability, reduced hypoxic damage, attenuated cytokine and catecholamine-induced cell damage and antiapoptotic actions. Oligodendrocytes in the periventricular white matter seem to benefit most from this protection and these have previously been shown to be the main site of injury in cerebral palsy. Three meta-analyses and a Cochrane review concluded that *magnesium* sulfate given to women at risk of preterm birth substantially reduces the risk of cerebral palsy in their offspring with a relative risk of 0.68 (95% CI 0.54–0.87). There is currently no consensus on dose or timing, but 4 g IV loading dose over 20–30 minutes followed by a 1 g/h infusion for 24 hours or until delivery has been adopted by many units. *Magnesium* sulfate IV can cause hypotension, flushing, nausea and vomiting, sweating and pain at the injection site.

Breastfeeding and anaesthesia

Mothers are often highly motivated to breastfeed their infant. Should they require anaesthesia during this period it is reasonable to assess the safety of continuing with breastfeeding. We can assess the dose of any given drug likely to be passed to the infant by knowledge of the concentration in the maternal plasma, the ratio of that concentration to the concentration in breast milk and the volume of milk taken by the infant.

Although most of the agents used in anaesthesia are highly lipid soluble there is a higher fat content in the human brain than there is in breast milk. So the conscious level of the mother can be used as an accurate guide to the concentrations of drugs such as induction agents, volatile anaesthetic agents, opioids, BZDs and local anaesthetics. Assuming that the mother is alert and conscious, there is unlikely to be unsafe levels in the plasma. Additional safety margins are provided by the usually low milk-to-plasma ratio and the fact that the infant will be taking any quantity of drug by the enteral route further reducing the likely blood concentration in the infant. Most authorities suggest that breastfeeding can continue as normal, assuming that the standard anaesthetic medications have been used and the mother feels well enough to continue.

Non-anaesthetic drugs

Anticoagulation

The normal enhancement of coagulation that accompanies pregnancy may have the unfortunate side effect of increased rates of deep vein thrombosis and thromboembolism. These conditions should be treated in a similar fashion in the pregnant population as the non-pregnant. Equally, some women will be anticoagulated prior to conception and require maintenance of therapy.

Warfarin is often the treatment of choice for long-term anticoagulation in non-pregnant patients. It is, unfortunately, not suitable during gestation. It is a well-documented teratogen; the characteristic features of chondrodysplasia punctata are similar to Conradi–Hunerman syndrome and are very likely a result of multiple microhaemorrhages during the course of development.

Heparins are large water-soluble polar molecules that do not cross the placenta to any great extent. This makes them the treatment of choice for anticoagulation. There is no evidence to suggest they are teratogenic and their effect can be reversed rapidly if so required.

Antibiotics

Coincident infections during pregnancy may require treatment. On the whole, antibiotics tend to be large water-soluble molecules that do not cross the placenta in great quantities. The *penicillins* are widely accepted to be safe and are used with reasonable frequency. Equally the *cephalosporins* and *erythromycin* can be used confidently.

Tetracyclines have not been shown to have teratogenic effects per se, but they are known to bind to tooth enamel and cause discolouration if given up to the sixth month of pregnancy. For this reason another agent should be sought where possible.

Aminoglycosides have been associated with ototoxicity in the newborn. This appears to be a dose-related phenomenon. Advice is against the use of these antimicrobials, but if no other choices exist then close monitoring of levels is advised and reduction of the therapeutic course to the minimum possible time.

Metronidazole has been used safely in pregnancy and no evidence exists that it is harmful. Only when animals were given toxic concentrations of the antimicrobial did any fetal effects arise.

Anticonvulsants

All anticonvulsants cross the placenta and teratogenicity is well recognized with a twofold increase in congenital malformations. Major malformations include orofacial cleft and congenital heart defects. Sodium valproate and carbamazepine have a higher incidence of neural tube defect (1–3.8% and 1% respectively). Fetal anticonvulsant syndrome may also present in a variety of ways, such as dysmorphic features, hypoplastic nails or developmental delay. Newer second-line agents may be preferable. Management should aim to control seizures at the minimum dose of anticonvulsants possible.

Caffeine

Caffeine has been examined in large population studies and has not been shown to cause any harm to the unborn child. Early concerns that it may be associated with increased rates of spontaneous abortion and low birth weight have been allayed as it seems this was an effect confused with that of tobacco smoking.

Key points

1. Drugs and therapeutics for the mother can be challenging. It is important for maternal and fetal health that appropriate treatments are continued or modified. Attention must be paid to minimize the potential for teratogenesis and maximize fetal wellbeing.
2. Factors that affect the extent and speed of placental transfer of drugs are lipid solubility, ionization, protein binding and amount of free unbound drug.

3. Metabolism of drugs is largely unaffected by normal pregnancy.
4. With drugs and breastfeeding, it should be noted there is usually a low milk-to-plasma ratio. There is a further reduction in infant blood concentration due to the enteral route of ingestion.

Further reading

Chestnut, D. H., Polley, L. S., Tsen, L. C. and Wong, C.A. (eds.) (2014). *Chestnut's Obstetric Anaesthesia: Principles and Practice, 5th edn.* Philadelphia, PA: Saunders.

Collis, R., Plaat, F. and Urquhart, J. (2011). *Texbook of Obstetric Anaesthesia.* Greenwich: Greenwich Medical Media.

Evers, A. S., Maze, M., and Kharasch, E. D. (eds.) (2013). *Anesthetic Pharmacology, 2nd edn.* Cambridge: Cambridge University Press. https://www.rcog.org.uk/en/guidelines-research-services/guidelines/

Peck, T. and Hill, S. (2014). *Pharmacology for Anaesthesia and Intensive Care, 4th edn.* Cambridge: Cambridge University Press.

Smith, S., Scarth, E. and Sasada, M. (2011). *Drugs in Anaesthesia and Intensive Care, 4th edn.* Oxford: Oxford University Press.

Suresh, M. S., Segal, B. S., Preston, R. L., Fernando, R. and Mason, C. L. (2012). *Shnider and Levison's Anaesthesia for Obstetrics.* Philadelphia, PA: Lippincott Williams & Wilkins

Yentis, S., May A. and Malhotra, S. (2007). *Analgesia, Anaesthesia and Pregnancy: A Practical Guide, 2nd edn.* Cambridge: Cambridge University Press.

Maternal morbidity and mortality

Kate O'Brien

Introduction

Until the mid-1930s maternal mortality was high in the Western world with the maternal mortality rate (MMR) about 450 per 100,000 births (UK); the current MMR is 8 per 100,000 births.

The vast majority of maternal mortality occurs in the developing world. The Millennium Development Goals is an initiative to improve maternal health in developing countries. The aim is to reduce the maternal mortality ratio by three quarters from 1990 to 2015.

National maternal mortality statistics have been recorded in the UK for over 150 years. The Maternal Death enquiries have been published every three years since 1952; this is the longest running continuous medical audit in the world. The enquiries review and assess maternal deaths and recommend service changes to make childbirth safer.

History of maternal mortality

The maternal mortality rate in England and Wales was fairly static from 1880 to the mid-1930s and the risk of dying in childbirth was the same as in the Victorian era. Mortality from infectious diseases and infant mortality started to fall in the late 1890s. This was due to an increased standard of living: better housing, hygiene and nutrition; however, this was not translated into lower rates of maternal mortality until the mid-1930s. After this there was a steep decline in maternal mortality rates, which continued for the next 50 years. This pattern was consistent throughout the developed world.

The exception was in northwestern European countries: Sweden, Norway, the Netherlands and Denmark. In these countries there were well-trained midwives who used aseptic techniques from their inception (1890–1900) and there was a tradition of minimal surgical intervention whether at home or in hospital. This led to low rates of maternal mortality.

Another success story was the midwives in the Kentucky Frontier Nursing Service. The midwives travelled on horseback to help with childbirth. Despite the fact that these women lived in poor rural communities the maternal mortality rates were ten times less than those in the city of Lexington.

Medical interference

The UK maternal mortality figures showed a significant trend upwards in the 1890s; the maximum excess of deaths was, at its worst, 250 per 100,000 births. This was in the main due to the use of chloroform and unnecessary forceps deliveries.

Medical interference causes iatrogenic mortality. In Kentucky the maternal mortality rate was highest when physicians were involved in the delivery (1925–1937):

- Kentucky Frontier Nursing Service — MMR 60–70 per 100,000 births
- White women of Kentucky — MMR 440–530 per 100,000 births
- White women delivered by physicians in hospital in Lexington — MMR 800–900 per 100,000 births

Factors for the decline in the UK maternal mortality rates 1930s onwards

1. Sulfonamides for the treatment of puerperal sepsis
2. Introduction of ergometrine
3. Blood transfusions
4. Introduction of penicillin

Core Topics in Obstetric Anaesthesia, ed. Kirsty MacLennan, Kate O'Brien and W. Ross Mcnab.
Published by Cambridge University Press. © Cambridge University Press 2015.

5. Improved training
6. Improved anaesthetic techniques
7. Less interference in normal labours
8. Improvements in maternal care.

Confidential Enquiries into Maternal Deaths (UK)

This is the longest running continuous medical audit in the world. The enquiries look at all maternal deaths whether they are directly or indirectly related to pregnancy. The enquiries initially only applied to women in England and Wales, but were extended to Scotland and Northern Ireland in 1985.

In the 1952–1954 enquiry:

- There were 1,403 direct maternal deaths (2,052,000 confinements)
- The risk of dying directly from a pregnancy-related condition was 1:1,500.

In the 2000–2002 enquiry:

- There were 106 direct maternal deaths (2,016,136 births)
- The risk of dying from a pregnancy-related condition was 1:19,020.

The aim of the enquiry is to improve the quality of maternal care by providing guidance and recommendations based on the assessment of each case.

The overall death rate has decreased over the years, but the number of deaths associated with substandard care has stayed static at about 60%. The recommendations from the reports advise ways in which maternity services can improve the quality of care to prevent maternal morbidity and mortality.

Recent advice includes conditions where poor care has been identified:

1. Sepsis: is often poorly recognized and managed. Before the previous report was published, an alert was published warning about the increased number of deaths due to community acquired β-haemolytic streptococcus A. The deaths had increased from 3 in 2000–2 to 13 in 2006–8.
2. Failure to recognize serious acute illness:
   a. Delay in contacting anaesthetists or critical care specialists
   b. Postpartum haemorrhage
3. Pre-eclampsia/eclampsia: treat systolic hypertension, consider early invasive arterial pressure monitoring

4. Increasing numbers of women with chronic illness and co-morbidity:
   a. These women need multidisciplinary planning prior to delivery
   b. Obesity
5. Specialist clinical care: women with serious medical conditions require prompt multidisciplinary care.

In 2012 the body Mothers and Babies: Reducing Risk through Audits and Confidential Enquiries across the UK (MBRRACE-UK) is to continue the Maternal Death Enquiries. The collaboration is under the umbrella of the Maternal, Newborn and Infant Clinical Outcome Review Programme (MNI-CORP), and has been appointed by the Healthcare Quality Improvement Partnership (HQIP).

The process

1. Identification of the cases:
   a. A maternal death for the enquiry is defined as 'all deaths of pregnant women and women up to one year following the end of their pregnancy'
   b. This is regardless of the place or circumstances of death
2. Information collection:
   a. All health professionals who cared for the woman write an unnamed summary of their involvement
   b. They are also asked to provide a reflection on the care given and any lessons learnt
3. A national panel of experts assesses the data. The case is assessed for the real cause of death and any remediable factors associated with the death
4. Findings and lessons learnt are collated to provide a triennial report; this contains recommendations and guidelines, using up-to-date evidence, to improve future practice.

The deaths are divided into categories:

1. Direct deaths:
   a. Maternal mortality rate for mothers who died from medical conditions that could only be a result of pregnancy
   b. For example, obstetric haemorrhage or pre-eclampsia

2. Indirect deaths:
   a. The mortality rate for mothers' deaths from indirect causes
   b. From pre-existing or new medical or mental health conditions aggravated by pregnancy e.g. heart disease, suicide
3. Coincidental deaths:
   a. Accidents, lightning strikes
4. Late deaths:
   a. Deaths that occur from 42 days after the end of pregnancy to one year later.

The recommendations of the Maternal Death Enquiries (MDE) have been a major influence in improving maternal care at a professional and governmental level. Since the MDE's first report there has been a significant decrease in the number of anaesthetic-related deaths; it was the third most common cause of death in the 1960s and is now an uncommon event. This is due to a number of factors, increased supervision of trainees, improved monitoring equipment, a huge shift to regional rather than general anaesthesia for operative intervention and the introduction of antacid prophylaxis.

In the last MDE (2006–2008) there were six direct deaths attributable to anaesthesia; two of these were airway-related deaths. One of the specific recommendations in the report was: 'Management of failed intubation/ventilation is a core anaesthetic skill that should be rehearsed and assessed regularly.'

National Audit Project 4, *Major Complications of Airway Management in the UK* (2001), also highlighted deficiencies in airway management and failure to alter airway management according to the situation. This data is very similar to an audit of failed intubation in one UK region where in half the women there was a failure to follow a 'failed intubation protocol'.

The last MDE report shows, for the first time in many years, a decline in overall maternal mortality. The rate for direct deaths has fallen from 6.24 to 4.67 per 100,00 maternities ($P = 0.02$); however, the indirect deaths have not changed significantly.

The commonest indirect cause of death is cardiac disease:

- Cardiomyopathy
- Ischaemic heart disease/myocardial infarction
- Aortic dissection.

The MDE reports do not just show in-hospital mortality, but show inequalities in healthcare provision, particularly in vulnerable women. There are also 'top ten' recommendations to emphasize to Trusts and other professional bodies that these require action as a top priority.

The first reports targeted better management of haemorrhage, sepsis and anaesthesia. More recently thromboembolism was highlighted and the deaths have significantly fallen from 41 deaths (2003–2005) to 18 deaths (2006–2008).

The report covering 2000–2002 showed startling statistics:

- Socially excluded pregnant women faced up to a higher than 20-fold greater risk of dying than the more privileged
- Black African women, particularly asylum seekers, were also at higher risk
- This resulted in redefining how maternity services are now provided, making sure that antenatal care is more accessible to these women (2006–2008)
- The result is a downward trend in maternal mortality in Black African women and also from women from White ethnic backgrounds
- Maternal mortality has been significantly reduced in relation to the area of the mothers' residence (deprivation score and postcode).

Maternal mortality in the developing world

There is a huge inequality in maternal mortality in the developed and developing world. Every day 800 women die of preventable causes; 99% of all maternal deaths occur in developing countries. In 2013, it is estimated that 289,000 women died during pregnancy or following childbirth. The majority of these deaths were in poorly resourced settings.

The greatest risk of maternal mortality is in adolescent girls aged 15 or younger. In this group pregnancy-related complications are the leading cause of death.

Data collected by the World Health Organization (WHO), in 2013, clearly shows these inequalities:

Country	Maternal mortality rate per 100,00 live births
Spain	4
United Kingdom	8
India	190
Cameroon	590
Sierra Leone	1100

The Millennium Development Goals (MDGs)

There are eight international development goals that were agreed upon at the Millennium Summit of the United Nations in 2000. All the UN member states committed to achieve these goals by 2015.

The MDG5 goal was to improve maternal health:

1. 5A: reduce the maternal mortality ratio (MMR) by three quarters between 1990 and 2015:
   a. Maternal mortality ratio
   b. Proportion of births attended by a skilled birth assistant

2. 5B: universal access to reproductive health by 2015:
   a. Contraceptive prevalence rate
   b. Adolescent birth rate
   c. Antenatal care coverage
   d. Unmet need for family planning.

At the time that MDG5 was instituted the maternal death rate per year was 529,000. The lifetime risk of dying with complications of pregnancy and childbirth was 1:4,000 women in a developing country and 1:16 in sub-Saharan Africa.

Between 1990–2013 maternal deaths have fallen by 45%. The MMR has fallen 2.6% per year; to achieve the MDG5 goal it should be 5.5% per year.

Other regions have had significant reductions in maternal mortality, particularly in North Africa and Asia.

Causes of death

In the developing world, 75% maternal mortality is related to pregnancy or childbirth. The commonest reasons are:

•	Haemorrhage – mostly after childbirth	27%
•	Infection – puerperal sepsis	11%
•	Hypertensive complications related to pregnancy	14%
•	Complications from delivery Obstructed labour Thrombotic complications	12%
•	Unsafe abortion	8%
•	Pre-existing disease Malaria HIV and AIDS, this is prevalent in sub-Saharan Africa	28%

•	AIDS-related indirect maternal deaths Botswana: MMR 170 per 100,00 live births	23.5%
	South Africa MMR 150 per 100,00 live births	41.4%

Access to healthcare in pregnancy

There are factors that prevent women from accessing adequate healthcare in pregnancy and in the peripartum period. This is seen in both sub-Saharan Africa and South Asia.

The factors are:

- Distance from healthcare facilities
- Inadequate healthcare facilities
- Poverty
- A lack of information
- Cultural beliefs
- Lack of trained skilled health workers – midwives, trained nurses and doctors.

UK Obstetric Surveillance System (UKOSS)

UKOSS is a 'national system to study rare disorders of pregnancy'.

The objective of the project is 'to develop a UK-wide Obstetric Surveillance System to describe the epidemiology of a variety of uncommon disorders of pregnancy'.

Maternal mortality is the tip of the iceberg compared to severe maternal morbidity. There are pregnancy-related conditions and indirect conditions that lead to this morbidity and mortality. Each individual maternity unit will have only limited exposure to these uncommon conditions. Aggregating clinical information using this reporting system should result in a greater understanding of the disease process with the aim to improve outcomes for these women.

UKOSS methodology is a monthly prospective case collection from each maternity unit; this is in the form of a reporting card, which includes a 'nothing to report box'.

The data is collected centrally from a data collection form, which is different for each study.

The criteria for a condition to be studied by UKOSS are:

- An important cause of maternal morbidity or mortality
- Uncommon < 1:2,000 births

- Methodology is suitable
- Other data sources exist to enhance case ascertainment.

UKOSS was launched in 2005 as a joint venture between the Royal College of Obstetricians and Gynaecologists and the National Perinatal Epidemiology Unit.

The first interim reports were published in 2007 and have been subsequently published yearly. The studies encompass all types of morbidity from 'Failed tracheal intubation in obstetric anaesthesia' to 'H1N1v influenza in pregnancy'.

Scottish Confidential Audit of Severe Maternal Morbidity (SCASMM)

For the last 10 years, data (2003–2012) has been collected on severe maternal morbidity in all consultant-led maternity units in Scotland. There are 14 definitions of maternal morbidity that are used in the audit.

Practice is assessed according to published guidelines and this is used to identify variance in practice and good practice. Two types of morbidity were analysed in more detail:

1. Massive obstetric haemorrhage
2. Eclampsia.

All other domains of morbidity were calculated and a 'National Rate per 1,000 births' was calculated.

The main findings in the last 10 years are:

1. An increase in the rate of massive obstetric haemorrhage
2. Overall rates of eclampsia have fallen, this may be attributable to the routine use of magnesium sulfate in severe pre-eclampsia
3. All other morbidities have remained stable.

Sadly the 10th Annual Report will be the last.

The reports have provided valuable data on the frequency of maternal morbidity. The results of the reports should be used to benchmark every maternity unit's practice. Analysis of severe morbidity can improve outcomes and is a valuable tool for teaching and training.

Key points

1. There are unacceptable differences in maternal mortality between the developed and developing world.
2. Midwives or other suitably trained birth attendants are the key to lowering maternal mortality rates.
3. The maternal death enquiries have an important role in maternal safety and aid in changing policy in maternal care.
4. The mortality rate in most of the developed world is small. Looking at maternal severe morbidity in detail can lead to further improvements in the quality and safety of maternal care, resulting in better maternal and perinatal outcomes.

Further reading

Loudon, I. (1986). Deaths in childbed from the eighteenth century to 1935. *Med. Hist.* **30**: 1–41.

The Confidential Enquiries into Maternal Deaths. https://www.npeu.ox.ac.uk/mbrrace-uk (accessed April 2015).

Millennium Development Goals (2013). New York: United Nations.

UKOSS: https://www.npeu.ox.ac.uk/ukoss

Scottish Confidential Audit of Severe Maternal Morbidity: 10th Annual Report: Healthcare Improvement Scotland. http://www.healthcareimprovementscotland.org/our_work/reproductive,_maternal_child/programme_resources/scasmm.aspx

Maternal critical care

Sarah Wheatly and Kate O'Brien

Introduction

Maternal critical care is an evolving sub-speciality, encompassing the multidisciplinary care of the pregnant or recently pregnant woman needing organ support and/or intensive monitoring. Whilst some unwell women will need to be admitted to a general critical care facility, it has been recognized that critical care can and should be provided within the maternity unit, and that this may be advantageous to both mother and baby.

It is estimated that approximately 5% of obstetric patients will require critical care either on the delivery unit or a general critical care facility.

The maternal population has changed significantly over the last 20 years:

- Increase in obesity and in particular morbid obesity
- Increase in numbers of type 2 and gestational diabetes
- Increase in number of women having children in their 30s–40s
- Increase in maternal co-morbidity e.g. congenital heart disease, ischaemic heart disease.

Level 2 care can generally be provided on the delivery unit; however, level 3 care usually requires transfer to a general intensive care unit. The standard of care provided must be the same whether the woman is managed on a delivery unit or general critical care unit.

The Critical Care Minimal Data Set (CCMDS) is the tool that defines the level of care required for the patient (see Table 5.1).

There are a number of conditions requiring critical care on a delivery unit, see Table 5.2, for example:

1. Complications related to pregnancy:
   a. Massive obstetric haemorrhage
   b. Hypertensive disorders (pre-eclampsia, eclampsia)
   c. Genital tract sepsis

Table 5.1 Levels of Care

LEVEL 0	Needing hospital admission
LEVEL 1	Recently discharged from a higher level of care In need of additional monitoring Requiring critical outreach service support
LEVEL 2	Needing preoperative optimization Needing extended postoperative care Stepping down from level 3 care Needing single organ support: • Basic respiratory • Basic or advanced cardiovascular (count as single organ support) • Renal • Neurological • Hepatic • Dermatological
LEVEL 3	Advanced respiratory support alone Support of 2 or more organs

2. Medical complications:
   a. Respiratory disease, e.g. pneumonia, asthma
   b. Cardiac disease, e.g. ischaemic heart disease, cardiomyopathy, congenital heart disease
   c. Sickle cell disease
   d. Renal disease.

The Intensive Care National Audit and Research Centre (ICNARC) [2005] reported on a subset of women aged 16–50, who were pregnant or recently pregnant, admitted to general critical care. The purpose of the study was to evaluate the APACHE II scoring system in obstetric admissions.

Core Topics in Obstetric Anaesthesia, ed. Kirsty MacLennan, Kate O'Brien and W. Ross Mcnab.
Published by Cambridge University Press. © Cambridge University Press 2015.

Table 5.2 Most likely criteria for organ support on a labour ward

Respiratory
Basic

- >50% O_2 via facemask
- Deteriorating respiratory function requiring close observation
- Recent extubation (within 24 hours) after >24 hours of mechanical ventilation

Cardiovascular
Basic

- CVP line for monitoring and/or access for delivery of titrated fluid boluses in hypovolaemia
- Arterial line for monitoring and/or sampling
- Single IV vasoactive drug to support or control BP, output or perfusion

  includes labetalol OR hydralazine, but not uterotonics e.g. syntocinon

Advanced

- Multiple IV vasoactive or rhythm-controlling drugs

  includes labetalol and hydrallazine used simultaneously

- Continuous cardiac output monitoring

Neurological

- Continuous IV medication to control seizures and/ or continuous cerebral monitoring

  at present includes use of magnesium to treat eclampsia, but not for prevention

- Intracranial pressure monitoring

The results were:

1. Direct obstetric admissions were 0.7% of the ICU population
   - The mortality was 1.7%
2. Indirect or coincidental admissions
   - The mortality was 4.2%
3. Non-obstetric female admissions
   - The mortality was 14.7%.

This data seems to show that pregnancy or recent pregnancy confers an increase in survival following critical illness. The reasons are not immediately clear; however, it may be due to the physiological changes of pregnancy combined with delivery of the fetus.

Background

Maternal critical care has developed with the increasing need to care for mothers who develop complications of pregnancy, new disease, or exacerbations of underlying disorders during or immediately after pregnancy. A number of national reports have been key in its establishment. These reports, and the resulting developments include the following.

UK Maternal Death Reports

These triennial reports are the longest running clinical audit study in the world. The enquiry looks into the causes and factors associated with all reported maternal deaths. Recommendations are made to improve care and patient safety to reduce deaths.

Causes of deaths are divided into direct, indirect, late and coincidental. Whist the number of deaths has fallen significantly over the years, there is concern that the percentage of deaths associated with 'substandard care' (meaning that the deaths may have been avoidable) has remained static at about 60%.

This has resulted in a recommendation since the mid-1990s that 'high-dependency' care should be available on the delivery unit; in addition there was a further recommendation that 'invasive monitoring should be used' more widely (2001).

Despite all these recommendations, there was no guidance from any professional body on how to implement this in clinical practice.

Comprehensive Critical Care

This review of adult critical care services in the UK was published in 2000 in response to the need to improve the provision of care for the critically ill. The recommendations were:

1. Integration of critical care services within each hospital:
   a. 'Critical care without walls'
   b. Care provided in the most suitable location for the patient
2. Network development both within and between hospital Trusts:
   a. Standardization of care
   b. Regional guidelines
   c. Care bundles
3. Workforce development to balance staff skill mix with level of care needed:
   a. The standard of care should be the same wherever the patient is cared for
   b. Competency-based assessment for staff looking after these patients

4. Data collection:

    a. Evidence base to support clinical governance

    b. Workforce and service planning.

Safer Childbirth

Published in 2007, from the Royal Colleges of Obstetricians and Gynaecologists, Midwives, Anaesthetists and Paediatrics and Child Health, this was a comprehensive report on recommendations for standards of care in labour.

Included within this were the recommendations that:

1. High-dependency care should be available on or near the labour ward
2. There should be a core of midwives with experience and expertise in the management of the critically ill woman
3. The Critical Care Minimum Data Set (CCMDS), the national format for data collection on critical care patients, should be used on labour wards.

However, this report did not define what was meant by high-dependency care, nor did it specify how midwives should be trained in the management of the critically ill woman.

Levels of Care

Published in 2009, this report from the Department of Health refined and updated the levels of care first described in 'Comprehensive Critical Care'. It followed the approach of allocating levels of care according to clinical need and not location or nurse-to-patient ratio (Table 5.1).

Basic and advanced organ support was defined with descriptive examples. The definitions reflect data needed for the CCMDS, which in turn supports funding for critical care. Critical care is now thought of as level 2 and level 3 care only.

Awareness of the definitions and recommendations in the above reports and concerns about the exclusion of obstetric patients led to a Department of Health meeting of the Critical Care Information and Advisory Group (CCIAG) with representatives from obstetrics, midwifery and anaesthesia in 2007. It was agreed that the definitions of levels of care could be used for obstetric patients. Following this, updated versions of the CCMDS have included obstetric patients and it became officially recognized that critical care could be provided on a delivery unit. Most importantly the term 'critical care' could be used for maternity patients. The term maternal critical care was used to reflect the fact that this care is provided by a skilled multidisciplinary team centred on the mother.

Providing Equity of Critical and Maternal Care for the Critically Ill Pregnant or Recently Pregnant Woman

This 2011 document was produced by a multidisciplinary working group commissioned by the Joint Standing Committee of the Royal College of Obstetricians and Gynaecologists, and the Royal College of Anaesthetists in response to concerns about the lack of national guidance on the care of the critically ill mother.

The remit of the Working Group was to summarize existing standards and recommendations relevant to the care of the critically ill parturient, and to provide guidance for the first time on the management of parturients who become critically ill.

The document included:

1. A definition of maternal critical care
2. An estimation of numbers of women needing maternal critical care
3. A description of different settings for provision of maternal critical care
4. An outline of relevant competencies required to provide maternal critical care
5. A list of appropriate equipment needed.

Importantly, the document emphasized the need for critically ill parturients to be cared for with their babies where possible, and to have the same standard of care, from professionals with the same level of competencies, whether in a general critical care area or a maternity unit.

Steps in starting a critical care facility in the delivery unit:

1. Champions:

    a. Need a group of like-minded people that want to set up the critical care facility

    b. Assess the burden of critical care on the delivery unit (DU). The data capture can be difficult and will almost always understate the numbers

    c. Once the baseline numbers are collected, then you produce a statement of need

    d. This is circulated to the directorate responsible for maternity to assess the application, consider funding and decide which model of care is required. This may well be different in high-volume units with tertiary referrals compared to smaller units.

2. Multidisciplinary team (minimum):
   a. Lead consultant obstetrician
   b. Lead consultant anaesthetist
   c. Midwifery lead
   d. Critical care consultant
   e. Critical care nurse:
      i. Lead nurse for critical care
      ii. Lead nurse responsible for critical care on the delivery unit
   f. Midwife education practitioners
   g. Representation from obstetric and anaesthetic directorates
      i. The directorates have to apply to the local critical care network to recognize the designated area in DU as a critical care facility

3. Identify triggers for admission and discharge to and from:
   a. Maternal critical care
   b. General critical care (see Figure 5.1)
   c. Other specialties e.g. cardiology and renal services

4. Identify a designated critical care area on the DU:
   a. This may be in single rooms or a 2–4-bedded unit
   b. These areas must have fixed monitoring to be designated as critical care rooms; they need to have:
      i. Enough space
      ii. Adequate lighting
      iii. Electricity supply
      iv. Piped oxygen and air
      v. Suction
      vi. Storage
      vii. Data points

MATERNAL CRITICAL CARE (MCC) FLOWCHART

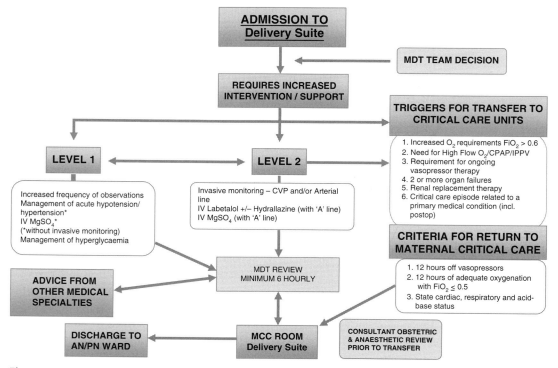

Figure 5.1 Maternal critical care flowchart.

c. The following should also be immediately available:

    i. Syringe pumps

    ii. Fluid infusion pumps

    iii. Intravenous fluid warmers

    iv. Forced air warmers e.g. Bair hugger

    v. Rapid infusor and warmer e.g. Belmont, Level 1

    vi. Airway trolley

    vii. Emergency haemorrhage trolley

    viii. Blood fridge

    ix. Eclampsia box

    x. Blood gas analyzer

    xi. Near patient coagulation testing e.g. TEG, ROTEM

    xii. Transfer monitor and ventilator

5. CCMDS collection:

a. This is an essential part of defining how many level 2/3 women are receiving maternal critical care

b. This needs to be part of general critical care data collection

c. The tariff for this is set by the CCMDS

d. Level 1 patients also are reported on; these are women that do not require level 2 care, but are at risk for deterioration and need to be intensively monitored. This hidden burden on the DU can be fed into the commissioning process to ensure that the tariffs are commensurate with the medical and midwifery time caring for these women.

e. Accurate coding of each maternal critical care episode

6. Benchmarking:

a. Assessment of severe maternal morbidity

b. Data incorporated into the critical care network data set.

Staffing

Nursing

It is essential for parturients requiring level 2 or 3 care to have their nursing needs met by staff who are trained and competent in critical care; midwives normally provide nursing care on the DU. Current midwifery training in the UK concentrates on normal pregnancy and labour, and does not require a general nursing background. Further training is therefore needed if midwives are to attain the knowledge, skills and competencies required to care for critically ill parturients. Several different courses with varying levels of practical experience are currently available, many now being university based. A useful framework for the skills and competencies required can be adapted from the DOH document 'Competencies for Recognising and Responding to Acutely Ill Patients in Hospital' and the 'National Competency Framework for Adult Critical Care Nurses'.

Recognition of critical illness is often poor, as highlighted in a number of Confidential Enquiries. Midwives benefit from undertaking 'acute illness management' training to pick up patient deterioration before overt maternal collapse; there are a number of these courses throughout the UK. This involves lectures and scenarios and then a competency assessment.

A combination of critical care nurses and midwives with enhanced competencies to care for level 2 women has been shown to work well in some units with both the critical care nurses and the midwives find that the combination of the two plays to their strengths.

All the critical care nurses have an induction programme; this includes lectures, sessions in clinics and simulation. The course is open to midwives who are gaining enhanced competencies to look after level 2 women and covers all aspects of maternal physiology, pathophysiology and common emergency scenarios (see Chapter 26).

Medical

Obstetricians in units providing level 2 critical care will need additional training in care of the critically ill as this is not currently included in speciality training. A number of general courses are available, though none specific to obstetricians or maternal critical care. This may be an area for development, using adaptations of existing intensive care courses, and core competencies in intensive care medicine as a framework.

Dedicated 24-hour anaesthetic cover from anaesthetists with a minimum of Step 1 intensive care competencies should be available for units providing critical care.

UK anaesthetic training includes a significant amount of intensive care at present, though most consultant obstetric anaesthetists do not have regular sessions in critical care. As maternal critical care evolves there is scope for consultants to have a dual role in both general critical care and maternity and this may also be an area for development.

The multidisciplinary team (MDT)

The MDT is an essential part of maternal critical care. There needs to be effective leadership, communication, including comprehensive handover, and appropriate referral to other specialties as required.

The MDT consists of midwives, obstetricians, anaesthetists and in some units critical care nurses. The ward rounds must be regular (4–6 hourly) to ensure that there is no deterioration of the patient's condition.

Transfer

There are many situations in which a critically ill parturient may need to be transferred: either within one hospital, or from one facility to another. This is most commonly either for:

1. Transfer to general or cardiac intensive care
2. Investigations e.g. CT scan.

Guidelines should be available for transfer of critically ill women. The triggers for transfer will be different for each unit, but these triggers must be clear for transfer to ICU and for discharge back to the DU (see Figure 5.1). The decision to transfer should be multidisciplinary, involving obstetricians, midwives, anaesthetists, intensivists and any other relevant speciality.

Key points

1. Women who have a need for maternal critical care generally have a good outcome.
2. The burden of maternal critical care will continue to rise from co-morbidity and the increasing caesarean section rate.
3. Midwifery and obstetric training should encompass illness recognition and management training. This needs to be urgently addressed by the RCOG and the RCM.
4. Transfer triggers, specific to the hospital, to general critical care need to be stated clearly.
5. The delivery unit often is the best place for many women with critical illness.

Further reading

Department of Health. (2000). Comprehensive Critical Care: A Review of Adult Critical Care Services. London: Department of Health.

Royal College of Obstetricians and Gynaecologists. (2007). Safer Childbirth: Minimum Standards for the Organization and Delivery of Care in Labour. London: RCOG.

Royal College of Obstetricians and Gynaecologists. (2011). Providing Equity of Critical and Maternity Care for the Critically Ill Pregnant or Recently Pregnant Woman. London: RCOG.

Department of Health. (2008). Competencies for Recognising and Responding to Acutely Ill Patients in Hospital. London: Department of Health.

Department of Health. (2012). National Competency Framework for Adult Critical Care Nurses. (2012). London: Department of Health.

Chapter

6

Obstetrics for the anaesthetist

Emma Ingram, Alex Heazell and Edward D. Johnstone

Intrapartum care at or near term gestation

Intrapartum care is a challenging and rapidly changing environment for all health professionals. As an obstetrician the key question is often 'Do I need to intervene? And if so, how much time do I have to do this?' Fetal monitoring, recommendation of mode and timing of delivery is aimed at reducing poor neonatal outcomes.

Within the scope of this chapter it is not possible to cover all potential intrapartum events that may require anaesthetic assessment and input. The aim of this chapter is to provide enough information on fetal monitoring to enable the anaesthetist to understand the urgency of a delivery and how this is determined in high-risk cases such as twins and vaginal breech delivery.

Intrapartum fetal monitoring

Intrapartum fetal monitoring techniques have enabled obstetricians to intervene and prevent the development of a severe hypoxia. However, these techniques are far from perfect. The mainstay of fetal intrapartum monitoring remains the cardiotocograph (CTG), which records the fetal heart rate (FHR) and the presence of uterine contraction activity using the tocograph. This is recommended by NICE for all 'high-risk' labours. Although not exhaustive, indications for continuous intrapartum CTG monitoring are listed below:

- Meconium-stained liquor
- Abnormal FHR detected by intermittent auscultation
- Maternal pyrexia of 38 °C on one occasion or 37.5°C on two occasions, 2 hours apart
- Fresh bleeding developing in labour

- Oxytocin use for augmentation
- Multiple pregnancy
- Vaginal breech delivery
- Maternal request
- Fetal growth restriction
- Preterm labour
- Maternal disease (pre-eclampsia, obstetric cholestasis).

The evidence for these recommendations is derived from observational studies rather than randomized controlled trials. The poor quality of these studies, which were performed more than 20 years ago, has resulted in a lack of evidence for CTG use in low-risk women. Therefore although it might seem counterintuitive to the anaesthetist to reduce the amount of monitoring information available to doctors and midwives caring for women in labour, current NICE guidance does not support the use of CTG in this group. A Cochrane review on continuous CTG during labour demonstrated a reduction in neonatal seizures, but no significant differences in cerebral palsy or infant mortality rates. This was offset by increases in caesarean section and instrumental vaginal birth rates.

Interpretation of CTG

The interpretation of a fetal heart rate (FHR) trace should take into consideration the presence or stage of labour, its progress, maternal observations and other risk factors present. CTG interpretation is subject to high intra- and interobserver variation related to experience, training and time of day. Computerized CTG interpretation software has been developed to support decision-making in the management of labour. Its use in labour is currently being evaluated in the multicentre randomized controlled INFANT study.

A documented interpretation of a CTG should be performed every hour, or with any clinical concern.

Core Topics in Obstetric Anaesthesia, ed. Kirsty MacLennan, Kate O'Brien and W. Ross Mcnab.
Published by Cambridge University Press. © Cambridge University Press 2015.

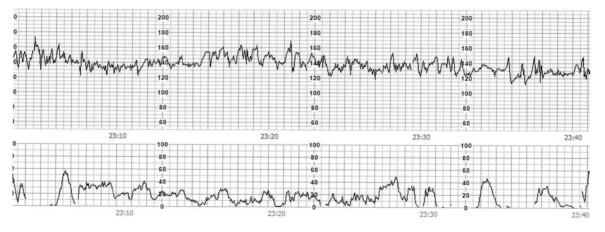

Figure 6.1a Normal and abnormal CTGs.
A normal cardiotocograph trace. The baseline is 135 beats/min variability 25 beats/min accelerations present and no decelerations.

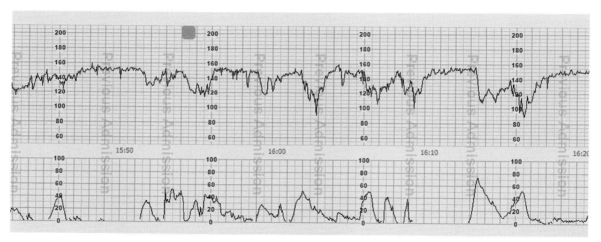

Figure 6.1b A pathological cardiotocograph trace demonstrating late decelerations. The radar of the deceleration and the peak of contraction are marked with arows.

Interpretation is based on four features – rate, variability, accelerations and decelerations. Based on these features the CTG can be classified as normal, suspicious or pathological (Table 6.1).

Baseline rate

The normal fetal heart rate is 110–160 bpm, with the mean tending to fall as gestation progresses. A low baseline (100–110 bpm) or a tachycardia (160–180 bpm), where accelerations are present and no other adverse features appear is not regarded as suspicious. This may represent a baseline reduction following opiate administration, or a tachycardia with an active fetus, both of

which may eventually settle. FHR is affected by maternal pyrexia and/or tachycardia and usually rises by 10–15 bpm. A slow rise in baseline over the duration of a labour may indicate increasing fetal acidosis and should be regarded as suspicious. A baseline rate of <100 or >180 is always abnormal.

Variability

Variability is defined as the beat-to-beat variation, and should be greater than 5 bpm; it represents the fetal autonomic nervous system function. A reduction in variability for up to 40 minutes may be normal with the fetal sleep cycle. A reduction in

Table 6.1 CTG parameters and interpretation

Feature	Baseline (bpm)	Variability (bpm)	Decelerations	Accelerations
Reassuring	110–160	≥5	None	Present
Non-reassuring	100–109 161–180	<5 for 40–90 minutes	Typical variable decelerations with over 50% of contractions, occurring for over 90 minutes Single prolonged deceleration for up to 3 minutes	The absence of accelerations with otherwise normal trace is of uncertain significance
Abnormal	<100 >180 Sinusoidal pattern ≥10 minutes	<5 for >90 minutes	Either atypical variable decelerations with over 50% of contractions or late decelerations, both for over 30 minutes Single prolonged deceleration for more than 3 minutes	

Category	Definition
Normal	An FHR trace in which all four features are classified as reassuring
Suspicious	An FHR trace with one feature classified as non-reassuring and the remaining features classified as reassuring
Pathological	An FHR trace with two or more features classified as non-reassuring or one or more classified as abnormal

variability has low sensitivity but high specificity for fetal acidosis.

Accelerations

The presence of accelerations in the FHR of greater than 15 bpm for 15 seconds is a reassuring feature suggesting fetal activity. The presence of accelerations has a high specificity for excluding fetal acidosis, although the absence of accelerations does not denote a suspicious or pathological CTG trace.

Decelerations

The presence of decelerations is a non-reassuring or abnormal feature on a CTG, and is classified according to the type (early, late and variable), duration and frequency. Early decelerations are uniform in size, shape and duration and are likely to represent head

compression in the late first or second stages of labour rather than hypoxia. Critically, early decelerations start with uterine contractions and the FHR has normally returned to baseline as the contraction finishes.

Late decelerations are so called because the deceleration in FHR starts to occur after the uterine contraction peaks, and persists after the contraction finishes. Late decelerations are more indicative of fetal hypoxia.

Variable decelerations are more common, accounting for more than 80% of decelerations seen. They are defined as a reduction from the baseline more than 15 bpm for 15 seconds with varying length, amplitude and uniformity. Commonly as a result of cord compression, variable decelerations are sub-classified into typical (which may be found near the end of the second stage of labour) or atypical. Atypical variable decelerations are more concerning and may show a loss of shouldering (accelerations before and after the

Table 6.2 FBS results and recommendations

FBS result (pH)	Interpretation	Appropriate action
≥7.25	Normal	Appropriate sampling should be repeated no more than 60 minutes later if the FHR trace remains pathological, or sooner if there are further abnormalities
7.21–7.24	Borderline	Sampling should be repeated no more than 30 minutes later if the FHR trace remains pathological, or sooner if there are further abnormalities
≤7.20	Abnormal	Consultant obstetric advice should be sought, with a view to an urgent birth

deceleration), a smooth decline, with a slow recovery to baseline which may overshoot, or be biphasic in shape.

When a CTG is normal the baby is very likely to be well, but the majority of abnormal CTGs occur in babies who are not distressed. A suspicious CTG requires review by an obstetrician for a management plan, which will depend on the overall clinical picture and the duration of concern. For example, the presence of variable decelerations in early labour is of more concern than near delivery. Suspicious features may respond to simple measures that can be performed to optimize placental perfusion.

These techniques may include:

- Changing of maternal position
- Adequate hydration with intravenous crystalloid fluid
- Avoiding uterine hyperstimulation by judicious use of oxytocin
- Reduction of maternal pyrexia by paracetamol and/or antibiotics.

If suspicious features persist, then consideration of further assessment with fetal blood sampling should be made. Unlike a CTG classified as suspicious, a pathological CTG requires action. This may mean expediting birth by instrumental delivery if imminent or by further assessment of fetal wellbeing by fetal blood sampling. If labour is not advanced enough to permit this (<3 cm dilated), or is contraindicated, then delivery by emergency caesarean section is required if pathological features persist.

Fetal blood sampling (FBS)

As an abnormal CTG has a relatively low positive predictive value (PPV) for acidosis, FBS is performed in most UK units in an attempt to reduce false positive diagnosis of fetal compromise and corresponding unnecessary intervention. Fetal blood sampling provides current fetal pH and base excess.

Serious adverse sequelae in the newborn period are rare after birth with umbilical cord pH greater than 7.0 or base excess less than −12 mmol/L.

FBS should be performed with the consent of the mother with full understanding that the subsequent result may influence the mode and urgency of delivery or that the FBS may need repeating should the CTG continue to be pathological. FBS is ideally performed in the left lateral position to optimize placental perfusion. Contraindications to FBS include gestation earlier than 34 weeks, maternal blood-borne infection (HIV, active hepatitis B and C) and potential inherited fetal bleeding disorders. Should there be a pathological trace where FBS is contraindicated, technically impossible due to dilatation, a failure of collection or the mother refuses the FBS, delivery should be expedited on the presumption of fetal acidosis.

FBS results should be interpreted in the context of the progress of labour (Table 6.2). FBS should not be performed with obvious fetal compromise as indicated by prolonged (>4 minutes) bradycardia or when vaginal delivery can be easily achieved using ventouse or forceps. In these cases immediate delivery should be expedited.

An abnormal FBS result requires urgent delivery. The delivery should be performed by the fastest and safest mode relevant to the operators' skill and experience.

Classification of urgency of delivery

The Sentinel Caesarean Section Audit suggested that in cases such as cord prolapse, a decision-to-delivery interval (DDI) of 15 minutes was feasible. However, in many Category 1 decisions, delivery within 30 minutes was not achieved. Once a decision to deliver has been made, delivery should be carried out with the urgency appropriate to the risk for that baby and the safety of its mother (Tables 6.3 and 6.4). Evidence suggests that delay is often associated with transfer to theatre.

In cases of suspected or confirmed acute fetal compromise, such as that of a pathological CTG or

Table 6.3 Classification of urgency for caesarean section

Category	
1	Immediate threat to the life of the woman or fetus
2	Maternal or fetal compromise that is not immediately life-threatening
3	No maternal or fetal compromise but needs early delivery
4	Delivery timed to suit woman or staff

Table 6.4 Suggested DDI target times

Category	Time from decision to delivery
1	30 minutes
2	75 minutes
3	24 hours
4	Timed to suit patient and staff

abnormal FBS result, delivery should be accomplished as soon as possible. Thirty minutes has become the accepted standard for Category 1 deliveries, and is often used as an audit tool to monitor performance.

Many units have implemented DDI timings to aim towards; this can aid in focusing the team on the urgency of the delivery, allow planning of the labour ward workload and allow auditing of key indicators. Although far from universal, commonly implemented target times are shown below.

Despite a DDI interval of 30 minutes being suggested, studies have demonstrated this was only achievable in two-thirds of emergency caesareans for fetal distress. A DDI interval of up to 75 mins had no significant increase in neonatal or maternal morbidity. However, during acute hypoxia, such as a fetal bradycardia, pH reduces by 0.1 units/min; the degree of acidosis will depend on the starting pH of a potentially already compromised fetus.

Fetal ECG (ST analysis)

Whilst the majority of units use CTG and FBS as their main methods of fetal monitoring, some units employ fetal ECG as an adjunct. Whilst, as with a CTG, an anaesthetist would not be expected to interpret a fetal ECG, it is important to understand the additional information it can provide and how this may alter clinical decisions. NICE suggests that fetal ECG may reduce intervention, but doesn't significantly alter neonatal outcome. The additional costs and complexities of staff training have meant it's not a common finding on delivery units at present.

The fetal ECG, like an adult ECG, displays P, QRS and T waves. Hypoxia during labour can alter the waveform of the fetal ECG. Repolarization of myocardial cells is sensitive to metabolic dysfunction caused by hypoxia. Hypoxia in the fetus changes the ST segment. Fetal ECGs are performed with ruptured membranes through a fetal scalp electrode (rather than an abdominal transducer, which is most often used for CTG) with computer analysis of the waveform. Progressive changes in the T/QRS ratio can be determined if applied before evidence of fetal stress, usually commenced at the beginning of labour to determine changes from the baseline (i.e. the fetal ECG cannot be applied once CTG abnormalities have commenced). Unlike CTG, fetal ECG does not require FBS to confirm hypoxia so delivery is indicated on the basis of fetal ECG analysis recommendation. Unfortunately, once a fetal ECG becomes abnormal then the safe delivery window is 20 minutes or less. This tight delivery window is another reason why many departments have not adopted the technology.

Instrumental delivery

Instrumental delivery is more common in primiparous women and those with epidural analgesia. The obstetrician will normally allow an hour of active pushing before considering intervening both to aid the mother and prevent prolonged second stage complications such as postpartum haemorrhage. Prior to performing an instrumental delivery the obstetrician will assess the cervical dilatation, fetal presentation (head = cephalic, bottom = breech), station of presenting part (relative to ischial spines), position, moulding (overlapping of fetal skull bones), presence of caput (fetal scalp oedema) and pelvic outlet capacity. In the UK, obstetricians will only perform instrumental deliveries at full cervical dilatation with the fetal head at or below the ischial spines. Having determined the suitability for instrumental delivery the obstetrician must determine the fetal head position using anatomical features felt on the fetal head. The occipito-anterior (OA) position presents the smallest relative fetal head diameter and is the easiest to deliver vaginally. Malposition occurs

39

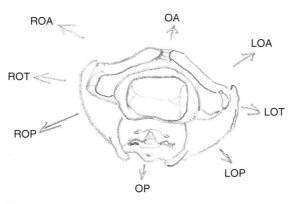

Presentation key

OA Occipito-anterior

OP Occipito-posterior

ROP Right Occipito-posterior

ROA Right Occipito-anterior

ROT Right Occipito-transverse

LOP Left Occipito-posterior

LOA Left Occipito-anterior

LOT Left Occipito-transverse

Figure 6.2 Diagrammatic representation of fetal presentation.

when the fetal head is not OA and is in an alternative position (See Figure 6.2). Occipito-posterior (OP) and occipito-transverse (OT) and variations on this (right occipito-posterior ROP= the occiput is 10–20° to the right, etc.) present a larger relative fetal head diameter and will often require rotation to OA by the obstetrician to achieve delivery.

The majority of instrumental deliveries are performed within the delivery room with the fetal head in the occipito-anterior (OA) position. However, if delivery is anticipated to be more complicated, instrumental delivery in theatre is recommended, the so-called 'trial of instrumental delivery'. Transfer to theatre allows adequate analgesia with either spinal or epidural, which improves associated pain and maternal concordance and allows a rapid conversion to Caesarean section if required. In general, deliveries that are anticipated to be more difficult or likely to fail, such as those with a high presenting part, malposition, macrosomic infant or a high maternal BMI, will be performed in theatre. Sometimes transfer to theatre is necessary for maternal analgesia alone. In cases of fetal distress when a difficult trial of instrumental delivery for malposition is considered it may be prudent to perform an FBS prior to transfer to provide an accurate assessment of fetal acidosis.

The choice of instrument depends on fetal head position, operator preference and experience. Whilst ventouse has a reduced incidence of perineal trauma, fetal traction is more limited than with forceps, meaning it is more likely to fail. Therefore, in situations with extensive caput, a large baby or poor maternal effort, forceps are usually the preferred choice even if the fetus is in OA position. If fetal head rotation is required to correct malposition then this can be achieved manually, with posterior cup ventouse or Keillands forceps. The success of attempts to rotate the fetal head and deliver the baby in theatre are very dependent on obstetrician experience and the anaesthetist should be prepared for sudden changes in the mode of delivery in such circumstances, particularly in dealing with less experienced staff. Further awareness of difficulty should also be raised if multiple instruments (i.e. ventouse and forceps) are used. Instrumental deliveries are also associated with perineal trauma including 3rd and 4th degree tears and postpartum haemorrhage. In theatre the anaesthetist can provide essential input with regards to the physiological signs of blood loss and take a lead role in co-ordinating its management.

Conversion to caesarean section after an unsuccessful attempted instrumental delivery presents the obstetrician with a high-risk surgical case where bleeding and uterine trauma frequently occur. As an obstetrician, a full dilation section after instrumentation creates a low impacted head, and a very friable vascular lower segment. It may be necessary to aid the delivery of the head by adjustment of the theatre table to a lower level or in reverse Trendelenburg position. Tocolytics or conversion to general anaesthetic may also be required. In these situations time is critical and anticipation or suggestion of these techniques by the anaesthetist can be helpful. Should the head remain impacted it may be necessary to push the head 'from below', which requires the cooperation of theatre staff in maternal positioning. Such deliveries may be stressful for the delivering obstetrician, particularly in the case of concurrent potential fetal compromise. Support from the anaesthetist including prompts about blood loss and any potential requirements for cross--matching can be helpful.

Intrapartum management of twins

Twins are regarded as high-risk pregnancies with a perinatal mortality rate five times higher than that of singletons. The increased perinatal mortality is largely related to prematurity, fetal growth restriction and complications of monochorionicity, such as twin-to-twin transfusion. However, intrapartum complications are also more common, especially with delivery of the second twin. Vaginally delivered second twins have a fourfold increased risk of intrapartum death, compared to planned caesarean section. An understanding of the types of twins, their subsequent management options and the potential intrapartum complications is essential.

For the purpose of mode of delivery, twins can be divided into those which share an amniotic sac and those which are separate. Dichorionic diamniotic twins, which have separate placentas and are within separate sacs, and monochorionic diamniotic twins who have a shared placenta but separate sacs, are potentially suitable for vaginal delivery. Monochorionic monoamniotic (MCMA) twins share both an amniotic sac and a placenta; therefore the bodies can become interlocked, preventing vaginal birth. Caesarean section is recommended for all monoamniotic twins and higher multiples.

Timing of twin deliveries is important due to increasing morbidity and mortality with advancing gestation. In this situation it's the shared placenta that becomes most significant. In dichorionic twin pregnancies delivery should be planned after 37–38 completed weeks and in uncomplicated monochorionic twins at 36–37 completed weeks. MCMA twins have the highest risk of stillbirth and cord entanglement and so should be delivered by 32–34 completed weeks. Due to the nature of twin pregnancy, one-third will go into spontaneous preterm labour before 37 weeks.

Mode of delivery remains a contentious issue. Some suggest that the risk of mortality and morbidity for the second twin advocates caesarean section in all cases. A Cochrane review suggests that caesarean section does not change neonatal outcome, whilst increasing maternal morbidity. A large randomized trial, the Twin Birth Study, aimed to answer the question of planned mode of delivery. Recent publication of the study demonstrated that planned caesarean delivery did not significantly decrease or increase the risk of neonatal death or serious morbidity, when compared with planned vaginal delivery.

Thus, the mode of delivery in uncomplicated twins is dependent on the presentation of the leading twin. With breech presentation of the first twin, which occurs in 20% of cases, the woman should be offered an elective caesarean section. Cephalic presentation of the leading twin would permit a trial of vaginal delivery.

To deliver twins, adequate experienced midwifery and obstetric staff is essential, and a theatre and anaesthetist should be readily available. Twins should have their fetal heart rate monitored throughout labour. As it is critical to differentiate between the two fetal heart rates this may be achieved by a fetal scalp electrode on twin one and an external CTG transducer on twin two. If CTG concerns arise in the leading twin an FBS can be performed as normal. CTG concerns with the second twin require a decision regarding operative delivery, as there are no measures to confirm whether twin two is acidotic. After delivery of the first twin, the second is stabilized to control lie and an ultrasound performed to confirm presentation, which can change in 20% of cases. Oxytocin should be ready for augmentation should contractions stop and the second twin should be allowed to descend into the pelvis before the membranes are ruptured. The second twin can deliver either cephalic or by breech extraction. During this technique internal podalic version is performed initially. The operator grasps the fetal foot within the uterus and gently and continuously pulls until in the pelvis. The breech delivery is then continued as described, but with continuous traction. Following delivery of the second twin, postpartum haemorrhage should be anticipated due to atony of the over-distended uterine myometrium.

Anaesthetic involvement in twin deliveries may involve placement of epidural anaesthesia, which can facilitate manoeuvres to deliver a breech second twin or provide anaesthesia for an urgent recourse to delivery. The anaesthetist should be readily available for emergency caesarean section and for management of postpartum blood loss.

Vaginal breech delivery

Breech presentation occurs in 3–4% of pregnancies at term. The Term Breech Trial recommended caesarean section as the safest mode of delivery for breech presentation at term in nulliparous women. This recommendation was based on a relative risk of neonatal mortality or serious neonatal morbidity of 0.33 for planned caesarean section compared to planned vaginal birth, although the absolute risks were small at 1.6% for planned caesarean section to 5% for planned vaginal birth. Recommendations were rapidly implemented and experience with vaginal breech deliveries has diminished amongst obstetricians and midwives since, with major implications on training. Options for a woman with a diagnosed breech at term are external cephalic version or caesarean section. Woman are counselled that vaginal breech delivery increases the risk of perinatal morbidity and mortality. Some women opt for a planned vaginal breech delivery, whilst some will present with an undiagnosed breech in labour. Vaginal breech deliveries can proceed as long as the woman is counselled appropriately and offered a caesarean section. There should be no other contraindications to vaginal delivery and essential conditions should be met throughout the delivery in order to optimize safety. The women should be:

- Labouring spontaneously
- On a consultant-led labour ward with suitable experienced staff onsite willing to perform or supervise the delivery
- Appropriately counselled with an understanding that early recourse to CS may be required (approx. 50% of breech labours in nulliparous women will end in CS)
- Have an appropriate sized fetus (weight not <2000 g or > 3800 g)
- Continuous CTG monitoring with no signs of fetal distress
- Progressing adequately in labour without the use of oxytocin augmentation.

A vaginal breech delivery requires one-to-one care. As the anaesthetist, regional analgesia may be helpful with possible delivery interventions. There needs to be a readiness to transfer to theatre for an emergency caesarean section should there be fetal distress, poor progress in labour or cord prolapse.

Once full dilatation is confirmed, the woman should be placed in the lithotomy position and the bladder emptied. The breech should be allowed to descend without traction or manipulation to the introitus, the fetus should be in the sacro-anterior position throughout. With distension of the introitus,

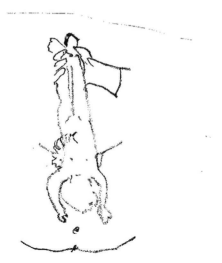

Figure 6.3 Breech delivery.

an episiotomy should be considered and maternal effort should allow steady advancement to the umbilicus. It may be necessary to manipulate the legs free with gentle pressure behind each popliteal fossa. As the body continues to descend with contractions, the scapula will become visible and the arms should deliver spontaneously if flexed. Lovset's manoeuvre may be required to deliver nuchal arms by rotation through 90° in either direction. The baby should be allowed to descend further until the nape of the neck is visible. Delivery of the head is now possible with flexion by pressure on the occiput (Mauriceau–Smellie–Viet manoeuvre) or by lifting the feet upwards in an arc (Burns–Marshall technique) (Figure 6.3). If neither of these manoeuvres is successful, forceps can be applied to deliver the head with the feet raised above. Breech delivery is more traumatic for the baby, and it's more likely to become cold. A paediatrician should be available after delivery for possible resuscitation and review.

Complications of breech delivery include cord prolapse, fetal distress or inadequate progress of labour, all of which require recourse to caesarean section. A more distressing and unusual situation is head entrapment, which more commonly occurs with preterm infants. This is an obstetric emergency, which requires senior multidisciplinary assistance. In this situation the head may be trapped by a bony abnormality or an incompletely dilated cervix. The initial aim is to increase the dimensions of the pelvic outlet by the McRoberts position and trying suprapubic pressure. Should this fail, tocolytics may be required or incisions to the cervix. In order to perform cervical incisions, adequate analgesia is required and haemorrhage may ensue. Drastic measures may require caesarean section with the baby being supported and pushed from below.

Key points

1. Interpretation of the CTG is based on rate, variability, acceleration and deceleration. It can be classified as normal, suspicious or pathological.

2. Normal fetal heart rate is between 110 and 160 beats per minute, a baseline rate of less than 100 and greater than 180 is always abnormal.

3. Suspicious CTGs require review and a management plan. This plan will depend on overall clinical picture, duration of concern and the consideration and results of further assessments.

4. Decision-to-delivery times can be used as a tool to monitor team performance and help towards improvements in the delivery of care.

5. Caesarean section after a failed instrumental delivery can be a challenging surgical procedure.

Further reading

Alfirevic, Z., Devane, D. and Gyte, G. M. L. (2013). Continuous cardiotocography (CTG) as a form of electronic fetal monitoring (EFM) for fetal assessment during labour (Review). *Cochrane Database Syst. Rev.*, **2013**(5), Art. No. CD006066.

Armstrong, L. and Stenson, B. J. (2007). Use of umbilical cord blood gas analysis in the assessment of the newborn. *Arch. Dis. Child Fetal Neonatal Ed.*, **92**(6), F430–F434.

Barrett, J., Hannah, M., Hutton, E. *et al.* (2013). A randomized trial of planned caesarean or vaginal delivery for twin pregnancy. *New Engl. J. Med.* **369** (14), 1295–1305.

Hannah, M. E., Hannah, W. J., Hewson, S. A. *et al.* (2000). Planned caesarean section versus vaginal birth at term: a randomised multicentre trial. Lancet **356**, 1375–1383.

National Institute of Health and Clinical Excellence (2011). Caesarean Section. CG132. 32–35.

National Institute of Health and Clinical Excellence (2007). Intrapartum care. CG55. 44–48.

Royal College of Obstetricians and Gynaecologists (2006). *The Management of Breech Presentation. Green-top guideline No. 20b*. London: RCOG Press.

Royal College of Obstetricians and Gynaecologists (2011). *Operative Vaginal Delivery. Green-top Guideline 26*. London: RCOG Press.

Shah, D. (2013) *Clinical Progress in Obstetrics and Gynaecology*. New Delhi: Jaypee Brothers.

Smith, G. C., Pell, J. P. and Dobbie, R. (2002). Birth order, gestational age and risk of delivery related perinatal death in twins: retrospective cohort study. *BMJ* **325**, 1004–1008.

Thomas, J., Paranjothy, S. and James, D. (2004). National cross sectional survey to determine whether the decision to delivery interval is critical in emergency caesarean section. *BMJ* **328**, 665.

Tuffnell, D. J., Wilkinson, K. and Beresford, N. (2001). Interval between decision and delivery by caesarean section: are current standards achievable? Observational case series. *BMJ* **322**, 1330.

Antenatal assessment

Allison C. L. Howells

In 2007 the Department of Health published *Maternity Matters: Choice, Access and Continuity of Care in a Safe Service*. The over-riding aim of any maternity service is to provide safe, high-quality care to women and their partners, thus enabling a safe pregnancy and birth for both mother and baby and to provide a confident start to family life.

For the majority of women, midwives and obstetricians will deliver care, but there are an increasing number of women whose pregnancy, labour or delivery require anaesthetic input.

Over the past decade the Centre for Maternal and Child Enquiries (CMACE), the Royal College of Obstetricians and Gynaecologists (RCOG), the Obstetric Anaesthetists' Association (OAA) and the Association of Anaesthetists of Great Britain and Ireland (AAGBI) have all produced guidance emphasizing the need for good communication between all the speciality groups providing antenatal care. Antenatal anaesthetic assessment is pivotal in planning peripartum care, particularly for those with co-existing disease, to ensure the best outcome for these women. The most recent guidance from the OAA/AAGBI states there should be an agreed system whereby the anaesthetist is given sufficient notice of all potentially high-risk patients. In the majority of obstetric units this would be done as a referral to an antenatal anaesthetic assessment clinic.

Antenatal anaesthetic clinic

There are increasing numbers of parturients presenting with co-existing, complex medical conditions. This may, in part, result from the advances in medicine that have rendered such conditions more stable and have seen these women surviving to childbearing age. Many women are now choosing to have children later in life, resulting in an increase in acquired co-morbidity. The prevalence of morbid obesity has significantly increased in the UK (1.4% in 1993, 2.9% in 2005). This was echoed by data published by the World Health Organization, demonstrating that the prevalence of obesity has nearly doubled between 1998 and 2008.

The anaesthetic service not only provides intrapartum analgesia and anaesthesia, but also assists in the delivery of peripartum care to women with complications related to their pregnancy or co-existing medical disease.

The aim of the antenatal clinic is to carry out a review of the woman's history, assess the impact of any co-morbidities and provide information. The outcome of the visit should be an individualized anaesthetic management plan for labour and delivery. Women with complex medical problems need to be discussed at a multidisciplinary forum, so that obstetricians, anaesthetists, midwives and other medical specialities are aware of the issues that might arise in the peripartum period.

In 1993 Rosaeg *et al.* published a review of patients seen in their anaesthetic clinic over a 6-year period. The review showed that the clinic provided a valuable service, not only to the pregnant woman, but also to the anaesthetist and other healthcare professionals involved in the woman's care. Another highlighted benefit was the provision of consistent advice and information regarding anaesthetic management that may impact on obstetric care to the obstetricians.

When setting up an anaesthetic assessment service it is essential that there is suitable infrastructure to support the clinic:

- Consultant time made available in job plans to run the clinics
- Consultation room dedicated to the clinic
- Setting appropriate referral criteria (see Table 7.1)
- Consultant review of referrals prior to booking

Core Topics in Obstetric Anaesthesia, ed. Kirsty MacLennan, Kate O'Brien and W. Ross Mcnab.
Published by Cambridge University Press. © Cambridge University Press 2015.

Table 7.1 Example of referral criteria taken from referral guidelines at St Mary's Hospital, Manchester

•	Anaesthetic	Previous difficulties with general or regional anaesthesia Severe reaction to drugs including anaesthetic agents or local anaesthetics
•	Cardiac	Congenital heart disease Coronary heart disease Previous cardiac surgery Arrhythmias/pacemaker or ICD in situ
•	Respiratory	Severe asthma Cystic fibrosis Restrictive lung disease
•	Musculoskeletal	Scoliosis Achondroplasia Previous spinal surgery/injury Muscular dystrophies
•	Neurological	History of brain injury/surgery Myopathy Multiple sclerosis Spina bifida Any spinal cord abnormality Stroke
•	Haematological	Haemaglobinopathy Coagulopathy
•	Endocrine	Thyroid disease/phaeochromocytoma/other endocrine disorder
•	Obstetric	Risk of major obstetric haemorrhage
•	Others	Severe obesity – BMI > 40 kg/m^2 Difficult venous access or needle phobia Refusal of blood products Learning difficulties or significant problems with consent Other severe disease

- Secretarial support
  - Booking women into the clinic
  - Appointment and clinic letters
  - Point of contact for the women
  - Retrieval of notes from other hospitals
- Interpreting services
- Dissemination of the findings from the clinic visit to all relevant personnel
- A system that ensures there is easy access to the clinic letters if a woman is admitted to the delivery unit out of hours
- Database of all the referrals
- Audit of the clinic service.

Who should be seen?

In an ideal world, all parturients would be reviewed in the antenatal period; however, personnel and financial constraints make this unworkable.

Locally agreed referral criteria enable patients at higher risk and women who have had problems with previous pregnancies to be referred to the anaesthetic antenatal clinic.

The recent OAA/AAGBI guidance on provision of obstetric services recommends that referral criteria for antenatal anaesthetic clinics should include:

- Women that might present difficulties should analgesia or anaesthesia be required (this could include women with poor venous access, e.g. due to intravenous drug use or severe burns, or those with learning difficulties or mental health problems)
- Women at high risk of obstetric complications
- BMI > 40 kg/m^2 at booking (as recommended by Joint CMACE/RCOG guideline on the management of women with obesity in pregnancy)
- Previous difficulty with or complications of regional or general anaesthesia
- Women with significant medical conditions.

This list is not exhaustive and should be tailored to the needs of each individual obstetric unit.

It is important to have formal referral criteria, regardless of whether the parturient is seen in an anaesthetic clinic or on an ad hoc basis, as it will increase the number of appropriate referrals and highlight the presence of the service. When introducing or amending referral guidelines it is vital to ensure that they are communicated to the healthcare professionals making the referrals and to provide a point of contact should there be any uncertainty over which patients to refer.

Once guidelines have been agreed and circulated, referrals can be made through an electronic booking system, written referral or standardized proforma, whichever is suitable for each obstetric unit. Referrals can be made either at the time of the booking visit or later in pregnancy, it is essential that there is clear guidance where the referral is sent to be reviewed by an anaesthetic consultant.

Where should they be seen?

A survey of UK obstetric units in 2005 showed that 70% of the units did not have formal anaesthetic clinics. This figure will have undoubtedly changed over the past 10 years, as with increasing pressure on the anaesthetic antenatal service, more obstetric units have changed from providing reviews on an ad hoc basis to a formal clinic environment.

Whether patients are seen on an ad hoc basis or in a clinic there should be a dedicated room available to allow the consultation to be conducted without interruption.

When should they be seen?

Once the referral has been made by the obstetrician or midwife and been reviewed by the anaesthetist, a decision needs to be made as to the timing of the antenatal anaesthetic assessment. The RCOG Good Practice Guideline 13 for Cardiac Disease and Pregnancy suggests that women with pre-existing cardiac disease should be seen by a multidisciplinary team at 32–34 weeks to discuss her delivery plan. While this recommendation is for women with pre-existing cardiac disease, it can be used to guide timing of an antenatal anaesthetic review for the majority of women. The timing of a woman's clinic visit will ultimately depend on the condition she is referred with; some women may well need to be assessed in the second trimester if their medical condition means they have a significant chance of preterm delivery.

If possible it is best to match the anaesthetic assessment with a planned antenatal clinic appointment, this prevents multiple visits to the hospital and improves non-attendance rates. Most women are referred in a timely manner; however, it is important to have some leeway in the clinic bookings for women who book late or who were not identified as high-risk earlier in their pregnancy.

Who should see the patient?

Recommendations and guidance from various bodies, including The Confidential Enquiries into Maternal and Child Health, RCOG, OAA and AAGBI, all suggest that a senior anaesthetist carries out the antenatal anaesthetic review. The clinics should be consultant led; if for any reason the consultant is not available, each case should be discussed with a consultant at the

earliest opportunity, to ensure appropriate advice has been given to the woman.

The clinic appointment

This appointment allows the anaesthetist to make a thorough assessment of the parturient and to plan for delivery, whilst giving the patient an opportunity to discuss any concerns they may have and make an informed choice about the options available to them during labour and delivery.

A full history of medical and obstetric conditions, and drug history, including any drug allergies, should be taken together with a full anaesthetic history. It would be a shame to miss the chance to elicit a history of suxamethonium apnoea in a woman referred with back pain due to a mild scoliosis. History-taking will always need to be focused on specific areas of concern, but should also take into account the physiological changes in pregnancy, which may significantly worsen any pre-existing condition.

Examination will be guided by the patient's condition, but should always include airway assessment, examination of the back, paying particular attention to the lumbar spine, and an assessment of venous access. Examination of the back should include visual inspection for scars, palpation of the vertebrae and where appropriate, ultrasound-guided estimation of the depth of epidural space. This can provide an invaluable source of information during labour or delivery when regional anaesthesia is required.

Discussion with the woman should be tailored to their reason for referral and how that may affect labour and delivery. Information should be provided and recommendations made regarding their choices for analgesia and anaesthesia and the need for any further investigations. Any specific concerns regarding their condition, analgesic options, mode and place of delivery can also be addressed. Patient information leaflets can be given for the patient to read at home and they need to have contact information should they require any further advice. [(www.oaaformothers.info) – translations of these leaflets are available in many languages on this website]

Once the consultation has finished, a detailed record of the history, examination, investigations, discussion and any outstanding issues should be made. Ideally this should be documented in the woman's notes, either in the form of a written entry or a dictated letter. A shortened version of the consultation should also be written in the woman's handheld notes in case of presentation at another hospital. It is also useful to keep a second copy of the consultation record on the delivery suite so that the information is readily available to consultant anaesthetists and anaesthetic trainees, in cases where there is a delay obtaining a patient's notes.

Depending on the co-morbidity, additional information or investigations can be requested; the appointment can also ensure that there is time to arrange other speciality involvement.

This includes:

- Further information from the GP
- Further information and discussion with other specialities
- Multidisciplinary review to decide timing and mode of delivery; this may need to be reviewed in light of any change in the woman's condition
- Arranging further investigations, e.g. echocardiography, spinal imaging
- Booking cell salvage for caesarean section e.g. placenta praevia, women refusing blood products
- Booking critical care and specialist theatre space, e.g. women with significant heart disease, women who may require respiratory support in the peripartum period.

Another important aspect of an anaesthetic assessment clinic is education. As previously mentioned, the antenatal anaesthetic clinic should be a consultant-delivered service. This environment provides the perfect educational opportunity for midwives, anaesthetists and obstetricians in training. Observers to the clinic will gain insight into the necessity for forward planning to ensure delivery of a safe and high standard of maternal care.

Key points

1. Anaesthetic antenatal assessment is critical in the planning of peripartum care in the presence of significant maternal co-existing disease.
2. An appropriate locally agreed referral criteria system is recommended.

3. A senior anaesthetist should carry out the review.
4. The timing of the visit will depend on the reason for referral, but most can be seen early in the third trimester.

Further reading

Centre for Maternal and Child Enquiries (CMACE). (2010). *Maternal Obesity in the UK: Findings from a National Project*. London: CMACE.

Centre for Maternal and Child Enquiries (CMACE). (2011). Saving mothers' lives: reviewing maternal deaths to make motherhood safer: 2006–08. The Eighth Report on Confidential Enquiries into Maternal Deaths in the United Kingdom. *Br. J. Obstet. Gynaecol.*, **118** (1), 1–203.

Cormack, C., Francis, S. and Yentis, S. (2007). Antenatal anaesthetic assessment of the pregnant woman. *Anaesth. Intensive Care Med.* **8**, (7), 269–272.

Department of Health. (2007). *Maternity Matters: Choice, Access and Continuity of Care in a Safe Service*. London: Department of Health.

Obstetric Anaesthetists' Association/Association of Anaesthetists of Great Britain and Ireland. (2013). *Guidelines for obstetric anaesthetic services*. London: AAGBI and OAA.

Rai, M. R., Lua, S. H., Popat, M. and Russell, R. (2005). Antenatal anaesthetic assessment of high-risk pregnancy: a survey of UK practice. *Int. J. Obstet. Anaesth.*, **14**, 219–222.

Rosaeg, O. P., Yarnell, R. W. and Lindsay, M. P. (1993). The obstetrical anaesthesia assessment clinic: a review of six years experience. *Can. J. Anaesth.*, **40**(4), 346–356.

Royal College of Obstetricians and Gynaecologists. (2008). *Standards for Maternity Care: Report of a Working Party*. London: RCOG.

Royal College of Obstetricians and Gynaecologists. (2011). *Cardiac Disease and Pregnancy. Good Practice no.13*. London: RCOG.

The Task Force on the Management of Cardiovascular Diseases during Pregnancy of the European Society of Cardiology (ESC). (2011). ESC Guidelines on the management of cardiovascular diseases during pregnancy. *Eur. Heart J.*, **32**, 3147–3197.

Chapter

8

Incidental anaesthesia during pregnancy

Desiree M. A. Choi and Kim G. Soulsby

Introduction

Parturients may require anaesthesia during their pregnancy in order to facilitate obstetric or non-obstetric surgical procedures. Common obstetric procedures required in pregnancy include cervical cerclage, ovarian cyst interventions and fetal surgery. The incidence of incidental or non-obstetric anaesthesia in pregnancy has been reported as ranging from 1:50–150 pregnancies, with appendectomy, cholecystectomy and pelvic laparoscopy being the most commonly encountered procedures.

Incidental anaesthesia must minimize the risk of interrupting the pregnancy and affecting fetal development. Alterations in maternal physiology accentuate anaesthetic risks and the approach to anaesthesia must be modified accordingly.

Fetal considerations

Anaesthesia may impact on the fetus in two ways: it may interrupt the pregnancy, resulting in either pregnancy loss or premature delivery, or it may impact on fetal development, either by teratogenic pharmacological effects or because of derangements in the physiological milieu.

The effects of a teratogenic insult depend on the gestation of the fetus at the time of exposure. Teratogens cause an 'all or nothing' effect in the early pluripotential developmental phase, such that the embryo will either die or be unaffected and develop normally. However, days 31 to 71 of human gestation correspond to the organogenesis phase, where exposure to teratogens may impair the structural development of organ systems. First trimester anaesthesia has been linked with increased neonatal central nervous system and eye malformation, particularly hydrocephalus and cataracts. In the phase following organogenesis, teratogen exposure is more likely to affect the fetal central nervous system, which undergoes development and maturation throughout pregnancy. These effects are likely to result in functional behavioural effects rather than structural malformations.

Drug teratogenicity

Organogenesis phase

There is theoretical reason to suspect that drugs used in anaesthesia may be teratogenic: the cellular mechanisms for differentiation and organogenesis include mechanisms known to be targeted by drugs used in anaesthesia. Neurotransmitter and receptor mechanisms, as well as signalling and second messenger systems are all known to be affected by drugs used in anaesthesia. This theoretical risk of teratogenicity has been difficult to quantify in a practical clinical context, because of difficulties extrapolating animal research data to human development (teratogenicity is species specific) and the obvious ethical and logistical problems of research on human fetal exposure to teratogens.

Later pregnancy

Drugs used in later pregnancy may have direct effects other than structural organogenesis impairment.

Benzodiazepines in late pregnancy may result in fetal benzodiazepine dependence and withdrawal (although unlikely in the short-term context of a single anaesthetic). Used peripartum, they are associated with fetal hypotonia, respiratory depression and hypothermia, and are probably best avoided in a viable gestation pregnancy.

Opioids have similar potential for fetal dependence and withdrawal, but again this is unlikely to result from short-term anaesthetic use. Peripartum opioid use results in reversible respiratory depression.

Core Topics in Obstetric Anaesthesia, ed. Kirsty MacLennan, Kate O'Brien and W. Ross Mcnab.
Published by Cambridge University Press. © Cambridge University Press 2015.

Non-steroidal anti-inflammatory drugs in the third trimester have been linked to premature closure of the ductus arteriosus, tricuspid incompetence and pulmonary hypertension. They have been associated with a range of fetal and neonatal effects consistent with their side-effect profile (including platelet dysfunction and intracranial haemorrhage, renal impairment and gastrointestinal bleeding), and their use should be avoided after 32 weeks' gestation.

Neuromuscular blocking agents are polar molecules that do not readily cross the maternal–placental barrier and are safe to use in late pregnancy.

The antiemetic prochlorperazine has been associated with neonatal jaundice and extrapyramidal side effects when used in high dose late in pregnancy.

Fetal effects of deranged maternal physiology

Organogenesis phase

There is some evidence that chronic hypercarbia and hyperthermia may be teratogenic, but it seems unlikely that anaesthesia would result in such exposure.

Later pregnancy

Derangements in maternal physiology that are precipitated or exacerbated by anaesthesia are likely to impact on the fetus by their effects on uteroplacental perfusion and oxygen delivery. Regardless of the cause of reduced uteroplacental perfusion, the fetal effects are similar: acidosis and fetal hypoxaemia will result. The insult may result in fetal injury, ranging from transient mild acidosis or hypoxaemia to brain injury, and ultimately to fetal death if the injury is unrecognized or untreated.

Uteroplacental blood flow

Reduced uteroplacental blood flow results most commonly from aortocaval compression, and is preventable with careful positioning during anaesthesia. Unrecognized and untreated reduction in circulating volume (whether absolute, as in haemorrhage, or relative as in sepsis) will reduce placental perfusion, and may do so without overt maternal hypotension because of the additional mobilized cardiac reserve in pregnancy.

Oxygen homeostasis

Fetal compensation to moderate, transient maternal hypoxaemia occurs by increased oxygen extraction, and may be well tolerated by the healthy fetus. This compensation is facilitated by fetal haemoglobin HbF, which has a high affinity for oxygen and which avidly binds maternal oxygen. However, an acidotic fetus will demonstrate a rightward shift in the oxygen dissociation curve, with reduced affinity for maternal oxygen. An acidotic fetus does not tolerate maternal hypoxia well.

In severe maternal hypoxia the maternal compensatory response is to divert flow to vital maternal organs, and away from the placenta. Uterine vasoconstriction results, reducing oxygen delivery to the fetus.

Carbon dioxide homeostasis

Carbon dioxide and its effects on acid–base balance may affect the fetus directly, by diffusing into the fetal circulation, and indirectly by the affecting uterine blood flow. Maternal hypercarbia results directly in fetal hypercarbia and respiratory acidosis. This results in a rightward shift in the fetal oxygen dissociation curve, with a consequent reduction in fetal oxygen extraction, leaving the fetus vulnerable to the effects of co-existent hypoxia. Fetal hypercarbia and acidosis also impair fetal myocardial contractility.

Maternal hypercarbia results in uterine vasodilation and increased uteroplacental flow, although severe hypercarbia may reduce uteroplacental flow by causing vasoconstriction. Maternal hypocarbia is poorly tolerated by the fetus, because hypocarbia and alkalaemia result in uterine vasoconstriction, reducing uteroplacental blood flow.

Miscarriage and premature delivery

The evidence for an increased risk of miscarriage following anaesthesia and surgery in pregnancy comes mainly from large retrospective studies of pregnancy outcomes following incidental surgery and anaesthesia. Further evidence is extrapolated from epidemiological studies linking occupational exposure to nitrous oxide and volatile anaesthetic agents with increased miscarriage rates.

Brodsky et al. showed an increase in the spontaneous abortion rate from the baseline of 5.1% to 8% in the first trimester pregnancies following anaesthesia and surgery. This seemed to be unrelated to the site of surgery, and abdominal and pelvic surgery was not more likely than remote surgery to induce miscarriage.

The increase in spontaneous abortion in the second trimester from 1.4% baseline to 5.9% was shown in pregnancies exposed to incidental surgery and anaesthesia, again irrespective of the anatomical site of surgery.

Once a pregnancy is of viable gestation, incidental surgery and anaesthesia may increase the risk of premature labour and delivery. This appears to be higher for gynaecological and abdominal surgery, which involves manipulation of the uterus. A systematic review found the rate of premature delivery following non-obstetric surgery to be 3.5%, with appendectomy carrying the highest risk of premature delivery. The trend towards the use of laparoscopic techniques in parturients has raised concerns regarding the risk of direct injury from laparoscopic instruments, and from indirect effects of hypercarbia and pneumoperitoneum. However, a number of subsequent studies have suggested that laparoscopy is not associated with increased risk of pregnancy loss or poor fetal outcome.

Maternal considerations and the conduct of anaesthesia during pregnancy

A detailed review of the physiology of pregnancy has been covered in Chapter 1. This chapter considers the changes relevant to anaesthesia and the conduct of anaesthesia in pregnancy. An appreciation of the normal physiology of pregnancy in each trimester is important, because maintenance of normal physiological parameters during anaesthesia is important for both the parturient and the developing fetus. Equally, the altered physiology of pregnancy impacts on the way the parturient responds to anaesthesia, and on the potential risks of anaesthesia and anaesthetic procedures including tracheal intubation.

Planning and preoperative preparation

Elective operations should not be undertaken during pregnancy, and should be postponed until after delivery where possible. If surgery is necessary, ideally it should be delayed until the second trimester in order to avoid the organogenesis phase. Surgery in the third trimester is associated with a risk of premature labour. Deferring surgery until six weeks post partum allows a return to the non-pregnant state, thus reducing the incidence of perioperative thromboembolism.

When consent is sought from a pregnant woman for incidental surgery, the risks of anaesthesia both to her, the pregnancy and the fetus should be discussed.

Consideration should be given to where the surgery is performed. If the pregnancy is viable, surgery should be conducted where facilities for obstetric and neonatal care are available. Planning should involve a multidisciplinary approach, and should include obstetric, midwifery and neonatology teams where appropriate. The pregnancy will require monitoring postoperatively, and might affect where postoperative care is delivered.

Preoperative assessment should include a thorough airway assessment. Prokinetics and antacid premedication should be administered.

Mode of anaesthesia

There is no evidence that regional anaesthesia is less likely than general anaesthesia to result in miscarriage or premature delivery. There are other reasons, however, to consider a regional or local anaesthetic technique where possible. Fetal exposure to drugs is less with a regional technique. Regional techniques avoid instrumentation of the airway and the risks of difficult and failed intubation, gastric contents regurgitation and aspiration, and the derangements in maternal oxygen and acid–base homeostasis that result from mechanical ventilation.

General anaesthesia
Respiratory and airway

The incidence of difficult or failed tracheal intubation is higher in the obstetric population than in the general population, with an estimated frequency of 1:224. For similar reasons, mask ventilation may be more difficult as pregnancy progresses. Nasal intubation is not recommended as nasal mucosal congestion increases the risk of bleeding.

Perioperative hypoxia can be attributed to increased maternal oxygen consumption, compounded by a reduced functional residual capacity that is further compromised in a supine position. Thorough preoxygenation and denitrogenation is therefore important.

The tendency to acid reflux from early in the second trimester results in an increased risk of aspiration of gastric contents during general anaesthesia. Protection of the airway by performance of rapid sequence induction with cricoid pressure and endotracheal intubation is advised from the second trimester in order to minimize the risk.

Cardiovascular –– Compression of the inferior vena cava by the gravid uterus in the supine position must

51

be avoided by anaesthetizing parturients in a left lateral tilt position, or by manual lateral displacement of the uterus.

As pregnancy progresses, cardiac output increases as a result of an increased stroke volume, heart rate and circulating blood volume. This increased cardiovascular reserve allows the healthy parturient to compensate efficiently for reduction in blood volume from haemorrhage. It is important to appreciate that a reduction in blood pressure may be a late sign of hypovolaemia.

Pregnancy is a prothrombotic state and measures to reduce the risks of perioperative deep venous thrombosis should be taken.

General anaesthetic drugs – – A reduction in blood flow to the uteroplacental unit can occur with intravenous induction agents that precipitate maternal hypotension. A comparison of the effects of propofol and thiopental can be found in Chapter 11. Studies have shown that propofol obtunds the maternal hypertensive response to laryngoscopy and intubation to a greater extent than thiopental. A study has shown that maximal noradrenaline concentrations are higher in parturients induced with thiopental compared with propofol (although adrenaline concentrations are similar). This could lead to uterine vasoconstriction and reduced uterine blood flow; however, in the study neonatal outcomes were the same. Ketamine may increase uterine flow in the third trimester, by increasing cardiac output and blood pressure, but there are concerns about its tendency to increase uterine tone, and its potential for causing persisting behavioural changes even after a single-dose fetal exposure. Etomidate has been used for caesarean section, but unproven concerns exist over its potential to suppress fetal cortisol production and render the fetus vulnerable to hypoglycaemia.

Volatile anaesthetic agents during pregnancy can reduce uterine perfusion by reducing maternal blood pressure; however, these effects are partially compensated by uterine vasodilation and relaxation, which tend to increase uterine blood flow. All volatile agents appear to be safe for use in pregnancy, although nitrous oxide is teratogenic in animals under certain conditions. Pregnancy increases sensitivity to volatile agents, reducing the minimum alveolar concentration value.

Neuromuscular blocking agents are safe to use in pregnancy, and cross the placenta only minimally. It should be borne in mind that their effects may be prolonged slightly by altered hepatic metabolism (rocuronium and vecuronium) or reduced plasma cholinesterase levels (suxamethonium) in pregnancy.

Uterine blood flow should be maintained by avoiding maternal hypotension. Phenylephrine has been shown at caesarean section to maintain uterine flow, while preserving fetal acid–base status, and is the suggested drug for treating maternal hypotension.

Intraoperative hypertension results in uterine vasoconstriction and reduced uterine flow, and should also be avoided. Labetalol, hydralazine, glyceryl trinitrate and magnesium sulfate are all safe alternatives for lowering blood pressure in pregnancy.

Postoperative analgesia should be optimized to avoid maternal catecholamine surges that can lead to a reduction in uterine blood flow. Regional anaesthetic techniques, opioids and simple analgesia are all safe. Non-steroidal anti-inflammatories should be avoided.

Regional anaesthesia

Regional anaesthesia is the preferred technique, where possible, for surgery during pregnancy. It may be precluded, however, by the nature of the proposed surgery, maternal refusal, sepsis or coagulation concerns (including pregnancy-induced thrombocytopenia which occurs in 1% of pregnancies). Amide anaesthetics bupivacaine, lidocaine and ropivacaine have been shown to be safe in pregnancy, and central neuraxial block techniques are widely used in obstetric anaesthetic practice. A smaller dose is required per dermatomal block in pregnancy. Fetal compromise may occur when maternal hypotension is untreated, and care must be taken to treat hypotension and maintain adequate circulating volume.

Fetal monitoring

Previability (23–25 weeks) it is good practice for fetal heart auscultation using hand-held doppler to be performed before and after elective surgery to reduce maternal anxiety and prevent any potential litigation.

After viability, fetal assessment with ultrasound or CTG may be appropriate. This depends on the nature of the surgery and whether it is elective or emergency. Intraoperative monitoring of the fetal heart is not necessary as if concerns regarding fetal wellbeing are present then obstetric involvement is needed, as delivery of the fetus may be necessary.

Key points

1. Surgery during pregnancy should be avoided and deferred where possible.

2. The risk of miscarriage is lowest in the second trimester, and the risk of premature labour and delivery is highest in the third trimester.

3. Most anaesthetic drugs appear to be clinically safe in pregnancy, and have been used with no apparent maternal or fetal harm.

4. Some drugs should be avoided in later pregnancy.

5. Careful maintenance of the normal physiology of pregnancy is important, both for maternal wellbeing and for fetal outcome.

6. Considered planning for incidental surgery in pregnancy should involve a multidisciplinary team approach, with thought for timing, location, personnel involved and the need for perioperative fetal monitoring.

Further reading

Boivin, J-F. (1997). Risk of spontaneous abortion in women occupationally exposed to anaesthetic gases: a meta-analysis. *J. Occup. Env. Med.*, **54**(8), 541–548.

Brodsky, J. B., Cohen, E. N., Brown, B. W. Jr, Wu, M. L., Witcher, C. (1980). Surgery during pregnancy and fetal outcome. *Am. J. Obstet. Gynecol.*, **138**, 165–167.

Cohen-Kerem, R., Railton, C., Oren, D., Lishner, M., Koren, G. (2005). Pregnancy outcome following non-obstetric surgical intervention. *Am. J. Surg.*, **190**(3), 467–473.

Hudspith, M. (2002). Anaesthesia during pregnancy. In Collis, R., Plaat, F., Urquhart, J. (eds.), *Textbook of Obstetric Anaesthesia*. London: Greenwich Medical Media Ltd.

Iwamoto, H. S. (1993). Cardiovascular effects of acute fetal hypoxia and asphyxia. In Hanson, M., Spencer, J. A. D., Rodeck, C. H. (eds.), *Fetus and Neonate: Physiology and Clinical Applications*. Cambridge: Cambridge University Press.

Mazze, R. I. and Kallem, B. (1989). Reproductive outcome after anesthesia and operation during pregnancy: a registry study of 5405 cases. *Am. J. Obstet. Gynecol.*, **161**, 1178–1185.

Mickley, G. A., Kenmuir, C. L., McMullen, C. A. *et al.* (2004). Long-term age-dependent behavioral changes following a single episode of fetal N-methyl-D-aspartate (NMDA) receptor blockade. *BMC Pharmacol.*, **4**(1), 28.

Reitman, E. and Flood, P. (2011). Anaesthetic considerations for non-obstetric surgery during pregnancy. *Br. J. Anaesth.*, **107**(1), 72–78.

Sadot, E., Telem, D. A., Arora, M. *et al.* (2010). Laparoscopy: a safe approach to appendicitis during pregnancy. *Surg. Endosc.*, **24**(2), 383–389.

Sylvester, G. C., Khoury, M. J., Lu, X. and Erickson, J. D. (1994). First-trimester anesthesia exposure and the risk of central nervous system defects: a population-based case-control study. *Am. J. Public Health*, **84**(11), 1757–1760.

Non-regional analgesia techniques for labour

Gordon Yuill

On 19 January 1847, James Young Simpson used diethyl ether to anaesthetize a woman with a deformed pelvis for delivery, to widespread opposition and consternation from his contemporaries, questioning its safety and his wisdom.

The controversy about the delivery of Queen Victoria's eighth child, Prince Leopold, in 1853 was such that her Court physicians publically denied that John Snow had anaesthetized her with ether to ease the pain. Four years later the issue was less controversial and it was widely acknowledged that Queen Victoria had received an anaesthetic to help her with the birth of Princess Beatrice, her ninth child. Anaesthesia for childbirth had become part of medical practice by 1860, in large part in response to the demands of women.

Our armamentarium for the management of labour has thankfully grown somewhat since the nineteenth century. This chapter will discuss the non-regional techniques (non-pharmacological and pharmacological) that are available in the UK.

The Cochrane Collaboration

In 2012 The Cochrane Collaboration summarized the evidence from Cochrane and non-Cochrane systematic reviews on the efficacy and safety of non-pharmacological and pharmacological interventions to manage pain in labour. This represented over 300 trials within 18 systematic reviews and they were able to categorize the interventions into: 'What works' (epidural, combined spinal and epidural, inhaled analgesia), 'What may work' (immersion in water, relaxation, acupuncture, massage, local anaesthetic nerve blocks, non-opioid drugs) and 'Insufficient evidence to make a judgement' (hypnosis, biofeedback, sterile water injections, aromatherapy, transcutaneous electrical nerve stimulation (TENS), parenteral opioids).

Non-pharmacological methods

Many non-pharmacological methods have been tried for the relief of labour pain, with varying success and much interindividual variability. Women may consider these options as an integral and important part of their labour experience, despite the benefits often being intangible and not easily documented by scientific method. It is important that the anaesthetic provider is aware of some of these techniques, their benefits and limitations, in order to be able to have a full and informed discussion with their patient. The 2012 Cochrane overview found some evidence to suggest that immersion in water, relaxation, acupuncture and massage may work, whilst there was insufficient evidence for hypnosis, biofeedback, sterile water injections, aromatherapy or TENS. Table 9.1 provides a useful summary.

Pharmacological methods

Although a whole array of drugs has been used for the pain of labour, parenteral opioids and inhalational analgesia have formed the mainstay of non-regional methods. Despite being less efficacious than regional analgesia, they are more widely available, cheaper, more simple to administer, less labour intensive and often more culturally acceptable. Thus, opioids and inhalational techniques are more widely used around the world, especially in areas where epidural availability is poor.

Parenteral opioids

Opioids have a long history as labour analgesics. They can be given via numerous routes (sub-cutaneous, intramuscular or intravenous), by either an intermittent bolus or patient-controlled technique. As μ-agonists that readily cross the placenta, they are all capable of

Core Topics in Obstetric Anaesthesia, ed. Kirsty MacLennan, Kate O'Brien and W. Ross Mcnab.
Published by Cambridge University Press. © Cambridge University Press 2015.

Table 9.1 Complimentary methods of pain relief.

	Mechanism of action	Advantages	Disadvantages	Evidence
TENS	Based on gate theory	Non-invasive, easy to use, good for back pain	Useful only in early labour, cost implications	Systematic review of eight RCTs failed to demonstrate analgesic effect
Immersion	Sensation of warm water inhibits pain transmission and supports gravid uterus	Popular, backed by Government Health Committee	Cannot use with other methods, limited accessibility, temporary	Cochrane review of three trials. No difference in pain relief between immersion groups. Systematic review of seven RCTs: mixed results
Massage	Inhibits pain transmission, provides support and distraction	Perceived as highly effective by those using it	Labour intensive	One RCT with 28 women showed physical and emotional benefits
Acupuncture (acupressure, laser acupuncture)	Stimulates specific points on body with fine needles (or pressure or laser); may inhibit pain transmission or produce natural endorphins	'Drug free'	Invasive, need trained therapist, can take 30 min for effect	One RCT with 100 women in Sweden comparing acupuncture suggested former group needed less analgesia, including epidurals
Waterblocks	Injection of 0.1 ml sterile water in four spots over sacrum. Action similar to TENS	Easy to perform, good for back pain	Temporary relief only (45–90 min), initial burning sensation	Two double-blind RCTs showed reduction in labour pain, but other work showed they were not rated by women as effective as other methods
Continous support	Presence of trained support person can improve the physiological and psychological aspects of labour	Popular, useful in any stage	None	Cochrane review of 15 RCTs involving 12,791 women. Those with continuous support, as opposed to conventional care, were less likely to have intrapartum analgesia, operative birth or be dissatisfied with their experiences
Hypnosis	Entering a hypnotic state to have better control over the pain	Non-invasive	Not all women susceptible (10–20% are not), time consuming, can be harmful	Cochrane review of three RCTs: one reported less anaesthesia and another less narcotic use, but overall meta-analysis showed no difference in the need for pain relief

Table 9.1 (cont.)

	Mechanism of action	Advantages	Disadvantages	Evidence
Aromatherapy	Use of essential oils of plants and flowers for therapeutic effect	Non-invasive	Individual sensation of smell, so oils need to be tested	One small (n=22) RCT compared ginger with lemongrass – no difference in pain scores or pharmacological pain relief
Homeopathy	A minute amount of a substance can be used to alleviate symptoms ('like cures like')		Needs to be individualized	No RCTS

RCT = randomized controlled trial, TENS = Transcutaneous electrical nerve stimulation
(Reproduced from Fortescue C, Wee MYK (2005). Analgesia in labour: non-regional techniques. *Continuing Education in Anaesthesia, Critical Care & Pain*; 5: 9–13 with permission from Oxford University Press.)

maternal sedation, respiratory depression, loss of protective airway reflexes, and the risk of neonatal depression.

The Cochrane overview in 2012 concluded that there was insufficient evidence that parenteral opioids were more effective than placebo or other interventions for pain management in labour.

Intermittent bolus

Pethidine (meperidine)

Pethidine was introduced into obstetric practice in the 1940s. It has remained the most widely used intermittent bolused opiate worldwide. It was first made legally available in 1950 in the UK for midwives to use independently. A survey of UK practice in 2008 found that 84% of UK units still used pethidine for labour analgesia despite significant doubts to its efficacy. This is probably due to familiarity, ease of administration, low cost and lack of evidence of a superior alternative. Some women find they are more able to cope with their labour pains due to its ability to provide sedation, dysphoria and amnesia.

It is a synthetic, phenylpiperidine derivative that is an agonist at μ- and κ-opioid receptors. It is used in a dose of 50–150 mg IM, which may be repeated 4 hours later. Onset of pain relief occurs within 45 minutes and lasts 2 to 3 hours.

The Cochrane overview in 2012 found that compared to other opioids more women receiving pethidine experienced adverse effects, including impaired capacity to engage in decision-making about care, sedation, hypoventilation, hypotension, prolonged labour, urine retention, nausea, vomiting and a slowing of gastric emptying.

It rapidly crosses the placenta, equilibrating within 6 minutes, and it has been shown to cause decreased fetal heart rate variability within 25 to 40 minutes that can last for an hour. It has a maternal half-life of 2.5 to 3 hours, but a more prolonged neonatal half-life of up to 18 to 23 hours. Pethidine is metabolized in the liver to its active metabolite norpethidine, which is a potent respiratory depressant with convulsant properties, which can accumulate with repeated doses, and has a half-life in the neonate of 60 hours. It should be used with caution in women with severe pre-eclampsia and other causes of renal impairment. The babies of women who have received pethidine in labour have been shown to be sleepier, less attentive, at risk of neonatal respiratory depression and hypothermia, and less able to establish breastfeeding, despite normal Apgar scores at birth. However, about 10% of neonates will have a 1 minute Apgar score of <6 if pethidine is given 2–3 hours before delivery, as this coincides with peak fetal concentrations. The incidence is reduced if given before or after this.

Diamorphine

Diamorphine is a synthetic derivative of morphine and is widely used as a labour analgesic in the UK. In the 2008 UK survey of practice it was found that diamorphine was used in 34% of units, and more frequently than pethidine in some areas. In other surveys it was rated better than pethidine and Entonox by both midwives and parturients. It is essentially a pro-drug that is rapidly metobolized to 6-mono-acetylmorphine, an active metabolite that is more lipid soluble than morphine, before further break-down to morphine. This increased lipid solubility accounts for its rapid onset, but also for its speed across the placenta, suggesting that infants born shortly after maternal diamorphine administration are at greater risk of respiratory depression. It is usually given in a dose of 5–7.5 mg IM. Most studies comparing pethidine and diamorphine find that neither drug works well, with almost 50% of women reporting poor pain relief and up to 40% of women requesting second-line analgesia. However, patients who receive pethidine are more likely to report no pain relief and the incidence of vomiting is lower in the diamorphine group. Pethidine was also associated with lower Apgar scores at 1 minute.

Morphine

Morphine is possibly the first opiate used as an analgesic in labour. Morphine is rarely prescribed in labour in the UK. Its dose is 2 to 5 mg IV or 5 to 10 mg IM. It rapidly crosses the placenta, but rapid maternal elimination decreases fetal exposure. Its side effects are dose-related and similar to those of pethidine, without having a pro-convulsant metabolite. Some studies have shown that neither pethidine nor morphine reduce pain scores, but they do both increase sedation. It was popular in the 1920s and 1930s, and used with hyoscine to induce 'twilight sleep' for labour and delivery. Women frequently had little memory of labour or of being in pain.

Fentanyl

Fentanyl is a tertiary amine, which is a synthetic phenylpiperidine derivative. It is a highly selective μ-agonist, is highly lipid soluble and has an analgesic potency 100 times that of morphine and 800 times that of pethidine. Its high lipid solubility gives it a rapid onset, which combined with a short duration of action and a lack of metabolites makes its use in labour attractive. However, it may accumulate after large or multiple doses and studies have shown it to have a similarly poor analgesic effect as pethidine.

Other opioids

Other opioids, including those with partial agonist and agonist/antagonist properties have been used in labour.

The systemic opioids that are used for labour analgesia are summarized in Table 9.2.

Patient-controlled analgesia

Patient-controlled analgesia (PCA) for labour has been used clinically since the 1970s, offering an attractive alternative when neuraxial anaesthesia is unavailable, contraindicated or unsuccessful. By giving the parturient a degree of control it offers high levels of satisfaction, despite only average reductions in pain scores. Concerns about the potential to cause harm should not be taken lightly though. Respiratory depression is a real possibility when the use of potent opioids and the reliance on safe administration, dosing and equipment are combined. Opioids such as pethidine, morphine, diamorphine, fentanyl, alfentanil and nalbuphine have all been used in this way, but the most appropriate drug, dose and dosing schedule has not been defined.

The introduction of remifentanil in the 1990s has led to an explosion in interest in using remifentanil patient-controlled analgesia for labour.

Remifentanil patient-controlled analgesia

Remifentanil is a 4-anilido-piperidine derivative of fentanyl, which is an ultra-short acting μ-1 opioid receptor agonist. It has a low volume of distribution, low lipid solubility, a terminal half-life of <10 minutes, and its context-sensitive half-life of 3.5 minutes is independent of the duration of the infusion. Blood–brain equilibrium occurs in 1.2 to 1.4 minutes and it is rapidly metabolized by plasma and tissue esterases to an inactive metabolite. In theory, the rapid onset of analgesia offers advantages for labour analgesia. The timing of delivery of each bolus is crucial: if it occurs at the beginning of a 70-second contraction it is likely to be effective for the following one. It crosses the placenta rapidly; however, the mean umbilical artery-to-umbilical vein concentration ratio is 0.29, demonstrating that the drug is rapidly metabolized and redistributed in the fetus. This pharmacokinetic profile gives remifentanil an advantage over other opioids used for labour analgesia. It has been shown to be superior to inhalational analgesia, pethidine IM and PCA, and fentanyl PCA in labour, with greater reduction in pain scores, lower rates of conversion to epidural analgesia and better overall satisfaction. It seems that remifentanil produces clinically effective, but not complete, analgesia, with about a 10% conversion rate to neuraxial analgesia.

Table 9.2 Systemic opioids for labour analgesia.

Drug	Usual Dose	Onset	Duration	Comments
Meperidine	25–50 mg IV 50–100 mg IM	5–10 min IV 40–45 min IM	2–3 h	Has an active metabolite with a long half-life Maximal neonatal depression 1–4 h after dose
Morphine	2–5 mg IV 5–10 mg IM	3–5 min IV 20–40 min IM	3–4 h	More neonatal respiratory depression than meperidine Has an active metabolite
Diamorphine	5–7.5 mg IV/IM	5–10 min IM	90 min	Morphine pro-drug More euphoria, less nausea than with morphine
Fentanyl	25–50 µg IV 100 µg IM	2–3 min IV 10 min IM	30–60 min	Usually administered as an infusion or by PCA Accumulates during an infusion Less neonatal depression than with meperidine
Nalbuphine	10–20 mg IV/IM	2–3 min IV 15 min IM/SQ	3–6 h	Opioid against/antagonist Ceiling effect on respiratory depression Lower neonatal neurobehavioural scores than with meperidine
Butorphanol	1–2 mg IV/IM	5–10 min IV 10–30 IM	3–4 h	Opioid against/antagonist Ceiling effect on respiratory depression
Meptazinol	100 mg IM	15 min IM	2–3 h	Partial opioid agonist Less sedation and respiratory depression than with other opioids
Pentazocine	20–40 mg IV/IM	2–3 min IV 5–20 min IM/SQ	2–3 h	Opioid against/antagonist Psychomimetic effects possible
Tramadol	50–100 mg IV/IM	10 min IM	2–3 h	Less efficacy than with meperidine More side effects than meperidine

IM, intramuscular; IV, intravenous; PCA, patient-controlled analgesia; SQ, sub-cutaneous
(Reproduced from Chestnut DH, Polley LS, Tsen LC, Wong CA (2009). *Chestnut's Obstetric Anesthesia: Principles and Practice, 4th Edition.* Philadelphia, PA: Elsevier. ISBN: 978-0-323-05541-3 with permission from Elsevier.)

Whilst no ideal regimen has been identified, the timing of dose administration, the rate of bolus delivery and the lockout interval are important to analgesia outcome. In the UK it is available in over one-third of units, with almost half of all other units expressing an intention to introduce it. One-third of those using remifentanil offer it as a routine method of pain relief, the remainder limit its use to those who cannot have regional analgesia. The most popular regimen in the UK is a 40 µg bolus with a 2-minute lockout. There is some debate about whether a 3-minute lockout would be more appropriate, as shorter lockouts allow additional doses to be received before maximal side effects (and peak analgesic effects) have occurred. There is a wide interindividual variability and tolerance has been shown to occur.

Maternal side effects are transient, and include sedation, hypoventilation, oxygen desaturation, nausea and vomiting. However, there is no room for complacency, as case reports of respiratory and/or cardiac arrest demonstrate. Thus, a strict protocol is mandatory. The most important criterion is continuous one-to-one care with a competency-assessed midwife. The other essential requirements include: a dedicated intravenous cannula, an antireflux valve on the administration line, monitoring of sedation level and respiratory rate and continuous oxygen saturation monitoring (see Table 9.3).

Table 9.3 Suggested guidelines for remifentanil PCA in labour.

Eligibility

  Informed consent
  No opioid use in the previous 4 h
  Dedicated IV cannula for remifentanil administration

PCIA protocol

  PCIA bolus: 40 μg
  Lockout interval: 2 min

Continuous observations

  SaO$_2$ (pulse oximetry)
  Nursing supervision: one-to-one

30-min observations

  Respiratory rate
  Sedation score
  Pain score

Indications for contacting the anaesthesia provider

  Excessive sedation score (not arousable to voice)
  Respiratory rate <8 breaths/min
  SaO$_2$ <90% while breathing room air

Sample guidelines adapted from those used by the Ulster Community and Hospitals Trust, Ulster, United Kingdom. Labour nurses must establish competency in the use of remifentanil PCIA before providing care.
PCIA – patient-controlled IV analgesia.
(Reproduced from Hinova A, Fernando R (2009). Systemic Remifentanil for Labor Analgesia. *Anesthesia and Analgesia* **109**: 1925–1929 with permission from Wolters Kluwer Health.)

Despite concerns about neonatal depression, fetal heart rate abnormalities and accumulation in the neonate, no study has identified an increased incidence of non-reassuring fetal heart rate recordings, and Apgar scores, neurobehavioural scores and umbilical cord gases have all been at least as good as those using pethidine or epidural analgesia.

Inhalational methods

As we have already seen, inhalational analgesia for childbirth has been used since the nineteenth century. The most commonly used agent is nitrous oxide, with some interest in halogenated agents.

Entonox

Entonox is the trade name given to a 50/50 mixture of oxygen and nitrous oxide. It was invented by Dr Mike Tunstall in 1961, approved for unsupervised use by midwives in 1965, and available in 99% of obstetric units in the UK in 1990, being used by 60% of parturients. It is uncommon in the USA, but is used in up to 86% of units in Canada. Its low blood-gas solubility (0.47) means that it equilibrates rapidly with blood, and as it washes out of the lungs rapidly there is minimal accumulation. At normal temperatures both components are present in pressurized cylinders in the gaseous phase (due to the Poynting effect); liquefaction of nitrous oxide and separation of the two components may occur at temperatures of −7 °C.

Evidence for the efficacy of Entonox is conflicting, although distraction, relaxation and sense of control all increase its subjective benefit. Technique of use and maternal cooperation are required. Parturients should be trained to time maximum effect with peak contraction pain, by inhaling from the very beginning of the contraction through to its end.

Adverse effects include drowsiness, disorientation and nausea. The risk of maternal hypoventilation, diffusion hypoxia and desaturation are increased with concomitant use of opioids. There is a theoretical risk of bone marrow suppression with prolonged use, and there may be an occupational risk to midwives if not scavenged or used in poorly ventilated rooms.

Halogenated agents

Up to the 1970s, chloroform, trichloroethylene, and methoxyflurane had all been used by midwives for labour analgesia. This is no longer allowed and an anaesthetist must now be present. This, and the need for specialized equipment, concerns for their tocolytic effects, environmental pollution, and the potential for maternal amnesia, altered consciousness and loss of protective airway reflexes, currently limits the routine use of inhaled halogenated agents.

Isoflurane

Isoflurane was first reported for labour analgesia in 1975, and at a level of 0.75% in air it produces better analgesia than Entonox, but with an increase in maternal sedation. Lower levels (0.25% in air) also produced better analgesia than Entonox, but maternal satisfaction was no better.

Desflurane

Desflurane has a lower blood-gas partition coefficient (0.42) than nitrous oxide, thus also allowing rapid onset and offset of action. When 1% to 4% desflurane in oxygen was compared to 30% to 60% nitrous oxide analgesia, scores were found to be similar, but at the expense of a high amnesia rate (23%).

Sevoflurane

Sevoflurane has been studied and found to have an optimal concentration of 0.8% for labour analgesia. At this level it is more effective than Entonox without desaturation, apnoea, or change in end-tidal CO_2. Apgar scores were unaffected. Its odour does have to be tolerated and subjective sleepiness seems to be increased compared with Entonox.

Key points

1. A wide variety of non-pharmacological pain-relief methods have been used with varying success. It is important to empower and support the parturient who wishes to utilize these methods.

2. Parenteral opioids have a long history as labour analgesics. They are easy to utilize, have well recognized side-effect profiles and so are commonly used worldwide.

3. PCA offers parturients a level of control that is reflected in its high satisfaction scores.

4. Remifentanil has many desirable characteristics as a labour analgesic, but the rigorous use of protocols is mandatory.

Further reading

Fairlie, F. M., Marshall, L., Walker, J. J. and Elbourne, D. (1999). Intramuscular opioids for maternal pain relief in labour: a randomised controlled trial comparing pethidine with diamorphine. *Br. J. Obstet. Gynaecol.*, **106**, 1181–1187.

Fortescue, C. and Wee, M. Y. (2005). Analgesia in labour: non-regional techniques. *CEACCP*, **5**, 9–13.

Fernando, R. and Jones, T. (2009). Systemic analgesia: parenteral and inhalational agents. In Chestnut, D. H., Polley, L. S., Tsen, L. C. and Wong, C. A. (eds.) *Chestnut's Obstetric Anesthesia: Principles and Practice, 4th edn.* Philadelphia, PA: Elsevier.

Harries, S. and Turner, M. (2008). Non-regional labour analgesia. In Clyburn, P., Collis, R., Harries, S. and Davies, S. (eds.) *OSH Obstet. Anaesth.* Oxford: Oxford University Press.

Smith, S., Scarth, E. and Sasada, M. (2011). *Drugs in Anaesthesia and Intensive care, 4th edn.* Oxford: Oxford University Press.

Hinova, A. and Fernando, R. (2009). Systemic remifentanil for labor analgesia. *Anesth. Analg.* **109**, 1925–1929.

Hughes, D. and Foley, P. (2013). The case for remifentanil PCA as labour analgesia. *RCA Bull.*, **78**, 6–8.

Jones, L., Othman, M., Dowswell, T. *et al.* (2012). Pain management for women in labour: an overview of systemic reviews. *Cochrane Database Syst. Rev.* **2012**(3), Art. No.: CD009234.

Muchatuta, N. A. and Kinsella, S. M. (2013). Remifentanil for labour analgesia: time to draw breath? *Anaesthiology*, **68**, 231–235.

Oloffson, C., Ekblom, A., Ekman-Ordeberg, G. *et al.* (1996). Lack of analgesic effect of systemically administered morphine or pethidine on labour pain. *Br. J. Obstet. Gynaecol.*, **103**, 968–972.

Tuckey, J. P., Prout, R. E. and Wee, M. Y. (2008). Prescribing intramuscular opioids for labour analgesia in consultant-led maternity units: a survey of UK practice. *Int. J. Obstet. Anesth.*, **17**, 3–8.

Regional analgesia techniques for labour

Lawrence C. Tsen

Introduction

Regional analgesia, which is pain relief delivered to a discrete region of the body, encompasses a variety of methods (Table 10.1), of which central neuraxial [e.g. epidural, spinal, combined spinal epidural (CSE) and dural puncture epidural (DPE)] techniques provide the most effective analgesia for all stages of labour and delivery (Box 10.1).

Patient benefits and concerns

The benefits of neuraxial techniques during labour include improved pain scores when compared to other forms of analgesia, minimal fetal exposure to analgesic medications, and improved maternal satisfaction with the overall birth experience. Biochemically, neuraxial techniques reduce maternal plasma concentrations of stress catecholamines, which may improve uteroplacental perfusion and the effectiveness of uterine contractions; hyperventilation is also reduced, which diminishes the leftward shift in the maternal oxyhaemoglobin dissociation curve and improves fetal oxygen delivery. Neuraxial techniques improve

the success of external cephalic versions, the delivery of multiple gestation infants and the removal of products of conception. Finally, the presence of catheter-based neuraxial techniques for labour *analgesia* can provide for the rapid conversion to *anaesthesia* should an emergent operative procedure occur; avoidance of the maternal airway, which can undergo significant engorgement during pregnancy and labour is a favourable action plan, given the untoward implications of a difficult intubation or extubation on maternal and fetal wellbeing.

Among the most frequent concerns vocalized by parturients is whether neuraxial analgesia affects the progress and outcome of labour. In parturients of mixed parity, a prolongation of the first and second stages of labour by 42 minutes and 14 minutes, respectively, has been observed with the use of epidural analgesia compared to parenteral opioids. Moreover, maintenance of epidural analgesia with intermittent boluses of 0.25% bupivacaine (which is more concentrated than that typically used in contemporary practice) has been associated with a higher proportion of instrumental deliveries, when compared to CSE techniques or parenteral opioids. However, the rate of

BOX 10.1 Stages of labour and delivery			
Stage	**Parameters**	**Source of Pain**	**Spinal Cord Level**
First	Onset of labour until complete cervical dilation	Peripheral nociceptors in the lower uterine segment and cervix	Visceral afferent neurons, enter 10th to 12th thoracic and 1st lumbar spinal segments
Second	Pushing and delivery of the fetus	Distention of vagina and perineum	Somatic afferent fibres in pudendal nerve, enter 2nd to 4th sacral spinal segments
Third	Delivery of the placenta	Distention of vagina and perineum	Somatic afferent fibres in pudendal nerve enter 2nd to 4th sacral spinal segments

Core Topics in Obstetric Anaesthesia, ed. Kirsty MacLennan, Kate O'Brien and W. Ross Mcnab.
Published by Cambridge University Press. © Cambridge University Press 2015.

Table 10.1 Regional analgesia techniques

Regional technique	Method	Obstetric stages of labour	Comments
Paracervical block	Nerve ganglion block by uterine cervix	1st stage	May cause fetal bradycardia from fetal absorption
Lumbar sympathetic block	In lumbar region	1st stage	Multiple, technically challenging injections
Pudendal block	Terminal pudendal nerve blockade	2nd stage	Not effective for uterine cavity, cervix or upper vaginal repair
Perineal infiltration	Terminal sensory nerves in perineum	2nd stage	Effective for blocking perineal sensation only
Neuraxial techniques		1st, 2nd and 3rd stages	Spinal opioids alone will provide analgesia limited to early 1st stage

caesarean delivery is not increased with the use of neuraxial techniques. Of interest, CSE techniques may have salutary effects on labour progress. In nulliparous parturients at less than 3 cm cervical dilation, the use of a CSE labour analgesia technique results in faster cervical dilation and delivery by an average of 30 minutes when compared to an epidural technique with 0.125% bupivacaine. Moreover, a significantly shorter median time from initiation of analgesia to complete dilatation has been observed with the CSE technique versus systemic analgesia (295 min vs. 385 min, P < 0.001); time to vaginal delivery was shorter as well (398 min vs. 479 min, P < 0.001).

An additional concern expressed by parturients is whether the fetus is affected by neuraxially administered medications. Indirectly, neuraxial techniques may affect uteroplacental blood flow through alterations in maternal blood pressure and uterine tone. Correction of blood pressure alterations can be remedied quickly, with minimal to no known adverse fetal effects. FHR changes, which are more commonly observed following spinal or CSE analgesia, can be minimized with the avoidance of higher opioid doses (i.e. fentanyl >50 μg, and sufentanil > 7.5 μg). Although most analgesic medications, including local anaesthetics and opioids, readily cross the placenta, the doses, when administered neuraxially, are very small, particularly in comparison to the amount of systemic medications required to provide similar analgesia; minimal, if any, direct effect of these agents on FHR activity or fetal wellbeing has been observed.

Indications and contraindications

Neuraxial techniques are particularly useful in patients with a difficult airway (e.g. high body mass index), worsening co-morbidities (e.g. pre-eclampsia), or the likelihood of an urgent operative delivery (e.g. placenta praevia, trial of labour after caesarean [TOLAC], high-order multiple gestation or breech presentation). Such patients may be suitable for an early ('prophylactic') placement of a catheter-based neuraxial technique; aside from a small test dose (3 to 5 mL of 1.5% to 2% lidocaine) to indicate a bilateral sensory block, the catheter need not be dosed until an analgesic or anaesthetic is requested or required.

The major contraindications to neuraxial techniques are patient refusal and the presence of an underlying infection (e.g. meningitis, abscess), cardiac issue (e.g. hypotension), coagulation issue (e.g. haematoma) or neurologic process (e.g. cranial herniation, puncture of tethered spinal cord) (Box 10.2). Severe obstetric haemorrhage in the antepartum period, including uterine rupture and acute, severe fetal distress, may also contraindicate neuraxial anaesthesia procedures because of the time necessary to establish a surgical anaesthetic. The most controversial conditions are those involving a decreasing platelet count, an evolving infectious process, or a fluctuating neurologic examination.

Ultimately, the risks and benefits of neuraxial analgesia should be individualized, with the patient engaged in an informed consent discussion. Included

BOX 10.2 Contraindications to neuraxial techniques

Absolute contraindications

- Patient refusal or inability to cooperate
- Localized infection at the insertion site
- Sepsis
- Severe coagulopathy
- Uncorrected hypovolaemia

Relative contraindications

- Mild coagulopathy
- Severe maternal cardiac disease (including congenital and acquired disorders)
- Neurologic disease (including intracranial and spinal cord disorders)
- Severe fetal depression.

in these decisions should be the experience of each individual anaesthetist and the environment in which care is being provided.

Types of neuraxial techniques

Epidural analgesia

Placement of a catheter into the epidural space provides an effective, reliable and titratable form of labour analgesia (Table 10.2) that can be converted to surgical anaesthesia for an instrumental or operative delivery, laceration repair or postpartum tubal ligation.

The selection of agents for epidural administration depends on the degree and duration of pain relief desired, with an overall goal of providing lumbar and sacral sensory analgesia with minimal motor blockade. Epidural opioids alone can provide analgesia during the early first stage of labour; however, a combination of opioids with local anaesthetic agents is necessary thereafter. Use of this combination minimizes the doses, and side effects, of each component, including pruritus (e.g. an opioid effect) and motor blockade (e.g. a local anaesthetic effect). An epidural bolus of fentanyl 100 µg, with or without local anaesthetic, can be of assistance during the second stage of labour when patchy analgesia or perineal sparing cannot be remedied with local anaesthetics alone.

Once the initial sensory blockade has been established, epidural analgesia can be maintained with dilute solutions of local anaesthetic agents with opioids, administered by intermittent bolus injections, continuous infusion, or both techniques simultaneously. The development of programmable infusion pumps has enabled patient-controlled intermittent bolus top-up injections, which reduces the total amount of medication used, decreases the amount of motor blockade, and increases patient satisfaction when compared to a continuous infusion or intermittent bolus methodologies alone.

Spinal analgesia

The finite duration of action of a single injection (i.e. 'single-shot') and the increased risk of post dural-puncture headaches with multiple injections, limit the utility of the spinal technique for labour analgesia. However, single injection spinal techniques can be used immediately prior to vaginal breech delivery, outlet forceps or vacuum extraction, or postpartum repairs of extensive tears or lacerations. Various doses and types of local anaesthetics may be used; however, the selection should consider the likelihood for caesarean delivery. Clear communication between the obstetrician and anaesthetist is essential for the appropriate technique and agents to be chosen.

The placement of a catheter into the spinal space (i.e. spinal catheter or continuous spinal technique) is particularly useful in patients where incremental dosing is desired (e.g. a cardiac disorder requiring adequate filling pressures) or the expected complexity or duration of the case is unknown (e.g. multiple gestation, morbid obesity, placenta accreta). A spinal catheter technique is also an attractive option when an inadvertent dural puncture occurs during a planned epidural technique.

A spinal catheter presents a significantly greater risk of a post dural puncture headache (PDPH), particularly when a 17 or 18 gauge epidural needle and a macro- (e.g. 19 or 20 gauge) epidural catheter is used. Smaller microcatheters (e.g. 27 to 32 gauge) allow the use of a smaller needle, but are associated with greater technical difficulties, failures, and complications (e.g. cauda equina syndrome, from repeated, generous dosing in an attempt to augment the level or density). Whether the spinal catheter should remain *in situ* for 24 hours following delivery in an attempt to reduce the incidence of a PDPH is controversial; the retained catheter should be knotted with the hub removed or taped to the skin under a transparent dressing to prevent inadvertent use.

Table 10.2 Selection considerations for neuraxial analgesic techniques for labour.

Technique	Advantages	Disadvantages	Comments
Continuous epidural	Ability to titrate duration, density and level of block	Technically more difficult, with possible inadvertent epidural needle dural puncture Slow onset Large drug doses Patchy, one-sided blocks can occur	
Continuous spinal	Ability to titrate duration, density, and level of block Rapid onset Low drug doses Ability to use puncture created inadvertently with epidural attempt	Large dural puncture with risk of headache if epidural needle used Possible adverse events if mistaken, and dosed, as epidural catheter	Complete analgesia for early 1st stage labour with opioid alone
Combined spinal-epidural (CSE)	Ability to titrate duration, density and level of block Rapid onset Low drug doses Rapid sacral spread Bilateral coverage	Delayed verification of epidural catheter functionality	Spinal needle can function as a 'finder' needle to minimize inadvertent dural puncture with epidural needle Complete analgesia for early 1st stage labour with opioid alone
Dural puncture epidural (DPE)	Ability to titrate duration, density and level of block Ability to verify functionality of epidural catheter Intermediate onset Intermediate sacral spread Improved bilateral coverage	Large drug doses	Spinal needle can function as a 'finder' needle to minimize inadvertent epidural needle dural puncture Technically similar to CSE, but spinal drugs are not given through spinal needle
Single-shot spinal	Technically simple Rapid onset Low drug doses Rapid sacral spread Bilateral coverage	Density and level cannot be augmented Pruritus	

Combined spinal-epidural technique

The CSE technique consists of the insertion of an epidural needle, placement of a longer spinal needle through the shaft of the epidural needle into the subarachnoid space (e.g. the 'needle-through-needle' approach), administration of spinal medications, removal of the spinal needle and placement of an epidural catheter. In comparison to the epidural technique, the CSE technique has a number of advantages, including a more rapid sacral sensory blockade (by approximately 6 minutes), smaller initial drug dose and lower incidence of epidural catheter failure (Table 10.2).

A lipid-soluble opioid (fentanyl or sufentanil) is an appropriate initial spinal drug during early labour; spinal opioid analgesia can preserve haemodynamic stability in preload-dependent cardiac patients.

Limitations with the CSE technique include spinal opioid-associated pruritus and fetal bradycardia, which can be reduced with fentanyl doses < 50 μg or sufetanil doses < 7.5 μg. The CSE technique also cannot determine if the epidural catheter is properly sited, until it is used to provide analgesia. Moreover, with any dural puncture, the risk for PDPH and infection is present, albeit uncommon with small-gauge (25–27 gauge) pencil-point needles and good aseptic technique, respectively.

The likelihood of a dural puncture with a 19–20 gauge epidural catheter passing through a 25–27 gauge spinal needle is low. However, drugs placed in the epidural space can pass through the 25–26 gauge spinal dural hole and improve sacral analgesia with very low risk for high spinal blockade (see DPE below).

Dural puncture epidural technique

The dural puncture epidural (DPE) technique consists of the insertion of an epidural needle, placement of a longer spinal needle through the shaft of the epidural needle into the subarachnoid space (e.g. the 'needle-through-needle approach), removal of the spinal needle and placement of an epidural catheter. No medications are directly administered through the spinal needle; instead, epidurally administered medications enter the subarachnoid space through the conduit made by the spinal needle.

In comparison to the epidural technique, the DPE technique has a number of advantages, including a faster sacral blockade, greater bilateral coverage and a lower epidural catheter failure rate (Table 10.2). In addition, the epidural catheter is immediately tested with medications for correct placement; this is the principal advantage over the CSE technique, particularly for parturients with a difficult airway or a high probability of an instrumental or operative delivery.

As with any dural puncture technique, the risk for a PDPH and infection is present, but uncommon.

Preparing for a neuraxial technique

History, physical, testing and informed consent

Prior to proceeding with any neuraxial technique, a focused review of the obstetric, anaesthetic, medical and surgical history should be performed, accompanied by a brief physical examination with vital signs. Routine platelet count and blood typing with screening or cross-matching are not necessary; however, lab and additional testing (i.e. electrocardiogram or imaging) should be dictated by the current condition of the patient and anticipated likely outcomes. Communication with the multidisciplinary team is encouraged.

A discussion of the potential risks and consent for the procedure should be undertaken antenatally if possible, or at the earliest possible convenience when in labour. The presence of labour pain does not preclude an informed consent; however, care should be taken to query and document the comprehension of the information discussed.

Medications, equipment and monitors

As expected and unexpected physiologic sequelae may occur following neuraxial techniques, intravenous access should be established, with medications and equipment available to respond to common (e.g. hypotension) and less frequent side effects and complications (e.g. high spinal, local anaesthetic toxicity; see below). Medications to have readily available include ephedrine and phenylephrine, but also atropine, epinephrine, naloxone, calcium chloride and lipid emulsion. Emergency equipment, including a self-inflating bag and mask, an oxygen source, a cardiac resuscitation

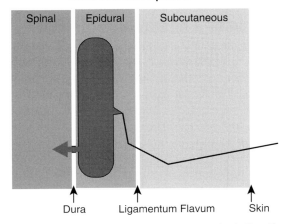

Dural Puncture Epidural

Spinal | Epidural | Subcutaneous

Dura | Ligamentum Flavum | Skin

Figure 10.1 Mechanism of dural puncture epidural effect. The dural puncture epidural (DPE) technique. Following the introduction of a 17 to 18 gauge epidural needle through the ligamentum flavum, a longer 25 to 26 gauge spinal needle is introduced through the epidural needle and punctures the dura (dural ligament or sac). The spinal needle is removed, and an epidural catheter is placed. Medication is dosed through the epidural catheter, which translocates though the spinal-needle-created passageway, into the subarachnoid space.

BOX 10.3 Sensory and motor assessment

Sensory evaluation
Cold, pinprick or touch sensation from caudad to cephalad orientation in the midaxillary line

Motor evaluation
Bromage scale (modified)-degree of blockade
None: Full flexion of knees and feet
Partial: Partial ability to flex knees, able to move feet
Almost Complete: Inability to flex knees, able to move feet
Complete: Unable to move knees or feet

trolley and a difficult airway trolley should be immediately available in a known, accessible location.

The maternal blood pressure should be measured between contractions at baseline, and every 1 to 3 minutes after neuraxial technique placement for approximately 20 minutes, or until haemodynamic stability has been demonstrated. Subsequently, throughout labour, maternal blood pressure should be measured every 15 to 30 minutes, or in accordance with local guidelines. Continuous pulse oximetry is useful to monitor maternal heart rate and saturation, and should be considered throughout labour in selected patients (e.g. sleep apnoea, cardiac disease, etc.). Assessment of the sensory level and motor ability should occur regularly (Box 10.3).

Fetal heart rate (FHR) monitoring should occur before and after the administration of neuraxial analgesia; opioid administration within the subarachnoid versus epidural space is associated with a higher incidence of non-reassuring FHR patterns. Continuous external FHR monitoring is often used for the remainder of the labour; however, it may not be necessary or possible in every clinical setting. In some cases, particularly when external monitoring proves difficult (e.g. high BMI), a fetal scalp electrode may be indicated.

Hydration and position

Insertion of an intravenous catheter (>18 gauge) is an absolute requirement prior to the placement of a neuraxial technique, to allow for correction of hypovolaemia and treatment of the sympathectomy-induced hypotension with fluids or vasopressors (e.g. phenylephrine 40 μg, or ephedrine 10 mg). A fixed volume of fluid prior to the administration of a neuraxial technique is not necessary, and recent investigations with spinal anaesthesia-induced hypotension during caesarean delivery indicate that fluid administration at the time of neuraxial technique administration (co-loading), versus in advance (pre-loading), is more effective. A balanced crystalloid solution (e.g. lactated Ringers or Hartmann's solution) without dextrose is the most commonly used fluid in labouring women; however, colloid solutions, which have a longer intravascular dwell time and consequently a more prolonged effect on preload and cardiac output, may be valuable, particularly when hypovolaemia is initially present or when the presence of even modest hypotension would be detrimental (e.g. aortic stenosis).

Although the sitting position is the most common position used for the initiation of neuraxial techniques, the lateral decubitus position may offer greater maternal comfort, less orthostatic hypotension, and improved ability to monitor FHR and maintain optimal maternal and fetal positioning. Moreover, the lateral position offers the option of providing a neuraxial technique in the setting of a presenting fetal part or cord prolapse. The sitting position may facilitate identification of the midline in high body mass index patients and improved respiratory mechanics in patients with respiratory issues. FHR monitoring during positioning may provide information on optimal positioning for fetal perfusion; aortocaval compression must be avoided at all times.

Insertion of a neuraxial technique

The timing of neuraxial technique insertion should be based on a conversation between the patient, the obstetric care team and the anaesthetist. The initiation of neuraxial analgesia early vs. late in labour does not affect the caesarean delivery rate. The choice of neuraxial technique, agents and dosages is based on a number of factors, including patient and provider preferences.

Prior to commencing the technique, the patient should be asked to confirm her identity and understanding of the anticipated technique, and the anaesthetist should verbally review aloud the relevant medical, obstetric and anaesthetic issues; these steps serve to improve patient safety.

The epidural space should be identified with a loss of resistance to intermittent or continuous pressure with either air, saline or their combination. Midline and paramedian approaches have been used. A specific epidural approach, method or medium used for loss of resistance has not been uniformly found to be better in ensuring successful placement, improving analgesia or minimizing risks.

If the epidural loss of resistance is equivocal, or the intent is to perform a CSE or DPE technique, a longer spinal needle (10 to 15 mm longer than the epidural needle when completely inserted) can be advanced as a 'finder needle' through the shaft of the epidural needle (needle-through-needle method) into the dural sac with cerebrospinal fluid (CSF) confirmed. If CSF is not obtained, the epidural needle may be of insufficient depth (thereby not allowing the spinal needle to reach the dural sac) or off the midline (allowing the spinal needle to miss the dural sac). If CSF is not confirmed, but the epidural catheter is threaded and dosed, a higher failure rate of the resulting analgesia or anaesthesia has been observed.

If during the epidural needle placement an inadvertent dural puncture (i.e. 'wet tap') occurs, an epidural catheter can be inserted into the subarachnoid space and used as a continuous spinal catheter technique. The patient, as well as the catheter itself and patient's chart, should be marked to clearly indicate the presence of a spinal catheter. Safety with the continuous spinal technique is reliant on all practitioners having familiarity and comfort in managing such a catheter; if accidentally dosed as an epidural catheter, a high spinal is likely.

Epidural catheters should be inserted 5 cm into the epidural space; catheter insertion less or greater than this amount may result in a greater incidence of failed block (due to movement out of the epidural space) or a one-sided block (due to the catheter residing towards one side), respectively. The spinal catheter insertion depth has not been well studied; however, most clinicians insert the catheter 3 to 5 cm into the subarachnoid space.

Test dose

Neuraxial techniques may be complicated by the inadvertent placement of the needle or catheter into intravenous, subdural or subarachnoid spaces. This typically occurs during the insertion process, although catheter migration may occur, perhaps through a defect created during the placement. To date, there is not an ideal test that can reliably distinguish the location of the needle or catheter.

A commonly used test dose is composed of 3 mL of 1.5% lidocaine with epinephrine (1:200,000 solution = 15 μg/3 mL). When given intravascularly, the lidocaine

component may provide limited symptoms (e.g. tinnitus, palpitations, light-headedness, dizziness), but the epinephrine should increase heart rate. However, the heart rate may increase by only 10 beats per minute (bpm) within 45 seconds, instead of 20 bpm in non-pregnant individuals; a transient decrease in FHR from uterine artery constriction may be observed as well. A test dose should be avoided during uterine contractions, when pain may also increase the heart rate. When a test dose enters the subarachnoid space, the lidocaine dose will provide a quick onset (within 3 minutes) sensory and motor blockade and an anaesthetic block within 10 minutes; this contrasts with a slower onset of less dense analgesia if the test dose is within the epidural space. Subarachnoid epinephrine will have minimal effects.

The best 'test' for an incorrectly placed needle or catheter is an astute clinician, who can critically assess haemodynamic and neuraxial blockade responses, as well as the often subtle symptoms parturients may experience. Good practice dictates that every clinician-administered bolus through any neuraxial catheter begins with aspiration, inspection of any aspirate, fractionation of the desired dose into smaller increments (0.5 mL spinal, 3 mL epidural), and evaluation of the effects.

Labour analgesia agent selection

Agents used to create labour analgesia include lipid-soluble opioids and long-acting local anaesthetic agents (Table 10.3). Opioids alone can provide sufficient analgesia for early first stage of labour in the intrathecal space only. A combination of opioids with local anaesthetics is necessary during this stage in the epidural space, as well as for later stages of labour in both the subarachnoid and epidural spaces. The combination of agents allows for smaller doses of both agents to be used, thereby minimizing undesirable side effects (e.g. opioid-induced pruritus, local anaesthetic-induced motor blockade), and provides faster onset.

The dermatomal spread of analgesia is dependent on the *total dose* of local anaesthetic agents in the subarachnoid space, and the *volume* of local anaesthetic administered is a more relevant factor in the epidural space. Opioids and local anaesthetic solutions have a lower specific gravity relative to CSF (i.e. hypobaric), which allow for cephalad extension of the sensory blockade. A T-10, sensory dermatome level is necessary for labour analgesia. Initiation of epidural analgesia with 15 to 20 mL of < 0.125% bupivacaine or

Table 10.3 Drugs for initiation and maintenance of labour analgesia

Drug	Epidural analgesia	Spinal analgesia
Local Anaesthetics[a]		
Initiation/Maintenance		
Bupivacaine	0.0625%–0.125%	1.25–2.5 mg
L-Bupivacaine	0.0625%–0.125%	1.25–2.5 mg
Ropivacaine	0.08%–0.2%	2.5–4.5 mg
Breakthrough/Delivery		
Bupivacaine	0.125%–0.25%	NA
L-Bupivacaine	0.125%–0.25%	NA
Ropivacaine	0.2%–0.4%	NA
Lidocaine[b]	0.75%–1.0%	NA
Opioids		
Initiation/Maintenance/Breakthrough		
Fentanyl	50–100 µg	15–25 µg
Sufentanil	5–10 µg	1.5–5 µg
Morphine	NA	0.125–0.25 mg

NA = not applicable.
[a] The volume used to initiate an epidural labour analgesic is 10–20 mL of local anaesthetic solution.
[b] Lidocaine and bupivacaine 0.25%, L-bupivacaine 0.25% and ropivacaine 0.4%

ropivacaine with sufentanil (0.2–0.3 µg/mL) or fentanyl (0.2 µg/mL) results in effective labour analgesia for vaginal delivery.

Maintenance of neuraxial labour analgesia

A variety of methods can be used to maintain analgesia, including intermittent bolus, continuous infusion or their combination. Intermittent bolus methods can be administered by the anaesthetist, the patient (e.g. patient-controlled epidural analgesia; PCEA) or a pump (e.g. timed bolus). Clinician-administered boluses are typically the most variable, given alterations in timing and therapy administered; by contrast, the PCEA method yields more control to the patient, resulting in more immediate delivery of the analgesia when desired and greater maternal satisfaction.

Typical epidural bolus doses of a dilute local anaesthetic with opioid combination (e.g. 0.125% bupivacaine with fentanyl 0.2 µg/mL) range from 5 to 8 mL or 8 to 12 mL in the presence or absence of a background infusion of 4–8 mL/h, respectively.

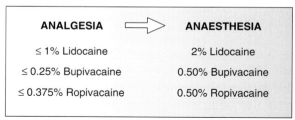

Figure 10.2 The continuum of epidural analgesia to anaesthesia effects due to anaesthetic concentration.

Lockout intervals are generally 10 to 15 min. The use of a background infusion, typically with one-third to one-half of the total hourly dose volume, provides better analgesia than a pure bolus-only approach, with fewer unscheduled interventions. Additional epidural top-up doses for breakthrough pain use higher volumes and/or concentrations of local anaesthetics; 0.25% bupivacaine or 0.375% ropivacaine 6 to 8 mL is commonly used. The requirement for concentrations of local anaesthetic agents sufficient for operative anaesthesia is typically unnecessary for labour analgesia (Figure 10.2) and may indicate a need for a replacement technique.

PCEA pumps should be locked to prevent tampering with the contents or settings and patients should be instructed to be the exclusive operator of the demand button. The labour and delivery suite should have clear policies on which personnel may adjust the content, rate or volume of pump settings or bolus doses. Records of the technique and all agents administered should be kept at the bedside.

Patient monitoring

The use of neuraxial analgesia, regardless of whether PCEA is used, mandates periodic (every 90–120 minutes) patient assessment to evaluate the quality and spread of analgesia, maternal symptoms and signs (blood pressure), and FHR responses. An inappropriately high level may suggest a subdural or subarachnoid migration of medication, whereas a low level may signal migration of the catheter intravenously or out of the intended space, or the administration of an inadequate dose. Assessments should be recorded on an analgesic record by the patient's bedside.

Neuraxial labour analgesia for peripartum interventions

The larger somatic nerve fibres that enter the spinal cord at sacral segments 2 to 4 frequently require the administration of a higher concentration or greater volume of local anaesthetic solution than that previously used for the visceral fibres during the first stage of labour. Because drug volume administered into the lumbar epidural space spreads mostly in a cephalad orientation, patients should be monitored for high sensory levels and associated haemodynamic and respiratory alterations.

Dense analgesia, and sometimes even anaesthesia, is required for delivery, particularly in the setting of an episiotomy, intended external or internal version, or forceps or vacuum-extraction delivery (Table 10.3; Figure 10.2). Postpartum, extensive vaginal and cervical repairs most often require anaesthesia, and may benefit from movement to an operating room for better obstetric visualization, surgical repair and response to postoperative issues. During this immediate peripartum period, open and clear communication between care providers is essential, so that relevant and timely expectations, plans and responses can be made.

Side effects

Hypotension

Neuraxial-induced sympathetic blockade results in peripheral vasodilation, increased venous capacitance and reduced venous return to the heart. Hypotension, defined as systolic blood pressure less than 100 mmHg or a 20% to 30% decrease from baseline, can be observed in approximately 10% of pregnant women following initiation of neuraxial analgesia. During pregnancy, hypotension may be compounded by aortocaval compression by the gravid uterus. Persistent hypotension may result in decreased uteroplacental perfusion, fetal hypoxia and acidosis, and thus the FHR should be monitored.

Preventive measures include maternal intravascular volume expansion (preloading with IV fluid, usually 500 to 1000 mL of crystalloid such as Hartmann's solution) and the avoidance of aortocaval compression by uterine displacement. Treatment includes assessment of the sensory and motor blockade (to rule out high blockade or inadvertent subarachnoid or subdural blockade), the titration of IV doses of vasopressors such as ephedrine (5–10 mg) and phenylephrine (40–100 μg) and the use of volume expansion. Vasopressor use can significantly reduce the nausea and vomiting following a spinal technique, which may be associated with reductions in sympathetic tone, blood pressure and cerebral blood flow.

Pruritus

The incidence and severity of pruritus is dose dependent and greater with the spinal vs. epidural administration of opioids. The aetiology is most likely related to sensory modulation, central opioid receptor activation and central inhibitory neurotransmitters (e.g. γ-aminobutyric acid [GABA] and glycine) antagonization. The co-administration of spinal bupivacaine appears to lower the incidence of pruritus.

Opioid-induced pruritus is typically self-limiting, although an effective treatment is the administration of a centrally acting agonist (which acts as a competitive antagonist; e.g. naloxone, naltrexone) or partial agonist–antagonist (e.g. nalbuphine). The use of these agents should be limited to prevent complete reversal of the desired analgesia. Because the release of histamine is not believed to be involved in the mechanism of opioid-induced pruritus, the observed benefit from the provision of antihistamines (e.g. diphenhydramine) is most likely due to the resulting sedation.

Nausea and vomiting

The anatomic and hormonal changes in gastric emptying associated with pregnancy can frequently result in nausea and vomiting; these symptoms may also be in response to neuraxial opioids or hypotension.

Treatment should be guided towards correcting hypotension if it exists. Antagonists to the 5-HT$_3$ (e.g. ondansetron), dopamine (e.g. prochlorperazine, metoclopramide), H$_1$ (e.g. diphenhydramine) receptors, as well as anticholinergics (e.g. hyoscine), benzodiazepines (e.g. midazolam) and steroids (e.g. dexamethasone) have been observed to be helpful in treating nausea and vomiting. Many of these agents should be administered slowly (over several minutes) to minimize extrapyramidal side effects or hypotension.

Fever and shivering

In some women with neuraxial labour analgesia, there is a small (< 1°C) increase in core temperature, particularly if labouring in a warm ambient environment. Shivering may also occur in this setting, independent of temperature increases. A non-infectious, inflammatory process appears to be the aetiology for the temperature increase, with a higher thermoregulatory sweating threshold and a reduction in pain-induced hyperventilation being partially involved. The clinical diagnosis of fever is a temperature greater than 38°C. Women with longer, more uncomfortable, dysfunctional labours (e.g. nulliparous, larger babies, non-vertex presentation) and infections (e.g. chorioamnionitis) are more likely to request neuraxial techniques and exhibit fever.

Maternal fever may result in both maternal and fetal infection/sepsis evaluations and result in exposure to antibiotics. Peripartum maternal fever should always prompt consideration and monitoring for an infectious aetiology. Acetaminophen (paracetamol) 650 to 1000 mg PO can be given to manage maternal fever, which provides some analgesia as well. Meperidine 12.5 mg IV can be administered for the treatment of shivering, acknowledging that increased sedation may occur; its use is most often relegated to the postpartum period, given the accumulation of normeperidine, which has been related to neonatal seizure activity with repeated *in utero* exposure.

Complications

Failed analgesia

The definition of analgesia failure can include an absence of analgesia, incomplete or patchy analgesia

or the need for a replacement technique. Neuraxial techniques that include a spinal component (i.e. spinal, spinal catheter, CSE, DPE) have a lower incidence of failed analgesia than the epidural technique. Obstetric factors (e.g. progress of labour, occiput posterior fetal presentation), maternal anatomic factors (e.g. distended bladder) and analgesic factors should be evaluated when significant changes in the quality of analgesia are reported. A sensory and motor evaluation should be conducted in the traditional caudad to cephalad direction, with adequate caudad evaluation to determine the presence of sacral blockade.

Treatment should be guided by the patient's symptoms and sensory evaluation. If an epidural, CSE, or DPE blockade spread is inadequate, one sided or patchy, administer 6 to 10 mL, remembering that the epidural space is volume sensitive, of a dilute local anaesthetic solution (e.g. 0.125% bupivacaine). If the sensory (and perhaps motor) blockade has been extended, and an interval analgesic improvement is observed, but remains inadequate, administer 6 to 10 mL of a more concentrated local anaesthetic solution (e.g. 0.25% bupivacaine). If interval analgesic improvement is again observed, but still inadequate, consider using a more concentrated local anaesthetic solution (e.g. 1% lidocaine), the addition of an opioid (e.g. fentanyl 100 µg) or replacement of the catheter. The requirement for even higher anaesthetic doses adequate for surgical interventions should prompt consideration of technique replacement (Figure 10.2). With a spinal catheter, CSF may not be able to be aspirated each time; however, the administration of 1 to 2 mL of 0.25% bupivacaine (or equivalent) should provide additional comfort; if analgesia remains insufficient, consider 1 to 2 mL of hyperbaric lidocaine 1.5%, and then, if insufficient, consider replacing the catheter.

All analgesic interventions should be considered in the context of the patient and obstetric needs; if the discomfort is intense or delivery imminent, the higher dose regimens may be employed earlier. However, administration of anaesthetic agents through neuraxial catheters should never sacrifice safety and should always employ the use of catheter aspiration before and between each dose; incremental, fractionated dosing; and appropriate pauses to evaluate intended and unintended (e.g. intrathecal or intravascular migration) effects.

High neuraxial blockade

A high 'total spinal' neuraxial blockade may be produced from local anaesthetic agents administered in

Table 10.4 Comparison of epidural, sub-dural and sub-arachnoid blockade during intended epidural technique

	Epidural	Sub-dural	Sub-arachnoid
Incidence		0.025 (0.017–0.033)	0.035 (0.02–0.04)
Onset	Slow	Intermediate	Rapid
Spread		Higher than expected, but with patchy sensory blockade	Higher than expected, but with present sensory blockade
Motor blockade	Minimal	Minimal	Dense
Hypotension	Less than spinal and subdural; dependent on height of sensory blockade	Less than spinal, greater than epidural; dependent on height of sensory blockade	Dependent on height of sensory blockade

the epidural, subdural and subarachnoid spaces. Subarachnoid and subdural injection occurs with an incidence of 1:2,900 and 1:4,200, respectively, with a high/total spinal occurring in 1:1,400 cases. Within the epidural space, large volumes (>30 mL) of local anaesthetic would be required to achieve a high spinal. By contrast, an inadvertent and unrecognized subarachnoid or subdural puncture may allow a relatively small volume of local anaesthetic to spread quickly.

Total spinal blockade manifests with rapidly ascending sensory and motor changes, bradycardia and hypotension, dyspnoea, with difficulty swallowing and limited ability to phonate, and loss of grip strength. Unconsciousness and respiratory depression may soon follow, most commonly as a result of hypoperfusion of the brain and brainstem. Medications within the subdural space may result in Horner's syndrome (i.e. anhydrosis, enophthalmos, ptosis and miosis) and a patchy sensory and motor blockade. A total spinal blockade with analgesic concentrations of local anaesthetic agents causes a more rapid and dense sensory and motor blockade than a subdural or epidural blockade (see Table 10.4).

Treatment includes assessment of the patient's symptoms and evaluation of the neuraxial catheter. Aortocaval compression should be avoided, 100% oxygen administered and the provision of positive pressure ventilation via an endotracheal tube if necessary. Maternal vital signs, EKG and FHR should be evaluated, with maternal circulation supported with vasopressor agents and fluids.

Inadvertent dural puncture

The incidence of an inadvertent dural puncture with an epidural needle or catheter is approximately 1% to 3%. When detected during the insertion of the epidural technique, the procedure may be re-attempted at another interspace, or the epidural catheter may be placed into the subarachnoid space for the provision of a continuous spinal analgesic technique for labour and delivery. This continuous spinal technique minimizes the risk of a repeat dural puncture at another site, particularly in the setting of anatomic or pathologic issues of the back (e.g. obesity, scoliosis), or passage of a sufficient amount of local anaesthetic agent or opioid through the dural puncture into the subarachnoid space, resulting in a high neuraxial blockade. A spinal catheter can be efficiently titrated for both analgesia and anaesthesia (see above).

The patient should be followed up for a post dural puncture headache, with pain relief provided by bed rest, hydration and the oral intake of caffeinated and analgesic products (including Fioricet or Fiorinal) for 24 to 48 hours. If correctly diagnosed as a PDPH, the administration of an epidural blood patch, whereby 10 to 20 mL of autologous blood is placed in the epidural space, is associated with a high (80%) success rate. Neurologic complications (e.g. peripheral neuropathy, subarachnoid bleed) as a result of spinal anaesthesia in the obstetric population are extremely rare; however, should these events occur, a consultation with a neurologist may assist in the diagnosis and management.

Intravascular injection of local anaesthetic

The incidence of intravascular injection during attempted epidural labour analgesia is 1:5000. Physiologic responses to intravascular injection are dependent on the amount and type of agents used. Initially, CNS symptoms (e.g. tinnitus, dizziness, restlessness, difficulty speaking, seizures and loss of consciousness) occur, which may be followed closely by cardiovascular signs (e.g. initial increases in blood pressure from sympathetic stimulation, followed by bradycardia, ventricular dysfunction, tachycardia and fibrillation) and collapse.

Prevention begins with meticulous attention to the technique and observation of the patient while delivering fractionated doses. Treatment includes suspension of further injection, calling for assistance, providing 100% oxygen with positive-pressure ventilation if necessary, avoiding aortocaval compression, monitoring and supporting maternal vital signs, monitoring FHR and preparing for emergency caesarean delivery within 4 minutes. The administration of 20% lipid emulsion (i.e. IV bolus 1.5 mL/kg followed by a continuous infusion of 0.25 to 5 mL/kg/min for 10 minutes or longer) should be considered; barbiturates or benzodiazepines may also be given to arrest seizure activity.

Key points

1. Neuraxial techniques, including spinal, epidural, combined spinal-epidural (CSE) and dural-puncture epidural (DPE) techniques, are commonly used in modern obstetric care for the provision of labour analgesia and anaesthesia for instrumental and operative deliveries.

2. The basic properties of spinal, epidural, CSE and DPE techniques may be advantageous for specific situations.

3. A catheter-based neuraxial technique can allow flexibility in titrating the onset and duration of the blockade; however, the spinal catheter technique is less commonly used due to the size of the dural puncture and the resulting high incidence of headache.

4. A number of analgesic and anaesthetic options exist for labour and delivery, including non-pharmacologic modalities, systemic agents and peripheral nerve blocks.

5. Whether neuraxial analgesia affects the progress and outcome of labour remains controversial, in part due to the complexity in study design. However, the majority of studies appear to indicate little overall effect of epidural analgesia on progress and outcome of labour. Anaesthetic and obstetric practice styles may influence who ultimately receives an instrumental or operative delivery.

6. Although the aetiology remains unclear, epidural labour analgesia appears to increase maternal temperature; however, a delay of 4 to 5 hours is observed prior to a mean increase of approximately 0.1°C/h following epidural initiation. The impact of these changes remains controversial, and deserves further investigation.

7. Awareness and communication of the indications and implications of neuraxial techniques among the entire obstetric care team, including obstetric, anaesthetic, neonatal and nursing care providers, remain of paramount importance to the continued welfare of the expectant mother and fetus.

Further reading

American Society of Anaesthetists Task Force on Obstetric Anaesthesia. (2007). Practice guidelines for obstetric anaesthesia: an updated report by the American Society of Anaesthetists Task Force on Obstetric Anaesthesia. *Anesthesiology*, **106**, 843–863.

Bucklin, B. A., Hawkins, J. L., Anderson, J. R. and Ullrich, F. A. (2005). Obstetric anaesthesia workforce survey: twenty-year update. *Anesthesiology*, **103**, 645–653.

Cappiello, E., O'Rourke, N., Segal, S. and Tsen, L. C. (2008). A randomized trial of dural puncture epidural technique compared with the standard epidural technique for labour analgesia. *Anesth. Analg.*, **107**(5), 1646–1651.

Leo, S., Ocampo, C. E., Lim, Y. and Sia, A. T. (2010). A randomized comparison of automated intermittent mandatory boluses with a basal infusion in combination with patient-controlled epidural analgesia for labour and delivery. *Int. J. Obstet. Anesth.*, **19**, 357–364.

Loubert, C., Hinova, A. and Fernando, R. (2011). Update on modern neuraxial analgesia in labour: a review of the literature of the last 5 years. *Anaesthesia*, **66**, 192–212.

Mercier, F. J. (2011). Fluid loading for caesarean delivery under spinal anaesthesia: have we studied all the options? *Anesth. Analg.*, **113**(4), 677–680.

Ngan Kee, W. D. (2010). Prevention of maternal hypotension after regional anaesthesia for caesarean section. *Curr. Opin. Anaesthesiol.*, **23**, 304–309.

Simmons, S. W., Taghizadeh, N., Dennis, A. T. and Cyna, A. M. (2012). Combined spinal-epidural versus epidural analgesia in labour. *Cochrane Database Syst. Rev.*, **10**, Art. No.: CD003401.

Halpern, S. H. and Abdallah, F. W. (2010). Effect of labor analgesia on labor outcome. *Curr. Opin. Anaesthesiol.*, **23**, 317–322.

Wong, C. A., Scavone, B. M., Peaceman, A. M. *et al.* (2005). The risk of caesarean delivery with neuraxial analgesia given early versus late in labour. *N. Engl. J. Med.*, **52**, 655–665.

Regional anaesthesia for operative delivery

Cathy Armstrong and Khaled Girgirah

Introduction

The rate of general anaesthesia (GA) for caesarean section (CS) has fallen from 55% (1989–1990) to 9.4% (2011–2012). Over the same time period there has been an increase in CS rates from 11.3% to 25%. Despite the rise in CS rate there are approximately 70% fewer obstetric GAs performed per year nationally.

The reasons for this include:

- Increasing awareness of the risks of general anaesthesia in the parturient. The UKOSS study demonstrated a 1:224 risk of failed intubation
- The introduction of pencil point spinal needles, which have reduced the risk of post dural-puncture headache to an acceptable level (0.25%)
- Changes in maternal demographics: increasing numbers of women with morbid obesity and other co-morbidities
- Alteration in maternal expectations. Better information antenatally regarding the risks and benefits of regional anaesthesia vs. general anaesthesia allows women to make informed choices.

Benefits of regional anaesthesia (RA) for the woman include:

- The partner can be present throughout the delivery
- Maternal/neonatal skin-to-skin contact at the time of delivery can facilitate bonding
- The drugs used to provide RA do not affect uterine tone and there is minimal, if any, direct effect of these agents on fetal heart rate activity or fetal wellbeing
- The addition of neuraxial opioids provides excellent postoperative analgesia
- A reduction in the need for general anaesthesia reduces risks e.g. failed intubation.

Audit standards from the Association of Anaesthetists are that the proportion of CS under regional anaesthesia should be:

- Category 1 CS   >50%
- Category 2–3 CS   >85%
- Category 4 CS   >95%.

Types of central anaesthetic neuraxial blockade

The CNB technique for delivery is dictated by:

- The experience of the anaesthetist
- The urgency of the decision-to-delivery interval (DDI):
  - Category 1: immediate threat to the life of the mother or fetus (< 30 minutes)
  - Category 2: no immediate threat to the life of woman or fetus (< 75 minutes)
  - Category 3: requires early delivery (> 75 minutes)
  - Category 4: at a time to suit the woman and the maternity service
- Co-morbidities, e.g.:
  - Obesity
  - Pre-eclampsia
  - Cardiac disease
  - Respiratory disease
- Whether the *in-situ* epidural is satisfactory enough to top-up.

The contraindications to CNB are detailed in Chapter 10.

The absolute contraindications are:

- Patient refusal
- Sepsis – local to the insertion site and systemic

Core Topics in Obstetric Anaesthesia, ed. Kirsty MacLennan, Kate O'Brien and W. Ross Mcnab.
Published by Cambridge University Press. © Cambridge University Press 2015.

- Coagulopathy:
  - Pathological
  - Iatrogenic.

There are a number of situations where there is a judgement that the risks of CNB are less than the risks associated with GA, e.g. a woman that has a stable platelet count of 70×10^9/L, with a normal coagulation screen. She may be considered unsuitable for a labour epidural, but an acceptable risk for siting a spinal for operative delivery.

The multidisciplinary team should be made aware of any woman with morbidities that could complicate the performance of CNB as this may result in a delay in decision-to-delivery time. Complex cases should be supervised by a senior anaesthetist.

Preparation for central neuraxial blockade is as follows:

1. Patient:
   a. A full medical history, to assess the woman's suitability for CNB
   b. Early identification of women who have an increased risk of operative delivery e.g. twin pregnancy, morbid obesity, medical co-morbidities, induction of labour
   c. Appropriate examination and review of relevant investigations in light of the history
   d. A full explanation of the procedure, including the benefits and risks of CNB (See Table 11.1)

Table 11.1 Risks of central neuraxial blockade

Risks	Epidural	Spinal
Hypotension	1:50	1:5
Failure of CNB, resulting in GA conversion	1:20	1:125
Post dural puncture headache	1:100	1:400
Neurological damage	1:1,000 (temporary)	
	1:13,000 (permanent)	
Epidural abscess	1:50,000	
Meningitis	1:100,000	
Epidural haematoma	1:170,000	
Accidental unconsciousness	1:5,000	
Severe injury, including being paralyzed	1:250,000	

e. Prompt access to translation services
f. Antacid prophylaxis

2. Equipment required prior to commencing CNB:
   a. Full standard monitoring
   b. A large bore cannula (16G or higher)
   c. Emergency drugs, including vasopressors, must be immediately available in the location (delivery unit room or theatre)
   d. A selection of different length Tuohy and spinal needles.

Spinal anaesthesia

Operative delivery encompasses caesarean section, forceps and ventouse deliveries. Spinal anaesthesia is the commonest way of providing anaesthesia for operative delivery and is the most reliable of CNB techniques. The woman can be positioned in the sitting or lateral position, this may be dictated by the patient, fetal monitoring requirements or uncommon events such as cord prolapse.

Skin preparation

Controversy remains over the most appropriate antiseptic solution with which to clean the skin prior to insertion of CNB. The Royal College of Anaesthetists, The American Society of Anesthesiologists and The American Society of Regional Anesthesia all recommend the use of chlorhexidine in alcohol as the skin disinfectant of choice for CNB. A UK working party review in 2014 (see Further Reading) recommend the use of 0.5% chlorhexidine in alcohol for CNB, this being the agent that gives the best balance for risk of neurotoxicity vs. the risk of infection.

Chlorhexidine gluconate has the following characteristics:

- Potent and broad spectrum
- Effective against bacteria and yeast
- Fast onset and long duration of action (when compared with povidone iodine)
- Efficacious even in the presence of blood
- Lower incidence of skin reactions (when compared with povidone iodine)
- Chlorhexidine in alcoholic solution has improved bacteriostatic profile when compared with chlorhexidine in aqueous solution
- There is an established risk of neurotoxicity in vitro and in animal studies; the risk of

developing chronic adhesive arachnoiditis is extremely rare

- There is limited in vivo evidence regarding the alterations in efficacy between 0.5% and 2% chlorhexidine
- Meticulous attention should be given to reducing the risk of contamination of CNB equipment with chlorhexidine. Some advocate the use of pre-soaked sponge applicators or sprays; time must be allowed for the solution to dry
- Hypersensitivity reactions have been described; most anaphylactic reactions have resulted from topical application to mucous membranes and the use of chlorhexidine-impregnated devices, although they can occur following contact with intact skin (see Chapter 23).

Other precautions (as per National Audit Project 3 recommendations) that should be employed at the time of CNB include:

- Thorough hand washing with appropriate preparation
- Hat, mask, sterile gown, gloves and drape

The recommended level for siting a spinal needle (25–27 gauge) is L3/4. Use of higher intervertebral spaces may result in damage to the cauda equina, particularly in view of the lack of reliability in confirming lumbar levels when using bony landmarks. See Chapter 18 for ultrasound of spine.

Spinal anaesthesia relies on distribution of local anaesthetic and/or opioids in the cerebrospinal fluid (CSF). Glucose levels in CSF are approximately two-thirds of that in venous blood. Use of a glucometer can help to confirm CSF if there is doubt. Whilst performing CNB, good communication with the woman is essential; it is important for the woman to report any issues with pain or paraesthesia on injection. If this occurs, then changing the direction of the needle can remedy the situation, if not then resiting the block is the safest option.

A reduced spinal dose of local anaesthetic (2.2–3.0 mL of 0.5% heavy bupivacaine) is required in the parturient as there is a smaller CSF volume in the lumbar region and greater sensitivity of nerve fibres to local anaesthetic. The cephalad displacement of CSF from the lumbar region is a result of caval compression and increased fat in the epidural space. Opioid analgesics are generally added to the local anaesthetic mixture to enhance the efficacy of the spinal block. The main contraindications to spinal opioid analgesia are opioid allergy and an active herpetic eruption.

Assessment of the block

The sensory block height should be assessed and documented prior to skin incision. Sensory examination should move caudad to cephalad bilaterally in the midaxillary or midclavicular lines.

The adequacy of regional anaesthesia for caesarean section has been assessed using a range of sensory modalities, including light touch, pinprick and cold. Absence of light touch sensation up to T5 dermatome is widely accepted to indicate an adequate level of block for caesarean section. Sacral anaesthesia is also essential as the S2–S4 dermatomes innervate the peritoneum overlying the lower uterine segment. Instrumental deliveries do not require the same height of block and can be commenced when certain of sacral anaesthesia and a block to T8. However, should the instrumental delivery be unsuccessful, the anaesthetist must assess the block height to ensure that it has reached an appropriate level to proceed to caesarean section under regional anaesthesia.

A survey of UK obstetric anaesthetists in 2010 showed that 74% still checked the block height with cold sensation to ethyl chloride alone. Concerns regarding the reliability of use of cold sensation to evaluate block height relate to the multimodal transmission of sensation. Cold, transmitted by Aδ fibres, may not be distinguished from cold discomfort, transmitted by C fibres. Aβ fibres may also be activated, transmitting light touch and possibly pressure sensation.

When sharp pinprick is used to assess block height, it is important to document the exact end point:

- Total loss of all sensation to the pinprick
- The pinprick is recognized as a touch
- The pinprick is recognized as being sharp, but is less sharp than normal
- The pinprick feels normal.

If the block is inadequate prior to skin incision then there are three options, which need to be discussed with the obstetricians:

- Repeat the spinal anaesthetic, the second dose is dependent on the block height from the previous spinal (1.0–2.2 mL 0.5% heavy bupivacaine)
- Postponement of the case in the elective setting
- Conversion to GA.

Pain during CS under regional anaesthesia is one of the most common causes of obstetric anaesthetic litigation. It is essential to document thoroughly the woman's concerns and offer alternative solutions, e.g. low-dose intravenous opioid analgesia, local anaesthetic infiltration by the surgeon or conversion to GA. Each step must be acted on promptly and the outcome of the intervention recorded.

Combined spinal epidural (CSE)

Indications for a combined spinal epidural approach for operative delivery include:

- Anticipated prolonged surgery with the potential to exceed the anaesthetic duration of a single shot spinal (e.g. multiple previous CS, obesity, combined CS and tubal ligation):
  - a standard intrathecal dose is administered; the epidural catheter is in place for intraoperative supplementation if the spinal block regresses over time
- Parturients with cardiac co-morbidities where sudden cardiovascular changes are undesirable:
  - a reduced intrathecal volume (1.0–2.0 mL) is injected to lessen the hypotension from sympathetic blockade; the block height can then be extended using the epidural catheter, thus minimizing cardiovascular instability.

There are two recognized techniques for CSE insertion:

1. Needle-through-needle technique: This is the commonest approach. The epidural space is located with a Tuohy needle, a spinal needle is passed through the Tuohy needle to puncture the dura and deposit medication in the CSF. The spinal needle is withdrawn and a catheter is then threaded into the epidural space. The risks of this technique include:
   a. Threading the epidural catheter through the dural puncture created by the spinal needle
   b. Failure to enter the intrathecal space with the spinal needle despite the Tuohy needle being located in the epidural space
   c. Potential problems threading the epidural catheter after spinal injection (i.e. blood in catheter, persistent pain on insertion), leading to abandonment of the epidural
   d. Reduced block height from the spinal anaesthetic due to increased time in sitting position while epidural catheter is placed.

2. Separate insertion of an epidural catheter and a spinal at different lumbar levels. The epidural is sited prior to spinal insertion. Risks include:
   a. The risk of damaging the epidural catheter on insertion of the spinal needle; however, this is minimized by insertion of the spinal at a level below the epidural site.

Both techniques rely on an epidural that is effectively 'untested' and may fail when attempting to extend the block.

Epidural 'top-up' for operative delivery

The maternity Hospital Episode Statistics (HES) shows that the risk of conversion to GA with epidural anaesthesia is 2.2%, whereas the risk of conversion with spinal anaesthesia is 0.8%.

Epidural analgesia is commonplace on consultant-led delivery units and the majority work well in labour. Epidural top-up for Category 1 and 2 CS in low- and high-risk women is an invaluable technique to ensure a prompt and effective anaesthetic block, e.g. difficult airway, morbid obesity and twin pregnancies. If the epidural block is inadequate there should be discussion with the woman about resiting the epidural.

It is vital that women with epidural analgesia are reviewed regularly. There are only two statistically significant factors that predict a failed anaesthetic top-up:

1. More than one anaesthetist top-up in the room
2. Increased maternal height.

An effective top-up requires:

- A good labour analgesic effect
- Testing to ensure there is a good sacral block
- Enough time to top-up safely.

This ensures that only epidurals that are working well are topped-up for operative delivery.

If there is doubt about the efficacy of the epidural, the catheter should be removed and a spinal anaesthetic sited in theatre. Cases must be assessed on an individual basis.

Top-ups for epidural anaesthesia can be performed in theatre or in a delivery room. If the top-up occurs in a delivery room it is mandatory that the anaesthetist remains in attendance. Full monitoring and access to emergency drugs is essential (see preparation for CNB).

Table 11.2 Examples of epidural top-up regimens

Lignocaine, adrenaline, bicarbonate (+/− fentanyl) mixture (LEB)
18 mL 2% lignocaine, 100 µg adrenaline (0.1 mL 1:1000) ±50–100 µg fentanyl
Pros: this is the fastest-acting mixture, almost halving the times of other mixtures, the addition of fentanyl further shortens the time to surgical anaesthesia
Cons: has to be mixed by the anaesthetist, this may result in drug errors, particularly with those unfamiliar in the technique. Increased analgesic supplementation during the CS

0.75% Ropivacaine
10–20 mL ±50–100 µg fentanyl
Pros: same time to surgical anaesthesia as levobupivacaine, but less supplementation during CS
Cons: slower onset to surgical anaesthesia

0.5% Levobupivacaine
10–20 mL ±50–100 µg fentanyl
Pros: widely used and familiar to most anaesthetists, no cardiotoxicity compared to racemic bupivacaine
Cons: slower onset of surgical anaesthesia

Intrathecal catheters

Indwelling intrathecal catheters used in labour and theatre have the potential to deliver the 'ideal labour analgesia/anaesthesia' with a reliable analgesic block in labour that could be topped up to provide a dense and fast anaesthetic.

Intrathecal catheters left *in situ* following inadvertent dural puncture at epidural insertion can be topped up for theatre using small volumes of local anaesthetic. However, intentional insertion and use of intrathecal catheters is currently not common practice in the UK.

Use of indwelling intrathecal catheters for labour & delivery was developed in the 1980s, however their safety was questioned following cases of cauda equina syndrome and nerve damage. There was also a high incidence of post dural puncture headache. However, recent development of microcatheters (26G–32G) has led to renewed interest and may change practice in the future. Further research into long-term complication rates needs to be completed before widespread use can resume.

Risks of CNB

The 3rd National Audit Project (NAP3) of the Royal College of Anaesthetists on major complications of central neuraxial block in the United Kingdom reported that CNB performed for obstetric analgesia or anaesthesia appears to be acceptably safe. Obstetric CNB was associated with fewer major complications than in other areas, likely as a result of a generally healthy patient population with short durations of epidural catheterizations. Although neurological complications in obstetric practice may be a result of the CNB, obstetric causes must also be considered. Risk factors for neuraxial infection following CNB include multiple attempts at insertion accompanied by massive obstetric haemorrhage. Post CNB headache should be investigated appropriately (see Chapter 26). Wrong route drug errors were more common in the obstetric group. Meticulous attention to epidural infusion connection and drug checking may help.

Less than 6% of all CNB reported in NAP3 were combined spinal epidurals. This group, however, accounted for over 13% of the reports of harm.

Hypotension

All types of CNB can cause maternal hypotension. Epidural and small-volume CSE blocks tend to take longer to provide surgical anaesthesia so the incidence is less frequent than for spinal anaesthesia. Approximately 80% of women will become hypotensive unless they are given a vasopressor; phenylephrine or ephedrine are commonly used.

The hypotension, due to preganglionic sympathetic blockade, causes a dramatic fall in systemic vascular resistance. In normal pregnancy the uterine arteries are maximally dilated, resulting in pressure-dependent blood flow. Studies have shown no adverse effects on oxygen supply to the fetus when phenylephrine infusion is used to maintain baseline blood pressure (BP).

Which vasopressor?

1. Phenylephrine:
   - Most effective drug to prevent hypotension associated with spinal anaesthesia
   - Most effective drug for prevention of nausea
   - Does not induce fetal acidosis
   - Decreases heart rate and cardiac output (clinically insignificant in low-risk pregnancies)

Table 11.3 Adjuvants table

Agent	Doses used and studied	Site of action	Information
Ketamine	0.5 mg/kg	Non-competitive NMDA antagonist	Limited data for post caesarean section analgesia Not recommended Would require further research
Clonidine	Intrathecal 75–400 µg Epidural 100–800 µg	α2 receptor: peripheral, spinal, brainstem	Can cause significant hypotension and sedation Analgesic benefit when used in combination with opiates
Neostigmine	Intrathecal 12.5–25 µg	Spinal nicotinic and muscarinic receptors	Limited use due to side effects Not enough data to use epidurally Requires more research
Magnesium	Intrathecal 50 mg Epidural 500 mg	Non-competitive NMDA antagonist	Requires more research Used in combination with local and opiates
Midazolam	Intrathecal 2 mg	GABA receptors	More research required Potential beneficial side effect profile
Epinephrine	Intrathecal 200 µg Epidural 2.5–30 µg	α receptors, local vasoconstriction	Prolongs duration of action

General advice: Adjuvants should always be reviewed in the context of risks and benefits. Agents can be used as sole agents, but are usually used in combination with opioids. All adjuvants have some benefits as an analgesic agent or on the duration of action of drugs. They will also alter the side-effect profile. More data is available for use as adjuvants in non-obstetric patients and all agents require further research to be able to give definitive advice.
NMDA N-methyl-D-aspartate, GABA

A suggested regime would be to commence a phenylephrine infusion (concentration 100 µg/mL) at a rate of 30 mL/h, titrated to blood pressure.

2. Ephedrine:

- Freely crosses the placenta
- Higher rate of nausea and vomiting, despite similar BP
- Can induce fetal acidosis; this is likely to be a direct β-adrenergic effect resulting in an increase in fetal metabolic rate.

Pre-eclampsia

The high systemic vascular resistance seen in severe pre-eclampsia (PET) often negates the need for vasopressor support following spinal anaesthesia.

Vasopressors must be immediately available, but should be given with caution owing to their exaggerated response in this condition.

Post dural puncture headache/ neurological damage

The management of these complications can be found in Chapters 26 and 22, respectively.

High central neuraxial block

The risk factors for a high block are:

- Epidural top-up:
  - The catheter can be intrathecal or subdural (see Chapter 10)
  - High concentration solutions of local anaesthetic
  - Too much volume of high concentration local anaesthetic
- Spinal anaesthesia: the following situations may lead to a quicker, more extensive spread of local anaesthetic. This is thought to result from lumbar

thecal compression resulting in rapid rostral spread.

- Following a recent epidural top-up, if the catheter has been removed for either speed or anticipated failure of top-up
- Women with raised BMI
- Multiple pregnancies.

Management

This is dependent on the height of the block and the woman's symptoms.

The block should be assessed as soon as possible after the patient has been positioned supine following regional anaesthesia.

The features of high block include:

- Bradycardia
- Hypotension
- Respiratory compromise
- Loss of consciousness.

Tilting the table early into reverse Trendelenburg may prevent any further extension of the block. Respiratory compromise or loss of consciousness necessitate prompt action, including securing the airway. Ventilation and sedation should be maintained until adequate spontaneous respiration is resumed. Hypotension and bradycardia are treated with:

- Intravenous fluids
- Vagolytics: atropine
- Sympathomimetics: ephedrine, adrenaline
- Vasopressors: phenylephrine, metaraminol.

Postoperatively, following a high block, it is important to debrief the woman. She should receive a full explanation of events and should have time to ask any questions that she might have.

Intraoperative side effects

Local anaesthetic (LA) toxicity

This can occur secondary to inadvertent intravascular administration of LA or epidural absorption of high volumes of high concentration LA agents. Management is supportive with administration of intralipid (Table 11.4).

Nausea and vomiting

This common side effect is most often seen in association with spinal anaesthesia. The most frequent cause of nausea and vomiting is hypotension: in studies looking at maintenance of BP using phenylephrine, if the BP is kept at 100% of baseline the incidence was 4%, compared to 16% when the BP is maintained at 90% of baseline.

Other factors include parenteral opioids, increased vagal activity, surgical stimuli and uterotonic agents.

The current evidence does not seem to favour either routine or rescue administration of antiemetics, so it would seem prudent to use them only if there is a specific indication.

Shivering

A significant number of women will experience shivering following CNB; some reports show this to be as high as 60%. The mechanism is unclear and is likely to be multifactorial, e.g. altered thermoregulation, intrathecal drugs and autonomic blockade. Shivering increases the metabolic rate and is often distressing for the parturient.

A study of shivering in parturients following institution of epidural anaesthesia for CS randomized parturients to receive either 50 mg pethidine or 0.9% saline intravenously post delivery. The results showed a decrease in shivering from 87% to 35% ($p < 0.01$) and a decrease in severe shivering from 57% to 0% ($p < 0.01$) in the pethidine group with no statistical change in those who received 0.9% saline. The effect of administering pethidine was apparent after 2 minutes.

Doses of 25 mg IV pethidine usually suffice. Tramadol has a similar effect, but causes more nausea and drowsiness.

Postoperative considerations

Analgesia

The management of postoperative pain should be multimodal. When time allows, addition of an opioid to the CNB will improve the quality of the anaesthetic block, postoperative analgesia and patient satisfaction.

In time-pressured caesarean sections, it may be safer to forego the addition of opioid to the CNB. An opioid PCA and transverse abdominal plane blocks should be considered (see Chapter 12).

Paracetamol and non-steroidal anti-inflammatory drugs (NSAIDs) are routinely prescribed regularly. A number of situations preclude the use of NSAIDs, e.g. renal dysfunction, lupus nephritis and pre-eclampsia; it is essential to perform an assessment of the woman's suitability for these drugs.

Oral opioid drugs should also be prescribed.

Table 11.4 AAGBI safety guideline: Management of severe local anaesthetic toxicity

1 Recognition	**Signs of severe toxicity:** • Sudden alteration in mental status, severe agitation or loss of consciousness, with or without tonic–clonic convulsions • Cardiovascular collapse: sinus bradycardia, conduction blocks, asystole and ventricular tachyarrhythmias may all occur • Local anaesthetic (LA) toxicity may occur some time after an initial injection
2 Immediate management	• Stop injecting the LA • Call for help • Maintain the airway and, if necessary, secure it with a tracheal tube • Give 100% oxygen and ensure adequate lung ventilation (hyperventilation may help by increasing plasma pH in the presence of metabolic acidosis) • Confirm or establish intravenous access • Control seizures: give benzodiazepine, thiopental or propofol in small incremental doses • Assess cardiovascular status throughout • Consider drawing blood for analysis, but do not delay definitive treatment to do this

3 Treatment	**In circulatory arrest** • Start cardiopulmonary resuscitation (CPR) using standard protocols • Manage arrhythmias using the same protocols, recognizing that arrhythmias may be very refractory to treatment • Consider the use of cardiopulmonary bypass if available	**Without circulatory arrest** **Use conventional therapies to treat:** • Hypotension • Bradycardia • Tachyarrhythmia
	Give intravenous lipid emulsion (following the regimen overleaf) • Continue CPR throughout treatment with lipid emulsion • Recovery from LA-induced cardiac arrest may take >1 h • Propofol is not a suitable substitute for lipid emulsion • Lidocaine should not be used as an antiarrhythmic therapy	**Consider intravenous lipid emulsion (following the regimen overleaf)** • Propofol is not a suitable substitute for lipid emulsion • Lidocaine should not be used as an antiarrhythmic therapy

4 Follow-up	• Arrange safe transfer to a clinical area with appropriate equipment and suitable staff until sustained recovery is achieved • Exclude pancreatitis by regular clinical review, including daily amylase or lipase assays for two days • Report cases as follows: in the United Kingdom to the National Patient Safety Agency (via www.npsa.nhs.uk) in the Republic of Ireland to the Irish Medicines Board (via www.imb.ie) If Lipid has been given, please also report its use to the international registry at www.lipidregistry.org. Details may also be posted at www.lipidrescue.org

Your nearest bag of lipid emulsion is kept: . . . . . .

This guideline is not a standard of medical care. The ultimate judgement with regard to a particular clinical procedure or treatment plan must be made by the clinician in the light of the clinical data presented and the diagnostic and treatment options available.

© The Association of Anaesthetists of Great Britain & Ireland 2010

Thromboprophylaxis

Thromboembolism is a particular risk for the parturient following caesarean section. Thromboprophylaxis is recommended for a minimum of 7 days or longer in those groups at high risk. In order to reduce the risk of spinal haematomas, thromboprophylaxis is prescribed 4 hours following instrumentation of the back, i.e. following insertion of a spinal needle or removal of an epidural catheter.

If there is concern about the coagulation status, then the multidisciplinary team will make an assessment regarding when to commence low-molecular-weight heparin. Pneumatic boots and compression socks can be used in the interim.

Follow-up

All patients who have had a CNB should be followed up by the anaesthetic team within 24 hours. Follow-up data records patient satisfaction and any untoward side effects of regional anaesthesia (see Chapter 26).

Enhanced recovery after caesarean section

Recent years have seen an increase in activity in the area of enhanced recovery after caesarean section. NICE guidance would support safe discharge of parturients 24 hours following elective caesarean section if they are recovering well, are apyrexial and do not have complications following CS. Many units are working towards this by embracing the principles of enhanced recovery:

- Focus on patient education antenatally
- Reduction in starvation times
- Preference for regional anaesthesia
- Reduction in the duration of urinary catheterization
- Active management of postoperative pain with regular oral pain-relieving medication
- Active management of postoperative nausea and vomiting
- Early reestablishment of oral intake and removal of intravenous cannula
- Encouragement of early mobilization.

Programmes such as these can only be instituted with good patient information, adequate community support and easy contact with the hospital should the need arise.

Key points

1. Regional anaesthesia for operative delivery is increasing.

2. A reduced spinal dose of local anaesthetic is required in the parturient owing to smaller CSF volume and greater sensitivity of nerve fibres to local anaesthetic.

3. Assessment and documentation of block height should be performed prior to commencement of surgery.

4. Combined spinal epidurals may offer prolongation of surgical anaesthesia and reduced cardiovascular instability.

5. Prior to top-up of a labour epidural for operative delivery ensure that the epidural is functioning well and that sufficient time is allowed.

6. Complications of CNB are rare; however, the anaesthetist must remain vigilant postoperatively.

Further reading

Allam, J., Malhotra, S., Hemingway, C. and Yentis, S. M. (2008). Epidural lidocaine-bicarbonate-adrenaline vs levobupivacaine for emergency caesarean section: a randomised controlled trial. *Anaesthesia*, **63**, 243–249.

Campbell, J. P., Plaat, F., Checketts, M. R. *et al.* (2014). Safety Guidelines: skin antisepsis for central neuraxial blockade. *Anaesthesia*, **69**, 1279–1286.

Goring Morris, J. and Russell, I. F. (2006). A randomised comparison of 0.5% bupivacaine with a lidocaine/epinephrine/fentanyl mixture for epidural top-up for emergency caesarean section after "low dose" epidural for labour. *Int. J. Obstet. Anaesth.*, **15**, 109–114.

NHS Information Centre. (2011–2012). HES online – NHS maternity statistics. Health and social care information centre (HSCIC). http://www.hscic.gov.uk/catalogue/PUB09202.

Royal College of Anaesthetists. (2012). *Raising the Standard: A Compendium of Audit Recipes, 3rd edn*. London: Royal College of Anaesthetists, 220–221.

Royal College of Obstetricians and Gynaecologists. (2015). Reducing the Risk of Venous Thromboembolism during Pregnancy and the Puerperium. Green Top Guideline No. 37a. London: Royal College of Obstetricians and Gynaecologists. https://www.rcog.org.uk/globalassets/documents/guidelines/gtg-*37a*.pdf

Royal College of Obstetricians and Gynaecologists. (2010). Classification of Urgency of Caesarean Section: A Continuum of Risk. Good Practice No. 11. London: Royal College of Obstetricians and Gynaecologists. https://www.rcog.org.uk/globalassets/documents/guidelines/goodpractice11classificationofurgency.pdf

Russell, I. F. (1995). Levels of anaesthesia and intraoperative pain at caesarean section under regional block. *Int. J. Obstet. Anaesth.*, **4**, 71–77.

Russell, I. F. (2004). A comparison of cold, pinprick and touch for assessing a level of spinal block at caesarean section. *Int. J. Obstet. Anaesth.*, **13**, 146–152.

Sanders, R. D., Mallory, S., Lucas, D. N. *et al.* (2004). Extending low-dose epidural analgesia for emergency caesarean section using ropivicaine 0.75%. *Anaesthesia*, **59**, 988–992.

Yentis, S. M. (2006). Height of confusion: assessing regional blocks before caesarean section. *Int. J. Obstet. Anaesth.*, **15**, 2–6.

General anaesthesia for caesarean section and transverse abdominal plane block

Suraj Jayasundera and Karen Butler

Introduction

Over the last 40 years, the caesarean section delivery rate in developed countries has increased substantially; 9% of deliveries were by caesarean section in England in 1980 compared with 24.6% in 2008–2009. The reason for the increase is likely multifactorial including:

- Advancing maternal age at first pregnancy
- Improved safety of the procedure (both surgically and anaesthetically with the increase in regional anaesthesia)
- Changes in women's preferences
- Increasing numbers of parturients who have had a previous caesarean section.

The variation in overall caesarean section rates in hospitals in England can mainly be attributed to the variation in rates of emergency caesarean section. The use of electronic fetal monitoring and fetal scalp blood sampling, partograms, active management of labour and consultant involvement in decision-making have all been shown to affect caesarean section rates.

General anaesthesia and caesarean section

The early Confidential Enquiries report anaesthesia as the third most common cause of direct maternal death, after hypertensive disease and thromboembolism; this was mainly attributed to general anaesthesia. General anaesthesia is now more than 30 times safer than it was in the 1960s.

Neuraxial anaesthesia, with its superior safety profile and improved patient experience, has largely replaced general anaesthesia as the technique of choice for caesarean section. The Royal College of Anaesthetists, in the *Compendium of Audit Recipes*, 3rd edition 2012, recommends that less than 15% of

Category 1–3 caesarean sections and less than 5% of elective caesareans, be performed under general anaesthesia. General anaesthesia was used for 8% of all caesarean sections in England and Wales in 2013 (Hospital Episode Statistics HES data).

General anaesthesia will always have a role in obstetric theatres and it commands special precautions, compared to general anaesthesia in the non-pregnant population.

Indications

One of the principal indications for general anaesthesia is speed. In the circumstance of a Category 1 caesarean section (immediate threat to life of woman or fetus), general anaesthesia is still the quickest and most reliable method of ensuring surgical anaesthesia.

Other indications include maternal preference, contraindication to neuraxial block, failure of neuraxial block and certain emergencies, including severe haemorrhage.

The advantages of general anaesthesia include speed of onset, definitive control of the airway and ventilation and reduced hypotension when compared with spinal anaesthesia.

Risks

General anaesthesia in the parturient poses its own particular risks. These are further exacerbated in the labouring woman.

Airway complications

The Confidential Enquiry into Maternal and Child Health 1976–1978 reported 16 deaths from failed intubation, oxygenation, and aspiration and airway problems compared with 2 deaths in 2006–2008.

Failed intubation remains a major cause for concern amongst obstetric anaesthetists. A recent surveillance

Core Topics in Obstetric Anaesthesia, ed. Kirsty MacLennan, Kate O'Brien and W. Ross Mcnab.
Published by Cambridge University Press. © Cambridge University Press 2015.

conducted by United Kingdom Obstetric Surveillance System (UKOSS), over a 2-year period, reported an estimated rate of failed intubation at 1 in 500 (up to four times that of the non-obstetric population). In 2013, Quinn *et al.* reported the incidence to be 1 in 224.

Although airway complications in obstetric practice are rare, a number of factors further add to the complexity, including:

- Alterations in physiology whilst pregnant with a reduction in respiratory reserve and increased oxygen consumption
- Altered anatomy with short neck, airway oedema and large breasts
- Increasing prevalence of obesity
- Isolated location
- Active labour.

Failure to oxygenate the patient not failure to intubate causes death. This was highlighted in the 8th CMACE report and further alluded to in the obstetric review in NAP4, both recommending that obstetric anaesthetists must maintain their airway skills such that they are able to effectively manage failed intubation. NAP4 further recommends the need for familiarization with a broad range of supraglottic airway devices that may reduce the risk of aspiration and facilitate the insertion of a definitive airway. Fibreoptic equipment and skill should be available when required.

Each trust will have a policy for managing failed intubation, including a failed intubation algorithm. The algorithm for managing an obstetric failed intubation should follow the DAS guidelines for 'unanticipated difficult intubation during RSI in the non-obstetric adult patient', with the emphasis on oxygenation and when to wake the mother up.

The decision to wake a mother, following a failed intubation, with ongoing fetal distress is difficult; abandoning GA may lead to fetal death, but arguably maternal wellbeing is paramount and waking the patient in order to proceed with a regional technique would be appropriate. NAP4 suggests that waking a mother should not be an automatic reaction should an airway difficulty be encountered, particularly if a supraglottic airway device is successfully being used that can also aid intubation. Ultimately, this will depend on the quality of the airway and the specific obstetric circumstances.

Aspiration

Mendelson's syndrome (described in 1941 by Mendelson, a New York obstetrician) refers to the chemical pneumonitis caused by aspiration during anaesthesia, particularly in pregnancy. Historically, aspiration pneumonitis is said to occur if greater than 25 mL of gastric content of pH < 2.5 enters the lungs, although there is little evidence supporting this. In pregnancy, the lower oesophageal sphincter tone is reduced and labour pains and opiates decrease gastric emptying, leading to increased gastric volumes. These factors, combined with the reduction of oesophageal sphincter tone during general anaesthesia, place the labouring parturient at significant risk of aspiration.

Rapid sequence induction

Performance of a rapid sequence induction with pre-oxygenation, cricoid pressure, rapid administration of induction agent and quick, short-acting muscle relaxant and tracheal intubation became standard practice by the 1960s. This initially led to a surge in deaths from failed intubation, failed oxygenation and other airway problems until the mid-1980s. This has now become rare, due to a combination of better training and assistance, and use of failed intubation drills along with capnography.

Critics allege that cricoid pressure provides no benefit in reduction of aspiration and can be detrimental to laryngoscopic view. Although it is difficult to demonstrate benefit, as many interventions were introduced at the same time (antacid prophylaxis, starvation in labour, tracheal intubation, capnography, improvement in training), it would also be difficult to demonstrate no benefit as trials would be unethical. Studies have shown that cricoid force, particularly in the optimum range of 20–30 N, does not distort the view at laryngoscopy. If, however, it is distorting the view, it is entirely acceptable to release, decrease or increase force. Other risks of general anaesthesia include:

- Awareness
- Respiratory complications
- Dental damage
- Corneal abrasion
- Anaphylaxis
- Sore throat
- Uterine atony secondary to anaesthetic agents
- Post operative nausea and vomiting
- Neonatal depression.

Preoperative assessment

In the emergency situation, time is limited and preoperative assessment must be comprehensive and

Obstetric Failed Intubation Algorithm

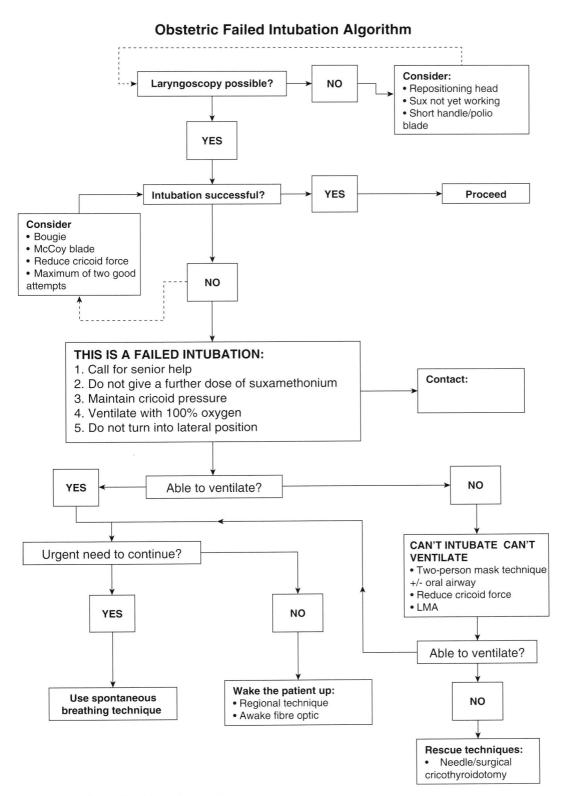

Figure 12.1 Obstetric failed intubation algorithm.

Table 12.1 Proposed template for obstetric preoperative assessment

- Problems with previous anaesthetics
- Family history of anaesthetic reactions
- Co-morbidities:
  - Most parturients are ASA 1. However, maternal age, co-morbidity and obesity are increasing and pre-existing cardiac or respiratory disease is not uncommon
- Obstetric history:
  - Pre-eclampsia being of particular relevance
  - Placental site
- Allergies
- Medications
- Airway assessment
- Starvation times
- Recent blood results including group and save or cross-match if appropriate

focused in order to reduce the risks from anaesthesia. See Table 12.1.

Premedication

Premedication aims to reduce the risk of aspiration and should be given to all parturients planned for, or at risk of, operative delivery.

Ranitidine (H_2 receptor antagonist) blocks the action of histamine on gastric parietal cells, decreasing gastric acid production. The oral preparation reaches peak plasma concentrations within 1–3 hours. There is a relationship between plasma concentrations of ranitidine and suppression of gastric acid production, but wide interindividual variability exists. Aim for oral administration 60–90 minutes prior to anaesthesia (or 30 minutes for IV administration). Its effects are sustained for up to 8 hours. It is recommended to be administered 6 hourly when in high risk labour.

Metoclopramide (dopamine antagonist) inhibits gastric smooth muscle relaxation. It accelerates intestinal transit, increases the lower oesophageal sphincter resting pressure, increases amplitude of oesophageal peristaltic contractions and raises the threshold of activity in the chemoreceptor trigger zone. Given orally it can take between 30 and 75 minutes to act, but 1–3 minutes when given IV. Its effects are sustained for 1–2 hours. Use of prokinetic agents in labour is not as widespread as it once was.

Sodium citrate 0.3 M 30 mL has the benefit of instantaneous efficacy as an acid-neutralizing agent; however, its effects are short lived. It is best used within 20 minutes of induction.

Anaesthesia

Induction

Successful performance of a Category 1 caesarean section under general anaesthetic requires the anaesthetist to maintain clear communication, with good leadership and team working skills.

Of UK obstetric units, 70% perform anaesthesia for caesarean section in the operating theatre rather than an anaesthetic room; this reduces the time from induction to delivery.

To minimize delay, intravenous induction is performed once the patient is catheterized, the abdomen draped and surgeons scrubbed. The patient is positioned with left lateral tilt to avoid aortocaval compression. Some practitioners also advocate a 30° head-up tilt, arguing improvement in maternal wellbeing through an increased functional residual capacity (FRC), reduced breast interference with intubation and reduced gastro-oesophageal reflux.

The ramped position, with the parturient sat up approximately 15°, with the tragus of the ear lying in the same horizontal plane as the sternal notch and the head extended, is particularly useful for the obese parturient; reducing the risk of acid reflux, pulmonary shunting and improving the view at laryngoscopy. Preoxygenation in this position is improved as FRC is increased compared to the supine position, prolonging the safe apnoeic time after induction.

Aside from the importance of a tight-fitting oxygen mask, there is little consensus regarding the conduct of preoxygenation. Described techniques include tidal volume breathing for 3 min or performing 4, 5, or 8 vital capacity breaths. Regarding adequacy of preoxygenation, there is debate that use of a set time period for preoxygenation should be abandoned in favour of a target F_EO_2 (>0.8).

Induction agent

Properties of an ideal induction agent for obstetric anaesthesia include:

- Fast onset
- Clear end point

- Reliable dose range
- Cardiovascular stability
- Minimal adverse maternal and neonatal effects
- Ample user experience
- Appropriate licensing
- Low cost
- No premixing.

In a survey of UK consultant OAA members 2011, 93% of obstetric anaesthetists favoured thiopentone as the induction agent of choice for an obstetric RSI with only 7% of respondents using propofol. Of those surveyed in 2013, 55% 'hardly or never' used thiopentone outside of obstetric practice.

See Table 12.2.

Opiates

Only 15% of UK consultant OAA members surveyed in 2011 routinely administer opiates at induction. To avoid neonatal depression, opiate administration is traditionally withheld until after umbilical cord clamping. Parturients with pre-eclampsia and cardiac disease require an individualized approach regarding predelivery administration of opiates in order to obtund the potentially hazardous hypertensive effects of laryngoscopy and to maintain maternal cardiovascular stability. Short-acting opioids (alfentanil, remifentanil) are used and clear communication with the neonatal team ensures anticipation of potential neonatal respiratory depression.

Total intravenous anaesthesia (TIVA)

One published case series, using TIVA with remifentanil infusions in the semi-elective setting, reported that 6 out of the 10 neonates required mask ventilation briefly. Time required for TIVA preparation may limit its use in elective general anaesthesia.

Muscle relaxants

Succinylcholine has a long association with obstetric general anaesthesia, producing excellent intubation conditions within less than a minute, with the additional benefit of rapid offset. However, under-dosing of suxamethonium may worsen intubating conditions; even a dose of 1.5 mg/kg may be inadequate due to the increased volume of distribution in pregnancy.

Its undesirable side effects include anaphylaxis, trigger for malignant hyperpyrexia and prolonged action in plasma cholinesterase deficiency. A reduction of up to 35% in pseudocholinesterase concentration can lengthen the effects of suxamethonium. Return of spontaneous breathing should be observed prior to administering a non-depolarizing muscle relaxant. Suxamethonium-induced fasciculations increase oxygen consumption and may hasten onset of hypoxia.

Rocuronium has less undesirable side effects. At doses of 1 mg/kg it produces equivalent intubating conditions at 1 minute. Sugammadex (ORG 25969) rapidly reverses rocuronium-induced neuromuscular blockade. With increasing familiarity this may become a more popular combination.

Maintenance

Anaesthesia is typically maintained with a volatile anaesthetic and nitrous oxide. There is limited evidence regarding volatile agent use for caesarean section. Sevoflurane, with its rapid offset, is commonly used. The sympathetic stimulation produced by desflurane should be considered prior to use in hypertensive or pre-eclamptic parturients. Concomitant use of nitrous oxide allows a lower concentration of volatile, thus reducing the potential for uterine atony. Of surveyed anaesthetists in 2010, 85% used nitrous oxide in obstetric cases. Minimum alveolar concentration is decreased by up to 40% for pregnant patients; however, sufficient end tidal volatile is necessary to avoid awareness.

Following umbilical cord clamping, 5 IU oxytocin is slowly administered intravenously as a uterotonic (as per NICE guidance).

Antibiotic prophylaxis should be administered within 60 minutes prior to surgical incision to reduce maternal infectious morbidity (specifically endometritis). In an emergency this should not delay surgery and should be administered when possible.

Postoperative analgesia

Opioids (morphine), paracetamol and NSAIDs can be administered if there are no contraindications following umbilical cord clamping. Antiemetics are administered as required.

TAP blocks

In an attempt to anaesthetize the abdominal wall, various techniques have been employed, including local anaesthetic wound infiltration, bilateral ilioinguinal blocks and more recently transversus abdominis plane (TAP) blocks.

Table 12.2 Summary of comparison of thiopentone compared with propofol for obstetric anaesthesia

	Thiopentone	Propofol
Availability	Sole UK manufacturer Long-term production of drug not guaranteed	No manufacturing or availability issues
Association with obstetric anaesthesia	Long history of association	Introduced into clinical practice in 1980s Comparatively short history of association. Most commonly used induction agent for general anaesthesia in obstetrics outside of UK (2013)
Awareness	No difference (although studies small with poor standardization and power). To minimize maternal awareness dose suggested not less than 5 mg/kg	Lack of evidence of increased awareness To minimize maternal awareness dose suggested 2.5 mg/kg
Neonatal outcome	Small number of studies showing better Apgar scores Longer-term studies of neurodevelopment post maternal GA lacking	No evidence that propofol advantageous Some studies show no difference in Apgar scores
Maternal haemodynamics	Higher maximal maternal noradrenaline concentrations Less hypotension	Less hypertension at laryngoscopy and intubation More hypotension In combination with suxamethonium can cause severe maternal bradycardia
User experience	Still extensively used for obstetric emergency anaesthesia. Largely replaced by other induction agents for non-obstetric emergencies owing to lack of familiarity	Extensively used for elective anaesthesia Good experience profile for all grades of anaesthetist
Drug error	Highlighted by the UK patient safety report as a risk in obstetric practice Reconstitution error Syringe-swap with antibiotics	Minimal risk Nil reconstitution Distinctive appearance
Summary of product characteristics	Reconstituted drug should be used within 7 hours Pre-filled syringes 90 day shelf life 'Can be used without adverse effects in pregnancy' (in doses not exceeding 250 mg)	'Should not be used for obstetric anaesthesia unless clearly necessary' However, used worldwide by countries where thiopentone not available e.g. USA

TAP blocks were first described by Rafi in 2001. Abdominal field blocks have long been used in clinical practice. TAP blocks, however, are unique in requiring a single injection site. Incisions below T10 derive most benefit from TAP blocks, thus it is ideal for the commonly used Pfannenstiel incision. For classical incisions, its utility may be questionable as local anaesthetic spread is variable above the T10 dermatome. Supplementation with sub-costal blocks may solve this problem.

TAP blocks do not negate the need for opiates altogether as they do not block visceral pain. Studies of analgesia outcomes in ultrasound-guided TAP blocks, for caesarean sections, have been mixed:

- Improved analgesia has been demonstrated in two clinical trials. Both of these showed that TAP blocks had significant benefits if primary analgesia was established with intravenous opioids.
- One trial, comparing TAP blocks to intrathecal morphine, demonstrated inferior analgesia. In another recent trial, combining TAP block with intrathecal morphine failed to demonstrate any improvement in analgesia.

Anatomy

The innervation of the anterolateral abdominal wall arises from the anterior spinal nerves T7–L1. Having arisen from the intercostal space, these nerves travel between transversus abdominis (TA) muscles and internal oblique (IO) muscles. There is a lateral branch at the mid-axillary line and anterior branches that pass through the rectus muscle to supply the overlying muscles and skin. Hence, the nerves may be conveniently blocked posteriorly in the plane that exists between the IO and TA muscles: the transverse abdominis plane (TAP). The ilioinguinal and iliohypogastric nerves (L1 with some contribution from T12) have a slightly different course in that they generally remain deep to the TA muscle and are not found in the TAP until a more anterior position (once medial to the anterior superior iliac spine).

Block technique

Rafi originally described a landmark 'double pop needle technique' through the triangle of Petit. This area can be identified caudally by the iliac crest, anteriorly by the external oblique muscle and posteriorly by the latissimus dorsi muscle. To improve reliability and arguably safety, the block should ideally be performed under ultrasound guidance. The TAP block

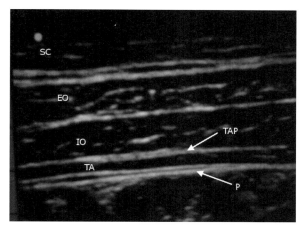

Figure 12.2 Local anaesthetic infiltrated into TAP layer. External oblique (EO), internal oblique (IO), transverse abdominis (TA) and peritoneum (P).

is typically described by placing a high frequency (5–10 MHz) ultrasound probe in the transverse plane between the lower costal margin and the iliac crest in the mid-axillary line. The structures readily identifiable are: sub-cutaneous fat, external oblique, internal oblique, transversus abdominis, peritoneum and bowel.

Using sterile precautions, a 50 mm needle is usually sufficient; however, a longer needle may be required in the obese parturient. The needle is inserted in plane, from the medial aspect, making sure that the needle tip is visible at all times. On entering the plane between IO and TA, a 'pop' is usually felt. When local anaesthetic is injected in this plane, the shape of a convex lens is created. There should be minimal resistance to injection. The block needs to be placed bilaterally for a caesarean section, hence a low concentration, high volume mixture (15–20 mL each side) of long-acting local anaesthetic is ideal.

For lower abdominal incisions (Pfannenstiel), injecting local anaesthetic at this mid-axillary site may miss blocking the L1 nerves and could account for the reported failure rate. These nerves do not enter the TAP until the anterior one-third of the iliac crest. To reliably block these nerves, it is important to perform the block near the iliac crest and not go too posterior, as described in the traditional approach.

Complications

Complications of TAP blocks are rare, particularly when guided by ultrasound; however, there has been a case report of liver injury using ultrasound

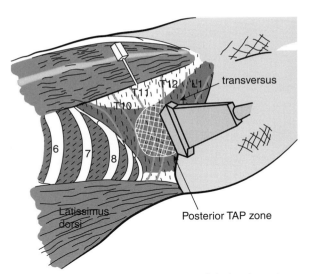

Figure 12.3 Diagrammatic representation of ideal probe and needle position.

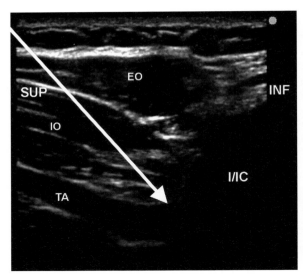

Figure 12.4 Ultrasound image demonstrating needle orientation when performing TAP block. Illustrations reproduced with permission from *Ultrasound Guided Procedures in Anaesthesia*, Barrington and Royse, www.heartweb.com.au

guidance. Reported complications of the blind technique include liver laceration, bowel perforation and intraperitoneal placement of a TAP catheter.

Extubation

Prior to emergence, consideration should be given to reduce gastric volume and pressure, with gentle in and out insertion of a wide-bore orogastric tube, if a full stomach if suspected (*Lessons Learnt from 8th Confidential Enquiry*). Ensure adequate reversal of neuromuscular blockade. Extubate once the parturient is awake, with full return of airway reflexes and in the left lateral position. In cases of morbid obesity or poor respiratory reserve it may be more suitable to extubate in the sitting position.

Postoperative care

The mother should be recovered in an appropriately staffed postoperative care unit. Further analgesia, if required, can be given in the form of titrated intravenous opioid. Opioid patient-controlled analgesia (PCA) systems are commonly used. Midwifery input is essential to support breastfeeding, bonding and care of the newborn.

Key points

1. Caesarean section delivery rates are increasing.
2. General anaesthesia is considered to be the quickest and most reliable method of ensuring surgical anaesthesia for caesarean section for immediate life-threatening cases.
3. Obstetric anaesthetists must maintain their airway skills to ensure safe management of failed intubation.
4. Antacid premedication is recommended for all labouring women at risk of operative intervention.
5. Thiopentone remains the most commonly used IV induction agent in the UK.
6. TAP blocks can be used as opiate-sparing adjuncts to analgesia.

Further reading

Centre for Maternal and Child Enquiries (CMACE) (2011). Saving mothers' lives: reviewing maternal deaths to make motherhood safer: 2006–2008. The eighth report on confidential enquiries into maternal deaths in the United Kingdom. *BJOG*, **118** (1), 1–203.

Hebbard, P., Barrington, M. and Royse, C. E. (2008). Ultrasound Guided Procedures in Anaesthesia. www.heartweb.com.au (accessed May 2015).

Knight, M., Spark, P., Fitzpatrick, K., Misztela D., Acosta, C. and Kurinczuk, J. J. on behalf of UKOSS (2011). *United Kingdom Obstetric Surveillance System (UKOSS) Annual Report 2011*. Oxford: National Perinatal Epidemiology Unit.

Levy, D. and Meek, T. 2006. Traditional rapid sequence induction is an outmoded technique for caesarean section and should be modified. *IJOA*, **15**(3), 227–232.

McDonnell, N. J. and Paech M. J. (2012). Editorial. The transversus abdominis plane block and post-caesarean analgesia: are we any closer to defining its role? *IJOA*, **21**(2), 109–111.

Murdoch, H., Scrutton, M. and Laxton, C. H. (2013). Choice of anaesthetic agent for Caesarean section: a UK survey of current practice. *IJOA*, **22**(1), 31–35.

Rafi, A. N. (2001). Abdominal field block: a new approach via the lumbar triangle. *Anaesthesia*, **56**(10), 1024–1026.

Royal College of Obstetricians and Gynaecologists (2004). Why Mothers Die 2000–2002. Report on Confidential Enquiries into Maternal Deaths in the United Kingdom. London: RCOG.

Van de Velde, M., Teunkens, A., Kuypers, M. *et al.* (2004). General anaesthesia with target controlled infusion of propofol for planned caesarean section: maternal and neonatal effects of a remifentanil-based technique. *IJOA*, **13**(3), 153–158.

Chapter 13

Anaesthesia for other obstetric indications: cervical suture, external cephalic version, controlled ARM, manual removal of placenta and perineal repair

John R. Dick

Cervical cerclage

Introduction

Preterm birth is defined as delivery before the 37th week of pregnancy and accounts for 7.6% of all live births. Prematurity is the leading cause for perinatal death and disability. With improvements in neonatal care, infants that reach 26 weeks' gestation have a survival rate of approximately 80%; however, up to 50% will have some form of disability, e.g. neurodevelopmental deficits, gastrointestinal and lung disease. The incidence of prematurity is increasing, in the UK from 7% (1995) to 8.6% (2010) and in the USA 9.5% (1981) to 12.8% (2006); this is mainly from an increase in medically indicated preterm delivery e.g. pre-eclampsia and fetal growth restriction. The economic burden as a result of prematurity is immense, in the UK it was £939 million/year (2009) and in the USA $2.9 billion/year (2007).

The causes of spontaneous preterm birth are multifactorial; however, one of the strongest predictors of spontaneous preterm labour is short cervical length.

Cervical insufficiency is characterized by recurrent painless cervical dilation and spontaneous mid-trimester birth; the diagnosis relies on previous clinical history. The Cochrane Collaboration reviewed the evidence for cerclage for preventing preterm birth in a singleton pregnancy in 2012. The nine randomized trials included showed that 'compared to expectant management the placement of cervical cerclage in women at risk of preterm birth significantly reduces the risk of pre-term births'.

However there is a lack of neonatal outcome and follow-up data.

Types of cervical cerclage

1. History indicated: should be offered to women with three or more previous preterm births and/or second trimester losses. Usually performed at 12–18 weeks gestation.
2. Ultrasound indicated: women with a history of one or more mid-trimester losses or preterm births who are undergoing ultrasound surveillance should be offered ultrasound-indicated cerclage if the cervix is 25 mm or less and before 24 weeks' gestation.
3. Transabdominal cerclage: this can be used following failed vaginal cerclage or extensive cervical surgery. This requires laparotomy or laparoscopy.
4. Rescue cerclage: the decision to perform rescue cerclage needs to be made by a senior obstetrician; the evidence of improved neonatal outcome in this situation is very limited.

Contraindications to cervical cerclage insertion:

1. Active preterm labour
2. Clinical evidence of chorioamnionitis
3. Continual vaginal bleeding
4. Preterm prelabour rupture of membranes
5. Evidence of fetal compromise
6. Lethal fetal defect
7. Fetal death.

Immediate complications for all types of cerclage include rupture of membranes, preterm labour and bleeding.

Core Topics in Obstetric Anaesthesia, ed. Kirsty MacLennan, Kate O'Brien and W. Ross Mcnab.
Published by Cambridge University Press. © Cambridge University Press 2015.

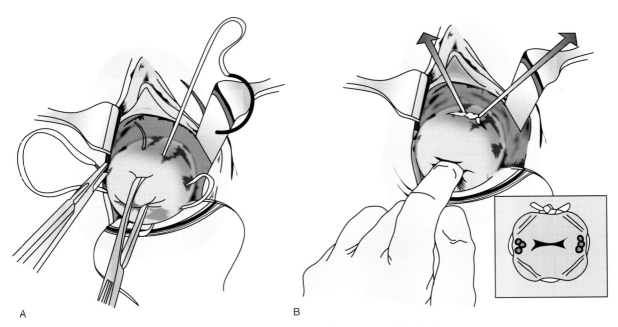

A   B

Figure 13.1 Insertion of McDonald suture. (Source Gabbe *et al.*, 2013, with permission of Elsevier.)

Transvaginal cerclage

Technique involves a transvaginal approach to the cervix and the placement of a sub-mucosal stitch at the level of the internal os of the cervix. The Shirodkar suture is harder to remove and is associated with a higher rate of caesarean delivery than the McDonald suture. The latter technique, which uses a purse-string of tape, has the advantage that it can be removed without anaesthetic either antepartum or intrapartum to allow for vaginal delivery (see Figure 13.1).

Abdominal cerclage

This is reserved for patients with an extremely short cervix or in patients with a history of failed transvaginal cerclage. This procedure is usually done by laparotomy or laparoscopy at around 12 weeks' gestation and requires a general anaesthetic. The suture is often left *in situ* and baby delivered by caesarean section.

Anaesthetic technique for transvaginal cerclage

For history-indicated cerclage there is a choice of spinal, epidural or general anaesthetic. There is one randomized trial comparing spinal and general anaesthesia for planned second-trimester cerclage. Yoon *et al.* measured oxytocin levels (as a surrogate of uterine stimulation) before, 1 hour after and 24 hours after the procedure and found no significant change in either group. A regional block will need to extend from T10 to S4 to cover both components of cervical innervations. The majority of practitioners use hyperbaric bupivacaine 0.5% (10–12.5 mg) with fentanyl (15–20 µg). In terms of intrathecal dose of bupivacaine, although a lower block height is required compared to caesarean section at term, spinal dose requirements are greater up to 20 weeks.

If the cervix is dilated and the membranes are prolapsing through the cervix, this may necessitate emergency cerclage. The choice of anaesthesia should be discussed with the obstetrician. General anaesthesia may confer some advantage if uterine relaxation is required; however, the risk of coughing and vomiting is increased compared to the use of spinal anaesthesia. In a rescue cerclage, especially with prolapsing membranes, the lateral position can be helpful in reducing intra-abdominal pressure and minimizing the risk of ruptured membranes during the procedure. If a regional technique is used then uterine relaxation can be achieved for 1–2 minutes with the use of nitroglycerin (GTN).

For general anaesthesia the patient's trachea should be intubated if there is an aspiration risk, but

93

for fasted subjects before 18 to 20 weeks' gestation, a laryngeal mask airway (preferably a 'second-generation' LMA with a gastric drainage tube) may be acceptable and may help to reduce coughing and straining on emergence. The choice of induction agent is between thiopentone and propofol, with propofol being best for laryngeal mask use and smoother recovery. There is no evidence to support the routine use of antibiotics for elective or emergency cerclage, although it is usual to provide cover for carriers of Group B streptococcus. For viable fetuses, usually defined as beyond 24 weeks, it may be wise to monitor the fetal heart rate periprocedure.

External cephalic version (ECV)

The incidence of breech presentation at term is about 3–4%. This has resulted in increases in caesarean section rate, due to concerns about and risks encountered with vaginal breech delivery (see Chapter 6). Breech presentation can be converted to a vertex presentation with ECV. Two recent meta-analyses published in 2011 concluded the success rate of ECV can be significantly improved if neuraxial block is utilized and there was no significant increase in fetal or maternal compromise.

Controlled artificial rupture of membranes (ARM)

This procedure is performed in theatre because of either polyhydramnios or unstable lie. This carries a risk of cord prolapse or malpresentation, which may lead to an emergency caesarean section. For safety, this procedure may be performed in theatre with fetal heart rate monitoring.

It is important to thoroughly discuss the options with the woman prior to the procedure:

1. No anaesthetic for ARM, then if there is a cord prolapse or malpresentation, the choice is either general anaesthesia or spinal anaesthesia if there is no fetal compromise.
2. Spinal anaesthesia, this may be appropriate if there are airway difficulties or other maternal morbidity, e.g. morbid obesity.
3. Combined spinal epidural technique, with a low-dose spinal for the ARM and an epidural catheter placed for labour. The CSE technique may allow the option to quickly extend the block for emergency caesarean in the event of cord prolapse.

In the event of a cord prolapse, available techniques to prevent the presenting part compressing the cord include manual displacement, filling the bladder and lateral position. These techniques can buy time to extend the epidural block for surgery, but the anaesthetist should be at all times prepared to induce general anaesthesia if requested.

Manual removal of placenta (MROP)

With active management of the third stage (i.e. uterotonic plus controlled cord traction), 95% of placentas will deliver within 15 minutes. A retained placenta is defined as failure to deliver within 30 minutes of birth. This increases to 60 minutes for passively managed third stage of delivery. Most commonly, the cause is placenta adherens, which is caused by a failure of contraction of the retroplacental myometrium. This type comes away easily with MROP. A trapped placenta occurs where the placenta is already separated, but is trapped by the cervix. There may also be placenta accreta (invasion of myometrium) that may require piecemeal removal. Ultrasound is useful for differentiating between the three types of retained placenta. It is recommended that a vaginal examination be performed just prior to transfer to theatre to assess for spontaneous delivery of the placenta if there is a delay between diagnosis and going to theatre.

Patients with retained placentas will continue to bleed from a failure of contraction of the placental bed, and can be significantly hypovolaemic. Whilst any delay in going to theatre increases blood loss, some patients will spontaneously complete the third stage at the expense of acceptable blood loss (a wait of 90 minutes prior to surgery resulted in a 55% placental delivery rate with estimated 400 mL blood loss), thus avoiding an intervention. Fortunately deaths associated with this condition are rare in the UK (two since 1967 from triennial reports) compared with less well-resourced countries (e.g. 13 deaths associated with retained placenta in 1999 alone), which is probably due to prompt diagnosis and management.

Anaesthetic management involves prompt assessment of patient for estimation of blood loss and volaemic status. Hypovolaemia should be corrected prior to theatre with timely planning for blood and blood products where indicated. If there is an epidural catheter *in situ* and the patient is haemodynamically stable then epidural anaesthesia can be used. A block from T10 extending to S4 is required. Similarly a spinal anaesthetic may be used to produce a similar block, but again this should only be used with extreme caution and after adequate resuscitation. In cases involving ongoing or major maternal haemorrhage a general anaesthetic is always preferred.

An oxytocin infusion is often started when the diagnosis of retained placenta is made; however, this can make MROP more difficult by causing the cervix to contract. GTN may be used to help relax the cervix and uterus (50–100 µg IV bolus or 1 mg sublingually) if a regional anaesthetic is being used. The use of direct umbilical vein injections of oxytocin has been the subject of a study, but showed no benefit. The role of intravenous prostaglandins may be beneficial in reducing the need for MROP in patients with retained placenta, although this trial used sulprostone, which is not available in the UK. There is an increased risk of infection from MROP and prophylactic broad-spectrum antibiotics should be used. An infusion of oxytocin is used to maintain uterine tone and hence minimize bleeding after the procedure.

Perineal repair

Perineal trauma occurs in most vaginal deliveries and will require a repair. The degree of tear needs to be identified post delivery.

Classification of perineal trauma:

1. First-degree lacerations: injury to the perineal skin and vaginal epithelium
2. Second-degree lacerations: extend into fascia and musculature of the perineal body, anal muscles are intact
3. Third-degree lacerations: extend into the fascia and musculature of the perineal body, involving some or all of the fibres of the external anal sphincter (EAS) and/or the internal anal sphincter (IAS). These are further subdivided according to which fibres are torn
4. Fourth-degree lacerations: involves all the perineal structures, EAS, IAS and the rectal mucosa.

Assessment before theatre

Perineal tears can cause massive haemorrhage; complex second-degree tears can often bleed profusely and may extend into the pouch of Douglas and the peritoneal cavity.

Local anaesthesia usually suffices for first- and straightforward second-degree tears, these normally being repaired in the delivery room.

Complex second-, third- and fourth-degree tears require repair in theatre. It is vital that the woman is adequately resuscitated prior to anaesthesia; women who are significantly hypovolaemic may require general anaesthesia. If the woman is euvolaemic, then spinal or epidural anaesthesia is preferable.

If an epidural catheter is *in situ*, then this can easily be topped up for perineal repair. Spinal anaesthesia has to be sufficient to cover uterine innervation, particularly when the woman has a complex vaginal tear.

All women who have a perineal repair in theatre should be given broad-spectrum antibiotics.

Third- and fourth-degree tears involve the anal sphincter and have significant associated morbidity, including faecal incontinence, rectovaginal fistula, infection and pain. These women should be referred to urogynaecology services 3–6 months after their perineal injury, for further assessment with regards to continence, sexual dysfunction and chronic pain of the lower genital tract.

Key points

1. If there is risk of preterm birth cervical cerclage will reduce the risk.
2. Neuraxial block can significantly improve the success rate of ECV.
3. Definition of retained placenta is failure to deliver the placenta after 30 minutes or 60 minutes if the third stage is managed passively.
4. Retained placenta is a leading cause of postpartum haemorrhage. The patient requires prompt assessment of volume status, estimation of blood loss and appropriate correction of any hypovolaemia.

Further reading

Arulkumaran, S., Regan, L., Papageorghiou, A. T. *et al.* (eds.) (2011). Preterm labour. In *Oxford Desk Reference: Obstetrics and Gynaecology*. Oxford: Oxford University Press, 350–351.

Berghella, V., Odibo, A. O., To, M. S., Rust, O. A. and Althuisius, S. M. (2005). Cerclage for short cervix on ultrasonography: meta-analysis using individual patient-level data. *Obstet. Gynecol.*, **106**, 181–189.

Gabbe, S. G., Niebyl, J. R., Galan, H. L. *et al.* (2013). Cervical insufficiency. In *Obstetrics: Normal and Problem Pregnancies*. Philadelphia, PA: Saunders, Chapter 27.

Hong, J.-Y. (2006). Adnexal mass surgery and anesthesia during pregnancy: a 10-year retrospective review. *Int. J. Obstet. Anesth.*, **15**, 212–216.

Jones, G. (2011). Late miscarriage and early birth. In Baker, P. and Kenny, L. (eds.), *Obstetrics by Ten Teachers*. Boca Raton, FL: CRC Press, 134–135.

National Committee for Confidential Enquiries into Maternal Deaths (NCCEMD). (1999). Second Interim Report on Confidential Enquiries into Maternal Deaths in South Africa. http://www.gov.za/sites/www.gov.za/files/interimrep_0.pdf (accessed May 2015).

Sultan, P. and Carvalho, B. (2011). Neuraxial blockade for external cephalic version: a systematic review. *Int. J. Obstet. Anesth.*, **20**, 299–306.

van Shalkwyk, J., van Eyk, N. and The Society of Obstetricians and Gynaecologists of Canada Infectious Diseases Committee. (2010). Antibiotic prophylaxis in obstetric procedures. *J. Obstet. Gynaecol. Can.*, **32**(9), 878–892.

Weeks, A. D., Alia, G., Vernon, G. *et al.* (2010). Umbilical vein oxytocin for the treatment of retained placenta (RELEASE study); a double blind randomized controlled study. *Lancet*, **375**, 141–147.

Yoon, H. Y., Hong, J. Y. and Kim, S. M. (2008). The effect of anesthetic method for prophylactic cervical cerclage on plasma oxytocin: a randomized trial. *Int. J. Obstet. Anesth.*, **17**, 26–30.

Chapter

14

Hypertension in pregnancy, pre-eclampsia and eclampsia

Suna Monaghan, Jenny Myers and Lorna A. Howie

Introduction

Hypertensive disorders of pregnancy are one of the most common antenatal complications, affecting 3–4% of all pregnancies:

- They are a leading cause of direct maternal death in the UK and USA, with a rate of 0.83 and 0.99 per 100,000 maternities respectively
- The necessity for urgent treatment of systolic hypertension (>160 mmHg) was one of the top ten recommendations in the last Maternal Mortality Report (CMACE 2006–2008):
  - There were seven deaths associated with inadequate control of systolic hypertension resulting in cerebral haemorrhage
  - Women with severe pre-eclampsia need to be managed by an effective multidisciplinary team
- There is fetal morbidity and mortality associated with pre-eclampsia:
  - Iatrogenic preterm delivery
  - Fetal death *in utero* and stillbirth
  - Fetal growth restriction
- There is also growing evidence of increased long term health risks in:
  - Women who have had pre-eclamptic pregnancies, including cardiovascular disease, type 2 diabetes mellitus and metabolic syndrome
  - Children of pre-eclamptic mothers also have an increased risk of hypertension and metabolic syndrome in later life.

Classification of hypertension in pregnancy

Hypertension in pregnancy is categorized according to gestation and cause (see Table 14.1). Before 20 weeks, it is likely to be due to chronic, pre-existing hypertension. Hypertension is often identified for the first time in early pregnancy and it is important to rule out any secondary causes. The commonest secondary cause is renal disease, but it is important to exclude vascular, endocrine and immunological causes. Approximately 20% of women with chronic hypertension will go on to develop superimposed pre-eclampsia.

Gestational hypertension complicates 10% of pregnancies and is defined as new-onset hypertension (>140/90 mmHg) after 20 weeks, without significant proteinuria or other features suggestive of multisystem disease.

Pre-eclampsia affects 3–4% of pregnancies, and is defined as new-onset hypertension with significant proteinuria: greater than 300 mg of urinary protein in 24 hours or a urinary protein:creatinine ratio (uPCR) > 30 mg/mmol.

Pre-eclampsia can occur at any time after 20 weeks' gestation, even into the postpartum period. Early-onset pre-eclampsia (<34/40) represents around 30% of cases and is often associated with more severe fetal compromise. Severe maternal disease can develop at any gestation. The only cure for the condition is delivery of the placenta.

Pre-eclampsia may take several days to resolve post delivery. Blood pressure and proteinuria should resolve within 12 weeks of delivery. Women with early onset pre-eclampsia have a 25% chance of ongoing hypertension and proteinuria; this suggests an underlying cause, usually related to a renal condition, which requires further investigation.

Definitions

Hypertension

This can be deemed mild, moderate or severe (NICE) (see Table 14.2). Blood pressure readings should be

Core Topics in Obstetric Anaesthesia, ed. Kirsty MacLennan, Kate O'Brien and W. Ross Mcnab.
Published by Cambridge University Press. © Cambridge University Press 2015.

Table 14.1 Hypertension in pregnancy

Condition	Diagnosis
Chronic hypertension	Hypertension (BP >140/90): • Present at booking • Present *before* 20/40 • Being treated at the time of referral to maternity services
Gestational hypertension	*New* hypertension (BP >140/90): • Presenting *after* 20/40 • *Without* significant proteinuria • Also known as pregnancy-induced hypertension (PIH) • Affects 1 in 10 pregnancies
Pre-eclampsia	*New* hypertension (BP >140/90): • *After* 20/40 • *With* significant proteinuria • Affects 2–3% of pregnancies • 2% can go on to develop eclampsia (worldwide)
Severe pre-eclampsia	*New* severe hypertension (BP >160/110): • *After* 20/40 • *With* significant proteinuria • +/− symptoms (see below) • +/− biochemical impairment • +/− haematological impairment • HELLP – severe expression of PET, associated with haemolysis, elevated LFTs and low platelets
Eclampsia	Convulsive condition associated with pre-eclampsia

Table 14.2 Definition of hypertension

Hypertension	BP reading
Mild	140–149/90–99
Moderate	150–159/100–109
Severe	>160/110

Pathogenesis

The cause of pre-eclampsia is not well understood; however, the placenta is the organ that drives pre-eclampsia.

The concept of a two-step model of trophoblast invasion has become widely accepted:

1. Invasion of the decidual segments of the spiral arteries (10–12 weeks)
2. Invasion of the myometrial segments (15–16 weeks).

In pre-eclampsia the second stage of the process is impaired and results in impairment of remodelling the spiral arteries. The outcome is a poorly perfused and poorly developed placenta. Placental ischaemia is thought to be the reason for release of placental factors and the resultant imbalance of angiogenic factors. The altered placental function is associated with changes in the production and secretion of a number of placental-derived factors, which cause widespread maternal vascular endothelial dysfunction.

Widespread changes in the maternal vascular endothelium are characterized by vasoconstriction, capillary leak and an activation of the maternal inflammatory and clotting cascades.

A number of placental factors have been investigated in relation to pathogenesis of pre-eclampsia and it is likely that there is more than one aetiological mechanism that leads to placental dysfunction and pre-eclampsia. Research has been focused on a number of angiogenic markers. Angiogenesis is essential for normal placentation and two factors contribute to this:

• Vascular endothelial growth factor (VGEF)
• Placental growth factor (PlGF).

There are two antiangiogenic markers that have been studied:

• Soluble FMS-like tyrokinase (sFlt-1): this peptide binds to and neutralizes the actions of VGEF and PlGF

made with manual sphygmomanometers instead of an automated machine, as these tend to underestimate systolic blood pressure.

Proteinuria

Significant proteinuria:

• Protein >300 mg/24 hours *or*
• Urinary protein:creatinine ratio (uPCR) >30 mg/mmol on a spot sample.

NB. A degree of proteinuria is a normal physiological change in pregnancy.

- Soluble endoglin (sEng): the levels of this peptide normally fall between the first and second trimesters; however, this is attenuated in women who go on to develop pre-eclampsia.

The result is an imbalance between proangiogenic and antiangiogenic peptides. These biomarkers may provide a way of detecting pre-eclampsia before the systemic signs of the disease appear. An elevation in sFlt and sEng with a reduction in VEGF and placental growth factor PlGF are currently being investigated as potential predictive, prognostic and diagnostic markers.

Risk factors

Many of the risk factors associated with pre-eclampsia identify a group of women with increased risk of vascular disease and these are the women at highest risk of developing the condition. It is likely that they are sensitized to the stressors of pregnancy and have an exaggerated response to placental dysfunction. The NICE guidelines recommend that women with risk factors for the development of pre-eclampsia should be prescribed 75 mg aspirin daily from 12 weeks until delivery. Aspirin is associated with a modest (around 15%) reduction in the rate of pre-eclampsia in high-risk groups. See Table 14.3 for risk factors related to development of pre-eclampsia.

Signs, symptoms and complications

Table 14.4 summarizes the diagnostic criteria for severe pre-eclampsia.

Table 14.3 Risk factors associated with pre-eclampsia

Moderate risk	High risk
• 1st pregnancy • Age > 40 • Pregnancy interval of > 10 years • Family history of pre-eclampsia • Multiple pregnancy • BMI ≥ 35	• Hypertensive disease during a previous pregnancy • Chronic renal disease • Autoimmune diseases (SLE, antiphospholipid syndrome etc.) • Diabetes • Chronic hypertension

Table 14.4 Diagnostic criteria for severe pre-eclampsia

Severe pre-eclampsia: hypertension and proteinuria in addition to any one of the following features:

CVS
- Severe hypertension (SBP >160 or DBP >110)
- Chest pain
- Sudden swelling of face/hands/feet

Renal
- Oliguria (decrease in GFR)
- Creatinine >100 mmol/L
- Cortical/tubular necrosis

CNS
- Severe frontal headache
- Visual disturbance including blurring and flashing in front of the eyes
- Cortical blindness
- Retinal oedema
- Clonus
- Eclampsia
- Cerebral haemorrhage/oedema

Respiratory
- Dyspnoea
- Pharyngeal/laryngeal oedema

GIT
- Nausea and vomiting
- Right upper quadrant pain (as a result of liver capsule tension)
- Epigastric pain
- ALT > 50 IU/L
- HELLP

Haematological
- Thrombocytopenia (platelets $<100 \times 10^9$)
- Falling fibrinogen
- Disseminated intravascular coagulation (DIC)
- Prolonged clotting times
- Microangiopathic haemolysis

Feto-placental
- IUGR
- Oligohydramnios
- Abruption
- Abnormal umbilical Doppler
- Preterm delivery (50% in severe pre-eclampsia)
- Still birth

Investigations

Pre-eclampsia represents a clinical syndrome and has a very variable presentation and progression. Although the most typical presentation is hypertension associated with proteinuria, many other clinical presentations exist.

In any woman with gestational hypertension or gestational proteinuria, a diagnosis of pre-eclampsia should be considered and multisystem disease should be investigated, e.g. altered renal function, altered liver function, activation of the clotting cascade and fetal growth restriction. The majority of women with pre-eclampsia and eclampsia will have normal blood tests.

1. *Proteinuria*: the diagnosis of gestational proteinuria is qualitative and once significant proteinuria has been established, there is no merit in repeatedly testing the urine, as protein excretion in pre-eclampsia is highly variable day to day and does not predict the development of maternal complications of severe pre-eclampsia. Women who are heavily proteinuric may also have hypoalbuminaemia, which is associated with an increase in thromboembolic risk.

2. Bloods: check daily in severe PET, more frequently if abnormal:

    a. *U+E* – an increase in serum creatinine is suggestive of worsening maternal disease

    b. *FBC* – a rapid fall in platelet count is suggestive of severe pre-eclampsia

    c. *LFT* – significant increases in the transaminases are suggestive of severe disease.

    d. *Clotting* – is rarely abnormal unless another condition is present, e.g. placental abruption. In severe pre-eclampsia, if the platelet count is rapidly falling, it can be useful to exclude DIC.

    e. *Urate* – this test has little value in the management of pre-eclampsia as it is not predictive of severe disease. It is occasionally grossly elevated as the first sign of renal involvement (prior to proteinuria) in association with hypertension and can therefore sometimes be useful as a diagnostic test. Gestational age-adjusted thresholds should be used.

Management

Women at high risk of developing the condition should be monitored more frequently with the aim of identifying signs of the condition early.

The management of pre-eclampsia involves:

1. Maintenance of hypertension at a safe level i.e. SBP < 150 mmHg (the absolute value will be dependent on any underlying chronic hypertension)

2. Using oral antihypertensives, e.g. labetalol, nifedipine and methyldopa

3. Regular monitoring of the mother and fetus for the development of adverse features.

Women with an established diagnosis of pre-eclampsia should be managed in the hospital setting to ensure regular monitoring of BP, blood tests and assessment of fetal wellbeing. Ultimately delivery of the baby and the placenta is the only curative treatment.

Women who develop severe pre-eclampsia (see Table 14.4) require level 2 care on a consultant-led labour ward and should be managed by an experienced multidisciplinary team comprising senior obstetricians, anaesthetists, critical care specialists, neonatalogists and physicians, if required.

The main principles for the management of severe disease are:

1. Maintenance of safe blood pressure (< 150/80–100 mmHg)

2. Fluid management

3. Cerebral protection

4. Thromboprophylaxis

5. Timely delivery.

Blood pressure

The most frequent cause of maternal death in association with pre-eclampsia is cerebral haemorrhage secondary to severe systolic hypertension. Prompt and effective treatment of severe hypertension has been highlighted by recent maternal mortality reports as a common area of sub-standard care.

Blood pressure should be measured manually at rest using Korotkoff V as the diastolic value, with an appropriately sized BP cuff. Manual sphygmomanometers are the most accurate way of measuring BP, as automatic devices tend to underestimate the systolic pressure. In severe disease, when intravenous antihypertensives are indicated and/or multiple blood samples are required, invasive arterial pressure monitoring may be beneficial.

Severe hypertension can be treated with oral or intravenous antihypertensives. Oral labetalol (200 mg doses) or nifedipine (10 mg doses) can be used in the first instance. If BP control is inadequate (SBP < 150, within 1 hour of antihypertensive medication), then intravenous labetalol and/or hydralazine should be given. Hydralazine is often more effective in certain ethnic groups, e.g. afrocarribean. There is no place for the administration of sublingual nifedipine; this can cause a precipitous drop in the BP (see Table 14.6).

Fluid management

Pulmonary oedema was a frequent cause of death in women with pre-eclampsia, but the widespread adoption of fluid restriction protocols has significantly reduced the frequency of this condition. Women with severe pre-eclampsia have significant intravascular volume depletion; this can be as much as 30–40% less than in normal pregnancy. The decrease in oncotic pressure coupled with widespread endothelial dysfunction and left ventricular diastolic dysfunction increases the risk of pulmonary oedema.

An intravenous fluid regimen of approximately 80 mL/h is advised for the management of women with severe pre-eclampsia. This should include all drugs and fluids (IV and oral).

If a syntocinon infusion is required, the diluent should be reduced to minimize fluid administration:

1. For augmentation of labour: 30 IU syntocinon in 500 mL 0.9% saline
2. Post delivery: 40 IU syntocinon in 50 mL 0.9% saline over 4 hours.

Urine output should be measured hourly, usually via a urinary catheter and urometer to ensure an accurate fluid balance. Diuretics should not be used to maintain urine output and their administration should be restricted to instances of pulmonary oedema. A urine output of 0.25 mL/kg/h can be tolerated for several hours and is rarely associated with acute renal failure unless another event occurs, e.g. haemorrhage.

Continuous saturation monitoring and regular chest auscultation should be performed to identify signs of pulmonary oedema. The postpartum diuresis will occur usually within 24–48 hours of delivery. Prior to this, in the presence of oliguria, regular monitoring of urea and electrolytes is mandatory and the use of NSAIDs must be avoided.

Haemofiltration may be necessary if there is persistent acidaemia, hyperkalaemia, uraemia or fluid overload. Central venous pressure monitoring can be misleading in pre-eclampsia as the constricted vasculature alters venous pressures and therefore does not give an accurate representation of intravascular fluid status.

Table 14.5 Eclampsia management

Eclampsia management
• **Call for HELP**
• Airway
• Breathing
• Circulation
• **Magnesium sulfate** Loading dose 4 g IV over 5 mins Maintenance dose 1 g/hr
• **For recurrent fits** Further 2 g magnesium over 10 mins (4 g if > 70 kg) Second line – diazepam 10 mg IV or thiopentone 50 mg IV Consider other causes of seizures May need CT scan once stabilized
• Intubation if failure to regain consciousness.

Cerebral protection

Eclampsia occurs in 1:2000 deliveries in the UK with 38% antepartum, 18% intrapartum and 44% postpartum. One in three fits occur before there is a measured rise in blood pressure or proteinuria; 1.8% are fatal and one in three will have ongoing neurological sequelae.

Neurological deterioration in eclampsia is secondary to cerebral vasospasm. The vasorelaxant effects of magnesium sulfate make it the drug of choice for the prophylaxis and management of eclampsia (Table 14.5).

In both instances a loading dose of 4 g IV over 5 min is followed by an infusion of 1 g/h (Collaborative Eclampsia Trial). Magnesium should be continued for 24 hours from the time of delivery or the last seizure, depending on which is later. If recurrent seizures occur, an additional 2 g IV magnesium should be administered. It should be appreciated that magnesium sulfate does not have significant antihypertensive effects nor does it treat the underlying disease process.

The potential of serum magnesium toxicity should be monitored using clinical signs (respiratory depression, reduced oxygen saturations, absence of deep tendon reflexes or ECG change). A diagnosis of magnesium toxicity can be confirmed by a serum level > 3.5 mmol/L and is a particular risk in the presence of oliguria as magnesium is renally excreted. The antidote is 10 mL 10% calcium gluconate IV, over 10 min.

Thromboprophylaxis

Women with pre-eclampsia are at increased risk of thromboembolic events secondary to a depletion of the intravascular compartment coupled with

101

Table 14.6 Antihypertensive agents

Drug	Labetolol	Nifedipine	Hydralazine	Magnesium sulfate	Methyldopa
Oral dose	up to 2.4g/day in 3–4 divided doses	10 mg (starting dose) Available in three different preparations: capsules, MR od and MR bd (check drug information carefully)	N/A	N/A	250 mg up to 1 g tds
Time to effect	30 min	60 min			
IV bolus dose	50 mg over 5 min repeated every 10 min to a max of 200 mg	N/A	2. 5 mg over 5 min repeated every 20 min to a max of 20 mg	4 g over 5–10 min	N/A
Time to effect	10 min		Within minutes	Within minutes	
IV infusion	4 mL/h doubled every 30 min to a max of 32 mL/h	N/A	1–5 mg/h	1 g/h	N/A
Class of drug	Beta blocker with alpha blocking properties	Calcium-channel blocker	Directly acting vasodilator		Centrally acting antihypertensive
Side effects	Caution in asthmatics and people with cardiac disease	Profound hypotension when administered with $MgSO_4$	Tachycardia Palpitations		Depression LFT abnormalities Sedation Haemolytic anaemia
Antidote				10 mL 10% calcium gluconate IV	

the hypercoagulable state of pregnancy. Thromboprophylaxis by pharmacological (low-molecular-weight heparin; LMWH) and physical (compression stockings) methods should be considered for all women with pre-eclampsia. The timing of therapeutic LMWH may need to be adjusted in relation to surgery and neuraxial analgesia/anaesthesia.

Timely delivery

Planned delivery should be done on the best day in the best way. The timing and mode of delivery is determined by a number of maternal and fetal factors. Maternal condition should always be optimized prior to delivery.

In cases of pre-term delivery it is necessary, if there is time, to give steroids to the woman to reduce the severity of respiratory distress of the newborn and enhance fetal lung maturity. The regime for gestation <34 weeks is dexamethasone 24 mg over 24–48 hours.

The timing of delivery in non-severe cases of pre-eclampsia is usually determined by gestation of the pregnancy. Before 34 weeks, conservative management with inpatient surveillance is recommended. It is good practice to have a care plan that outlines the circumstances that require prompt delivery; these include evidence of progression of maternal disease or significant fetal compromise. Delivery should take place in a unit that has adequate neonatal facilities. Between 34 and 37 weeks, the indications for delivery are less clear. If the maternal disease is stable and there is no fetal compromise, timing of delivery should be agreed between the obstetric and anaesthetic teams, following discussion with the mother.

After 37 weeks, there is little benefit associated with continuing the pregnancy from a fetal perspective and therefore delivery is recommended within 48 hours of diagnosis.

Mode of delivery

The mode of delivery will be determined by several factors, including maternal condition (e.g. rapid progression of disease), obstetric history (e.g. previous caesarean section) and fetal condition (e.g. prematurity, growth restriction, abnormal Doppler).

Irrespective of the mode of delivery, syntometrine is absolutely contraindicated and the use of carboprost should only be used after discussion with the obstetric team.

Labour

Epidural analgesia is often beneficial as it is associated with a reduction in the pain-mediated hypertensive response and may aid vasodilatation of the uteroplacental bed. It also has the advantage of allowing top-up for surgical intervention if required. Preloading with fluids is not recommended. A maternal platelet count should have been performed within the preceding 4 hours, or more recently if there has been a downward trend. Prophylactic LMWH should not have been administered in the preceding 12 hours (24 hours for treatment dose). It is not possible to be certain of the lowest acceptable platelet count using current evidence; however, in the absence of other coagulation abnormalities, a platelet count of $>80 \times 10^9$/L is considered to be acceptable for epidural analgesia. In the presence of thrombocytopenia, platelet transfusions may be considered to cover potential surgery or haemorrhage. The use of thromboelastography (TEG) is valuable if available, giving a real-time assessment of coagulation function. In cases of severe coagulopathy, regional anaesthesia is contraindicated and PCA opioids should be considered as an alternative.

Caesarean section

Maternal safety should not be compromised to allow emergency delivery. It is vital that maternal condition is stabilized prior to surgery. It is particularly important that severe hypertension is treated and maintained within safe limits (<150/80–100 mm Hg).

In the absence of other contraindications, regional anaesthesia is preferable as it avoids the potential fluctuations in BP often encountered during intubation and extubation. Spinal anaesthesia has been shown to be safe in pre-eclampsia with less hypotension than that experienced by women without pre-eclampsia. With increasing use of TEG some anaesthetists may accept lower platelet counts (50×10^9/L) for spinal anaesthesia if the TEG is reassuring, particularly if there are other maternal co-morbidities. In severe pre-eclampsia there is often an enhanced response to conventional doses of vasopressors and less hypotension during regional anaesthesia. It is prudent to use titrated doses of ephedrine (3 mg boluses) or phenylephrine (50–100 μg boluses) rather than an infusion of phenylephrine.

General anaesthesia may be necessary in certain circumstances, e.g. thrombocytopenia coagulopathy, pulmonary oedema, haemorrhage, acute fetal compromise, failed regional anaesthesia and eclampsia. Eclampsia often resolves after one episode treated with magnesium sulfate; however, if there is a decreased conscious level after one eclamptic fit, recurrent fits or concern about signs of cerebral oedema, there is a need to intubate to stabilize the woman and then decide on further management.

Obtunding the hypertensive response to intubation and extubation in pre-eclampsia or eclampsia is essential to avoid the risk of cerebrovascular compromise, cardiac ischaemia or arrhythmias.

This may be achieved with the use of one or a combination of drugs:

- Alfentanil 10–20 μg/kg
- Remifentanil 1 μg/kg
- Labetolol 10–20 mg
- Magnesium sulfate 30–40 mg/kg
- Lignocaine 100 mg IV
- Esmolol 1 mg/kg (only use after delivery, high risk of fetal bradycardia).

The choice of drug(s) will depend on familiarity and availability. If opioids are used, neonatologists should be made aware of the possibility of neonatal effects. Magnesium sulfate can prolong the effect of non-depolarizing neuromuscular blockers, contribute to uterine atony and potentiate the effect of calcium-channel blockers, e.g. nifedipine.

Pre-eclampsia accentuates the pharyngeal and laryngeal oedema that occurs in the latter stages of pregnancy, it is essential to anticipate the potential for a difficult airway.

Postnatal care

It is important that women are appropriately monitored in the immediate postnatal period and that hypertension is treated where necessary. Close attention to fluid management and cerebral protection should also be continued. Thromboprophylaxis and analgesic regimes may need modification in instances of coagulopathy, haemorrhage, renal or hepatic dysfunction.

Women frequently require antihypertensive treatment for several weeks post delivery and this should be gradually reduced in response to blood pressure measurements. Women who have had severe disease or early onset disease should be offered a secondary care postnatal review to ensure that the hypertension and proteinuria has resolved by 12 weeks. In women with persistent hypertension and/or proteinuria, underlying disease should be investigated.

All women who develop pre-eclampsia should have the opportunity to be counselled about the risk of recurrence in a future pregnancy (10–50%, dependent on severity and gestation at onset). Women should also be informed that they are at increased risk of developing hypertension and cardiovascular disease in later life.

Key points

1. Pre-eclampsia is a leading cause of maternal death worldwide.

2. Management is supportive until the definitive treatment of delivery. Timing of delivery should depend on severity of the condition and gestational age.

3. Blood pressure should be accurately recorded and managed. Systolic blood pressure >160 mmHg requires urgent treatment.

4. Dysfunction of maternal vascular endothelium results in the systemic disease process of pre-eclampsia.

5. Magnesium sulfate is the drug of choice for the prophylaxis and management of eclampsia.

6. Regional anaesthesia is preferable for caesarean section, in the absence of any contraindications.

7. If general anaesthesia is required, care must be taken to manage the hypertensive response and the potential for a difficult airway with oedema recognized.

Further reading

Cantwell, R., Clutton-Brock, T., Cooper, G. *et al.* (2011). Saving mothers' lives: reviewing maternal deaths to make motherhood safer: 2006–2008. Eighth report of the confidential enquiries into maternal deaths in the United Kingdom. *BJOG*, **118**(1), 1–205.

Dennis, A. T. (2012). Management of pre-eclampsia: issues for anaesthetists. *Anaesthesia*, **67**, 1009–1020.

Duley, L., Meher, S. and Abalos, E. (2006). Management of pre-eclampsia. *BMJ*, **332**(7539), 463–468.

Li Wan Po, J. and Bhatia, K. (2013). Pre-eclampsia and the anaesthetist. *Anaesth. Intens. Care Med.*, **14**(7), 283–286.

National Institute for Health and Care Excellence (2010). Hypertension in pregnancy: the management of hypertensive disorders during pregnancy. NICE guidelines CG107. http://www.nice.org.uk/nicemedia/live/13098/50418/50418.pdf (accessed May 2015).

Rana, S., Karumanchi, A. and Lindheimer, M. D. (2014). Angiogenic factors in diagnosis, management, and research in preeclampsia. *Hypertension*, **63**, 198–202.

Sepsis and influenza in pregnancy

Tim Holzmann and Dougal Atkinson

Sepsis

Introduction

Sepsis is defined as SIRS (systemic inflammatory response syndrome) caused by suspected or proven infection. SIRS is the body's response to an insult. The physiological hallmarks of SIRS are generalized vasodilatation and increased microvascular permeability. These changes can be triggered by both non-infective insults (e.g. burns) and infection. The development and progression of SIRS and sepsis are thought to be due to uncontrolled release of pro-inflammatory mediators and dysregulation of the inflammatory response, leading to widespread tissue injury. Sepsis is a dynamic process and can progress to severe sepsis and septic shock. Despite mortality rates improving over the last 10 years, mortality from septic shock remains high at approximately 24%.

Sepsis in obstetrics

In 2005, the World Health Organization (WHO) reported that infection and sepsis were responsible for 15% of global maternal deaths. In the latest UK Confidential Enquiry into Maternal Deaths sepsis was the leading cause of direct maternal death. Maternal mortality from sepsis has increased almost threefold in the last 25 years.

Sepsis can occur at any time during pregnancy and the puerperium. Sources of infection include both obstetric and non-obstetric causes (Table 15.1). The physiological changes of pregnancy can mask signs of sepsis and provide diagnostic difficulty. In addition, maternal deterioration can rapidly result in fetal compromise. Prompt diagnosis and management are essential. Close liaison between with obstetricians, anaesthetists, microbiologists, physicians and critical

care is important to ensure a good outcome for mother and baby.

The general principles of sepsis management discussed below apply to the obstetric patient, but must also take into account the physiological changes of pregnancy and associated conditions (e.g. pre-eclampsia).

Definitions

The following definitions have been developed to improve the ability to diagnose, monitor and treat sepsis:

Infection: the invasion of normally sterile tissue by organisms.

Bacteraemia: the presence of viable bacteria in the blood.

Systemic inflammatory response syndrome (SIRS): the presence of two or more of the following:

- Temperature >38.3 °C or <36 °C
- Heart rate >90 beats/min
- Respiratory rate >20 breaths/min or $PaCO_2$ <4.3 kPa
- WBC >12,000 cells/mm³ or <4000 cells/mm³.

Sepsis: SIRS due to a suspected or proven infection.

Severe sepsis: the combination of sepsis and at least one organ dysfunction (Table 15.2).

Septic shock: severe sepsis plus hypotension (MAP < 60 mmHg or < 80 mmHg if pre-existing hypertension) despite adequate fluid resuscitation (defined as a minimum of 30 mL/kg of crystalloids).

Pathophysiology of sepsis

The normal host response to infection is a complex process aimed at containing and controlling bacterial

Core Topics in Obstetric Anaesthesia, ed. Kirsty MacLennan, Kate O'Brien and W. Ross Mcnab.
Published by Cambridge University Press. © Cambridge University Press 2015.

Table 15.1 Causes of sepsis in obstetrics

Obstetric:
Chorioamnionitis
Endometritis
Wound infection
Septic abortion

Non-obstetric:
Upper and lower urinary tract
Pneumonia
Meningitis

Table 15.2 Examples of organ dysfunction

Capillary refill time > 3 seconds

Urine output < 0.5 mL/kg for at least one hour, or renal replacement therapy

Lactate > 2 mmol/L

Confusion (new onset)

Platelet count < 100,000 platelets/mL

Disseminated intravascular coagulation

Acute lung injury or acute respiratory distress syndrome (ARDS)

Cardiac dysfunction defined by echocardiography or direct measurement of the cardiac index

Table 15.3 Physiological targets for the first 6 hours of resuscitation

CVP 8–12 mmHg

MAP > 65 mmHg

Urine output > 0.5 mL/kg/h

Haematocrit > 30%

Superior vena cava oxygenation saturation ($ScvO_2$) 70% or mixed venous oxygen saturation (SvO_2) 65%

invasion, as well as initiating tissue repair. The physiological processes to combat infection are initiated when immune cells, particularly macrophages, recognize and bind to microbial components. This process involves specific cell-surface receptors, including TLR, NOD, MDL-1 and TREM-1. Binding of microbial components to these receptors activates intracellular cascades leading to the release of pro-inflammatory cytokines (e.g. TNFa, IL-1, ICAM-1 and NO). At the same time, interactions between polymorphonuclear leucocytes (PMN) and the vascular endothelium enable migration of PMNs to the site of injury. The release of mediators by these cells results in local vasodilatation, increased microvascular permeability and a protein-rich oedema.

This process is regulated by the complex interactions of pro- and anti-inflammatory mediators resulting in tissue repair and healing when the opposing elements are balanced. In SIRS and sepsis, the above processes become generalized, with normal tissues also becoming involved. The exact cause of this is unknown, but is likely multifactorial, including genetic susceptibility, excessive release of pro-inflammatory mediators and specific properties of individual micro-organisms. Mechanisms underlying the resulting organ dysfunction include tissue ischaemia from a combination of imbalances between coagulation, anticoagulation and endothelial abnormalities, direct cell injury by pro-inflammatory mediators and widespread apoptosis (programmed cell death) of various cells, including lymphocytes leading to immunosuppression.

Management of sepsis: the essentials

Initial resuscitation

This focuses on the timely delivery of goal-directed therapy. The Surviving Sepsis Campaign has developed guidelines to reduce mortality from sepsis and recommends the use of specific care bundles and physiological targets for the initial phase of resuscitation (Table 15.3).

Within the first or 'golden' hour of resuscitation, application of the 'Sepsis six' care bundle introduces the cornerstones of diagnosis (blood cultures), treatment (high-flow oxygen, IV antibiotics, fluids) and monitoring (haemoglobin and lactate, hourly urine output). Early delivery of antibiotics is a priority with mortality from severe sepsis and septic shock increasing with every hour administration of antibiotics is delayed. The key principle of resuscitation is to improve oxygen delivery to hypoperfused tissues, targeting factors of the oxygen delivery equation:

$$DO_2 = [1.39 \times Hb \times SaO_2 + (0.003 \times PaO_2)] \times CO$$

DO_2 = oxygen delivery, Hb = haemoglobin, SaO_2 = oxygen saturation, CO = cardiac output.

Both serum lactate and superior vena cava oxygenation saturation ($ScvO_2$) are surrogate markers of tissue perfusion and can be used as resuscitation targets. Poor lactate clearance in sepsis is associated with increased mortality.

Diagnosis

Appropriate cultures should be taken before antimicrobial therapy is initiated. However, the early administration of antimicrobials is paramount and attempts to achieve cultures should not cause delay in administering antibiotics (> 45 minutes). Current recommendations are to obtain at least two sets of blood cultures (aerobic and anaerobic bottles) before antimicrobial therapy. In the presence of vascular access devices (e.g. Hickman line) it is recommended to draw at least one set of blood cultures percutaneously and another through each vascular access device *in situ*. Cultures from other potential sources of infection (e.g. urine, placenta) should also be obtained where possible.

Antimicrobial therapy

Early administration of intravenous antibiotics reduces mortality and should be completed within the first hour of sepsis management. Broad-spectrum antibiotics should be commenced to cover the most likely source of infection. Early discussion with microbiology is recommended in critically ill patients. De-escalation of antibiotics can take place following identification of a causative microorganism.

Source control

When a source of infection is potentially amenable to intervention (e.g. retained products) urgent investigation is indicated, either using radiology or by surgical exploration. Any intervention to achieve source control should take place as soon as possible (and < 12 hours) following diagnosis. This may require both resuscitation and treatment to take place in parallel. Initial intervention may not necessarily aim for definitive management, but instead aim to minimize the physiological impact on the patient (e.g. percutaneous vs. open surgical drainage).

Fluid therapy

The quantity of fluid required for resuscitation is less when colloids rather than crystalloids are used. However, the use of certain colloids, especially the hydroxyethyl starches, is associated with increased morbidity (renal impairment) and mortality.

In view of this, crystalloids are the recommended resuscitation fluid for severe sepsis and septic shock. An initial fluid challenge of 30 mL/kg should be given to patients with sepsis-induced tissue hypoperfusion who are suspected to be hypovolaemic.

There is no evidence to support the superiority of either Ringer's lactate or 0.9% saline. The high chloride content of 0.9% saline can, however, result in a significant hyperchloraemic metabolic acidosis. The use of albumin in fluid resuscitation is safe, equally effective as 0.9% saline, but is more expensive. Current recommendations are to use albumin only when patients require substantial amounts of crystalloids.

Vasopressors

Current guidelines recommend a target mean arterial pressure (MAP) of > 65 mmHg. In life-threatening hypotension vasopressors may be required to maintain organ perfusion.

Noradrenaline is the recommended first-choice vasopressor. Dopamine now has only a limited role in septic shock, e.g. patients also presenting with bradycardia. When hypotension is severe it may be necessary to add an additional agent to achieve target MAP. Adrenaline is the recommended agent and can either be added to noradrenaline or used as a substitute.

Vasopressin is also effective in raising MAP when used in conjunction with noradrenaline and can reduce noradrenaline requirements.

Phenylephrine is not recommended in the treatment of septic shock; the exceptions are when noradrenaline use is associated with serious arrhythmias, blood pressure is persistently low when cardiac output is known to be high and as salvage therapy when combined inotrope/vasopressor drugs and low-dose vasopressin have failed to achieve the MAP target.

Although there are concerns regarding uteroplacental flow and the use of vasopressors, the importance of restoring maternal blood pressure and hence organ perfusion is paramount to fetal wellbeing and survival.

Inotropes

Dobutamine can be added to a vasopressor and is recommended in the context of myocardial dysfunction and ongoing signs of hypoperfusion, despite achieving adequate intravascular volume and adequate MAP.

Dobutamine can be used to normalize cardiac index and improve oxygen delivery. The targeting of supra-normal values is no longer recommended.

The early use of non-invasive cardiac output monitoring (e.g. LIDCO, oesophageal Doppler) and imaging of the heart with echocardiography is recommended in septic shock to guide fluid resuscitation and inotrope/vasopressor use.

Corticosteroids

Although the use of corticosteroids in septic shock results in haemodynamic improvement, a beneficial effect on patient mortality is limited to patients at high risk of death.

The exact mechanism of corticosteroid action in sepsis is unknown. One possible mechanism is to increase noradrenaline receptor sensitivity. In addition some patients with septic shock are thought to have relative adrenal insufficiency. The ACTH stimulation test does not predict response to treatment and should not be used to guide which patients receive hydrocortisone.

Intravenous hydrocortisone in the treatment of adult septic shock patients should only be given when adequate fluid resuscitation and vasopressor therapy have failed to achieve the haemodynamic targets. Intravenous hydrocortisone 200 mg per day should be given as a continuous infusion rather than in traditional bolus doses.

Etomidate suppresses the adrenocortical axis and has been associated with increased mortality in septic shock patients when used to facilitate endotracheal intubation. It should not be used in adult patients with septic shock.

Blood product administration

The optimal haemoglobin concentration for patients with septic shock is unclear. The haemoglobin level recommended for critically ill patients (70 to 90 g/L) can be safely applied to septic shock patients once tissue hypoperfusion has resolved, unless the patient has severe hypoxaemia, acute haemorrhage or myocardial ischaemia.

Abnormal clotting studies (e.g. elevated prothrombin time) are common in sepsis, but should not be corrected unless the patient is bleeding or invasive procedures planned. Newer technologies like the thromboelastogram (TEG) provide a more functional analysis of coagulation and can be helpful in selecting the required components.

Thrombocytopenia is a common finding in sepsis due to a combination of decreased production and increased consumption. Current thresholds for prophylactic platelet transfusions are counts $< 10,000/\ mm^3$ in the absence of bleeding, and $< 20,000/mm^3$ when the patient has a significant risk of bleeding. In active bleeding or where invasive procedures are planned, platelet counts should be $> 50,000/mm^3$.

Activated protein C is involved in both inflammatory processes and coagulation and was thought to be beneficial in patients with severe sepsis and septic shock with a high risk of death. It has not been possible to reproduce the initial positive study results and in view of significant side effects (bleeding) and high cost, the product has been withdrawn from clinical use.

Mechanical ventilation

Patients with severe sepsis and septic shock may require mechanical ventilation and their illness may be complicated by development of the acute respiratory distress syndrome (ARDS).

A lung-protective ventilation strategy can not only prevent the development of ARDS, but also reduce mortality in patients with established ARDS. Strategies utilizing tidal volumes of 6 mL/kg, predicted ideal body weight and limiting plateau pressure to < 30 cmH$_2$O are associated with better outcomes, independent of the mode of ventilation (volume or pressure) used. Permissive hypercapnia is an acceptable result of this ventilatory approach.

Positive end-expiratory pressure (PEEP) should be applied to minimize alveolar collapse and atelectotrauma. Current guidelines recommend strategies based on higher rather than lower levels of PEEP. Two different approaches to PEEP are described: titration to lung compliance or matching to oxygenation deficit guided by FiO$_2$.

In septic patients with severe refractory hypoxaemia due to ARDS (PaO$_2$/FiO$_2$ < 100 mmHg), recruitment manoeuvres, including prone ventilation, may improve oxygenation and patient outcome. In extreme situations, extracorporeal membrane oxygenation (ECMO) may be considered. High-frequency oscillatory ventilation (HFOV) has not demonstrated benefit in sepsis patients with ARDS.

Patients with established sepsis-induced ARDS who do not have evidence of tissue hypoperfusion benefit from limiting extravascular lung water. This can be achieved with a conservative fluid strategy and/or diuretic use. β$_2$-Agonists have not been shown to improve outcomes in ARDS.

Sedation, analgesia and neuromuscular blockade in sepsis

Minimizing sedation levels and daily interruption of sedation improves patient outcomes in sepsis. Neuromuscular blockers are associated with the development of critical-care neuromyopathy and should be avoided where possible in patients without ARDS. If required, they can be given by intermittent bolus or continuous infusion guided by neuromuscular junction monitoring. Depth of anaesthesia monitoring should also be considered when using neuromuscular blocking agents.

A 48-hour infusion of cisatracurium in patients with early, moderate to severe ARDS (PaO_2/FiO_2 < 150 mmHg) has been shown to reduce mortality without causing an increase in neuropathy.

Glucose control

Blood glucose levels in septic patients should be maintained < 180 mg/dL (10 mmol/L), using intravenous insulin where necessary. Strategies using tighter glucose control are associated with an increase in adverse incidents (hypoglycaemia) and do not improve outcomes.

Renal replacement therapy

Both continuous and intermittent renal replacement therapies can be used in the management of sepsis-induced renal failure, depending on local practice. Continuous therapies are recommended in haemodynamically unstable septic patients.

Deep vein thrombosis prophylaxis

All septic patients should receive both appropriate pharmacoprophylaxis and intermittent pneumatic compression devices, unless contraindicated.

Stress ulcer prophylaxis

All septic patients with bleeding risk factors should receive stress ulcer prophylaxis with proton pump inhibitors. These should be stopped once risk factors are no longer present to reduce the risk of ventilator-associated pneumonia and infection with *Clostridium difficile*.

Nutrition

Enteral nutrition should be started as early as possible in order to maintain integrity of gut mucosa and prevention of bacterial translocation. The use of immunomodulating nutritional supplements is not recommended.

Influenza

Influenza is a common viral infection that can pose a significant threat to pregnant women and their babies.

Virology and structure (Figure 15.1)

Influenza viruses are single stranded RNA viruses that make up three genera (Influenza A, B and C) of the family orthomyxoviridae.

Structurally the influenza virus consists of the following key components:

1 Central core of RNA (eight segments for A) genome and other viral proteins
2 Viral envelope containing two major types of glycoproteins:

Haemagglutinin (HA) enables virus binding to the target cell surface receptor sialic acid, enabling entry of the viral genome into target cells by membrane fusion. Sialic acid-presenting carbohydrates are present on several cell types in the respiratory tract, gastrointestinal tract, heart and brain.

Neuraminidase (NA) acts as an enzyme, cleaving sialic acid from the HA molecule and therefore facilitating release of viral progeny from infected host cells.

Both cell-surface proteins initiate host antibody responses and allow serotyping of virus. NA is also a target for antiviral treatment.

Influenza A

This genus has one species (influenza A virus). Natural hosts include wild aquatic birds, poultry, pigs and humans. Transmission of the virus to other species can result in devastating outbreaks (e.g. poultry and human pandemics). Influenza A is the most virulent human pathogen, causing both epidemics and pandemics. The virus is divided into multiple serotypes based on the antibody response to the surface glycoproteins HA and NA. Human infection is restricted to H1–3, N1–2 serotypes.

Influenza B

This genus has one species (influenza B virus) with one serotype. It affects predominantly humans, but is less common than influenza A and results in milder illness. Its limited host range and limited antigenic diversity means influenza B can cause epidemics, but not pandemics.

Influenza C

This genus has one species (influenza C virus) and results in only occasional human infection.

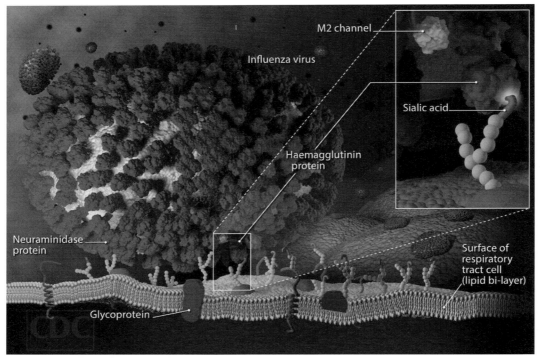

Figure 15.1 Structure of influenza virus (http://www.cdc.gov/flu/images/influenza-virus-fulltext.jpg (accessed 25/2/2013). For the colour version, please refer to the plate section.

Transmission

Infection is normally transmitted in three ways:

1 Airborne – aerosols produced by coughing or sneezing
2 Direct transmission of infected mucus with infected nasal secretions
3 Contaminated surfaces and bird droppings – hand-to-eye, hand-to-mouth and hand-to-nose.

Virus shedding when a host individual is infective starts the day prior to symptom onset and continues for approximately 5–7 days.

Antigenic drift and epidemics

During viral replication, no RNA proofreading takes place with point mutations occurring approximately once every newly replicated RNA. This leads to subtle changes in viral surface antigen, helping to evade previously acquired host immunity. This results in seasonal variation in virus. Seasonal flu is normally caused by influenza A and B and peaks in December–March each year in the UK. A new vaccine is required each year.

Antigenic shift and pandemics

Influenza virus RNA is made up of 7–8 segments. If different influenza A viruses infect one cell it can lead to a re-assortment of RNA segments and a whole new sub-type of surface antigen can result. This provides pandemic potential. Pandemics are infrequent, but recurrent worldwide outbreaks of influenza. They are caused by antigenic shift or direct transmission of an avian virus to humans.

There were three twentieth-century influenza pandemics resulting in millions of deaths, e.g. Spanish influenza (1918–20, H1N1 sub-type, 40+ million deaths), Asian influenza (1957–58, H2N2 sub-type, 1+ million deaths), Hong Kong influenza (1968–9, H3N2 sub-type, 1 million deaths).

Influenza A H1N1 2009

This influenza A virus emerged in Mexico in February 2009 and was the result of multiple re-assortment events between swine viruses leading to a novel gene mix not previously reported in swine or human influenza viruses. Pandemic status was declared by the WHO in June 2009 and lasted until August 2011.

The pandemic was considered mild with the majority of infected individuals experiencing a self-limiting illness (50% symptom resolution within 7 days). However > 16,000 individuals died. Pneumonia was present in up to 40% of cases admitted to hospital in the USA with viral pneumonitis or ARDS evident in nearly half of patients admitted to ICU in Australia and New Zealand and secondary bacterial pneumonia present in 20%.

H1N1 remains one of the seasonal influenza viruses in circulation globally.

Influenza in pregnancy

The increased risk of influenza during pregnancy is well recognized. In the 1918 pandemic and in a series of 1350 pregnant women, over 50% developed pneumonia and over half of these died with an overall case fatality of 27%. Half of those women of childbearing age who died were pregnant in the 1957 pandemic.

Pregnant women do not have a higher incidence of seasonal influenza but hospitalization rates are 18-fold that of healthy non-pregnant women of childbearing age.

In the 2009 H1N1 pandemic there was a fivefold higher rate of hospital admission in pregnant women vs. the general population, with the risk of mortality for pregnant women sevenfold that of non-pregnant women of the same age. The WHO reported pregnant women accounted for 7–10% of all hospital admissions with influenza. There were 12 maternal deaths in the UK between April 2009 and January 2010.

Infection is more common in the second and especially third trimesters and risk is further increased in the presence of other risk factors (see later). Pregnant women are more likely to deliver preterm and their babies are more likely to be stillborn or die in the first week of life if admitted to hospital with influenza.

Clinical features

Uncomplicated influenza

Influenza presenting with fever, coryza, generalized symptoms (headache, malaise, myalgia, arthralgia) and sometimes gastrointestinal symptoms, but without any features of complicated influenza.

Complicated influenza

Influenza requiring hospital admission and/or signs of lower respiratory tract infection (hypoxaemia, dyspnoea, lung infiltrate), central nervous system involvement and/or significant exacerbation of an underlying medical condition.

Risk factors for complicated influenza

1. Pregnancy
2. > 65 years old
3. Chronic cardiac, pulmonary, renal, hepatic or neurological disease
4. Morbid obesity (BMI ≥ 40)
5. Immunosuppression

   - severe primary immunodeficiency
   - current or recent (< 6 months) chemotherapy or radiotherapy for malignancy
   - solid organ transplant recipients
   - bone marrow recipients
   - high dose systemic corticosteroids (≥ 40 mg prednisolone per day for ≥ 1 week and within 3 months of stopping)
   - currently or recently (< 6 months) receiving other immunosuppressive therapy
   - HIV infection.

Diagnosis

In uncomplicated cases this is often on clinical grounds. Diagnostic tests include viral culture, serology, rapid antigen testing, PCR and immunofluorescence assays dependent on local protocol. Samples include nasopharyngeal (NP) swab, nasal swab and nasal wash or aspirate. For rapid detection techniques e.g. PCR, NP specimens are generally more effective.

Management

General principles

1. Low threshold for hospital assessment of pregnant women with suspected influenza and risk factors for, or clinical symptoms of complicated influenza.
2. Standard infection control measures should be instituted as per local guidelines (patient isolation, use of personal protective equipment) in suspected cases.
3. Follow local guidelines for diagnostic testing for influenza virus.
4. Start treatment in suspected cases before confirmation if clinically indicated and if signs of complicated influenza present.

Table 15.4 Clinical triggers for critical care review

Severe dyspnoea
Patients with influenza-related pneumonia or who have bilateral primary viral pneumonia
PaO_2 < 8 KPa despite maximal oxygen administration
Progressive hypercapnia
Refractory hypotension (excessive fluid administration may further exacerbate respiratory compromise)
Septic shock
Severe acidosis (pH < 7.26)
GCS < 10 or deteriorating conscious level

5. Exclude other pathologies (e.g. pneumonia), which may present with a similar clinical picture.

6. Manage exacerbations of pre-existing co-morbid disease (e.g. asthma)

7 Early involvement of relevant medical specialties in complicated cases including obstetric, anaesthetic, general medical, microbiology/virology. This will ensure an appropriate management plan is established for antiviral treatment, the location of ongoing treatment, timing of steroid administration and delivery of the baby where necessary.

8. Early involvement of the critical care team in complicated influenza. This should be based on clinical assessment, local EWS policy and clinical triggers (Table 15.4).

Antiviral therapy for treatment of influenza in suspected or confirmed influenza in pregnancy

Current recommendations for treatment of influenza (both A and B) in the UK are for oseltamivir and zanamivir. Both are selective inhibitors of neuraminidase (NA) preventing new virion release from infected cells.

1. Uncomplicated influenza

   Previously healthy – oseltamivir PO 75 mg within 48 hours of symptoms, where possible for 5 days

   Immunosuppressed – zanamivir INH (Diskhaler) 10 mg bd or if unable to take inhaled preparation oseltamivir PO 75 mg bd

2. Complicated influenza

   Previously healthy – oseltamivir PO/NG 75 mg bd with zanamivir INH, NEB or IV as second-line treatment

   Immunosuppressed – zanamivir INH, NEB or IV.

Early administration of oseltamivir within 48 hours appeared to confer a mortality benefit in the recent H1N1 pandemic. Critically ill patients may have the dose of oseltamivir increased to 150 mg bd or if enteral absorption is compromised, IV zanamivir administered. This is an off-licence indication available on compassionate grounds. Treatment courses may also be extended beyond 5 days. Discuss treatment with your local microbiologist or virologist. Both oseltamivir and zanamivir can be administered to breastfeeding patients where clinically indicated.

Complications of influenza

These include the following:

- Septic shock and multiple organ failure
- Disseminated intravascular coagulation
- Myocarditis
- Encephalitis and cognitive impairment
- Venous thromboembolism
- Bacterial superinfectiom
- Physical and psychological complications of prolonged critical illness.

Vaccination

The Health Protection Agency (HPA) recommends seasonal flu vaccination for all pregnant women in the UK. Vaccination also protects the baby before and after delivery and can result in a significant reduction in hospitalization rates for neonates in the first 6 months of life.

Key points

1. The incidence of sepsis and maternal mortality related to sepsis appears to be increasing.
2. The physiological changes of pregnancy can mask signs of sepsis and present challenges in diagnosis.
3. In sepsis management appropriate cultures should be taken prior to early administration of suitable antimicrobial agents.
4. There should be a low threshold for hospital assessment of pregnant women with suspected influenza.

Further reading

Department of Health and the Royal College of Obstetricians and Gynaecologists (2009). Pandemic H1N1 2009 Influenza: Clinical Management Guidelines for Pregnancy. Guidelines for Pregnancy prepared by the Department of

Health and the Royal College of Obstetricians and Gynaecologists (http://www.dh.gov.uk/en/Publicationsandstatistics/Publications/PublicationsPolicyAndGuidance/DH_107770).

Levy, M. M., Fink, M. P., Marshall, J. C. *et al.* (2003). 2001 SCCM/ESICM/ACCP/ATS/SIS International Sepsis Definitions Conference. *Crit. Care Med.*, **31**(4), 1250–1256.

Dellinger, R. P., Levy, M. M., Rhodes, A. *et al.* (2013). Surviving Sepsis Campaign: International Guidelines for Management of Severe Sepsis and Septic Shock: 2012. *Crit. Care Med.*, **41**(2), 580–637

Lucas D. N., Robinson P. N. and Nel M. R. (2012). Sepsis in obstetrics and the role of the anaesthetist. *Int. J. of Obstet. Anesth.*, **21**(1), 56–67.

Chapter 16

Cardiac disease in pregnancy

W. Ross Macnab, Anita Macnab and Akbar Vohra

Cardiac disease is a significant cause of maternal mortality worldwide. In the last UK maternal mortality report, cardiac disease was the leading cause of maternal death (2.3 deaths per 100000 maternities). Some mothers are waiting to have a family later in life and present with a variety of acquired heart conditions. There is a 1% incidence of heart disease in pregnant patients in the UK, which has reduced from an estimated 3% incidence due in part to a reduction in rheumatic heart disease. However, it is expected to increase as the number of patients with corrected congenital heart disease surviving to childbearing age increases and may also increase further as immigration patterns change. The incidence of cardiac disease is in the order of 0.2–4% in the Western industrialized countries and is about 4% in the United States. Congenital heart disease accounts for 75–80% of cardiac disease in pregnancy in the western world. Outside Western Europe and North America congenital heart disease accounts for only 9–19% of the cardiac disease in pregnancy. In non-Western countries rheumatic valvular disease causes 55–89% of cardiovascular disease in pregnancy.

Of patients with congenital heart disease, 96% will live for at least 15 years if they survive infancy. It is therefore essential to have a good knowledge of these cardiac conditions and a good understanding of the stresses on the cardiovascular physiology caused by pregnancy. These patients can turn up on any delivery suite in any hospital at any time.

Physiology

Important physiological changes in the cardiovascular system need to occur during pregnancy in order to facilitate the increased demand for oxygen and nutrients by the uteroplacental unit, and that of the growing fetus. Blood flow to the uterus increases from 50 mL/min at 10 weeks' gestation to 850 mL/min at term. This is accomplished by a 50% rise in cardiac output (CO) and blood volume. There is an increase in heart rate from 6 weeks. There is a reduction in systemic and pulmonary vascular resistance due to vasoactive prostaglandins and nitric oxide production, thus preventing a rise in pulmonary artery pressure from the increased circulating volume. The systolic and diastolic pressures decrease, reaching their lowest values during the second trimester, before increasing as term approaches, although never reaching prepregnancy values. Therefore, there is a risk of cardiac decompensation as pregnancy progresses. If the cardiac output does not increase adequately, placental insufficiency will occur, which will lead to fetal growth retardation. Changes in vascular resistance can lead to changes in flows through shunts. In patients with Marfan's, repaired coarctation or bicuspid aortic valve with ascending aortopathy, the increase in cardiac output can lead to aortic dilatation leading to dissection and rupture.

There is also a 15% reduction in colloid osmotic pressure during pregnancy, which can increase the risk of pulmonary oedema in patients with cardiac disease.

During labour CO increases by a further 25–50% with up to 500 mL autotransfusion of blood from an increased return from the intervillous spaces during contractions. There is a further increase in blood volume after delivery due to uterine contraction in the third stage. This can result in a clinical deterioration in patients with cardiac disease due to the associated rise in ventricular filling pressure and end-diastolic volume.

Core Topics in Obstetric Anaesthesia, ed. Kirsty MacLennan, Kate O'Brien and W. Ross Mcnab.
Published by Cambridge University Press. © Cambridge University Press 2015.

General approach to cardiac disease in pregnancy

Ideally, preparation should occur before pregnancy occurs. The responsible cardiologist and obstetrician should undertake preconceptual counselling. Risks involved to the patient should be discussed openly so informed decisions can be made. Cardiac function can be quantified with cardiopulmonary exercise testing. Cardiac function should be optimized, which may include surgical interventions such as valve replacement. Known teratogenic medications should ideally be discontinued. Women should be seen early in established pregnancy in joint cardiology and obstetric clinics. A multidisciplinary care plan can be made, including consideration of the services required at the intended delivery unit such as cardiology, cardiothoracic surgery and cardiac or general intensive care. An anaesthetist should review the woman at an early stage to develop a plan for delivery and postpartum care.

In general, predictors of a primary cardiac event during the pregnancy include:

- Prior cardiac event or stroke
- Prior arrhythmia
- New York Heart Association (NYHA) functional class >2
- Left-sided heart obstruction (mitral valve area <2 cm^2, aortic valve area <1.5 cm^2 or outflow tract gradient >30 mmHg
- Left ventricular ejection fraction <40%.

Congenital heart disease

At almost 1% (7/1000), congenital heart disease is the most common inborn defect, with 60% diagnosed before 1 year of age, 30% as children and 10% after 16 years of age. Of those surviving infancy, 96% will live for at least 15 years, with the majority of deaths occurring after 20 years age. There are approximately 150,000 patients with CHD in the UK and this number is increasing as surgical and medical management improves. At least 17% are recognized as having a genetic basis. The common defects are illustrated in Table 16.1.

In most cases of congenital heart disease the diagnosis, functional status and any therapeutic strategies will be well established prepregnancy. Depending on the condition, pregnancy could be well tolerated or be classified as risk class 4 in the modified WHO

Table 16.1 Incidence of congenital heart disease.

Defect	Incidence of CHD
VSD	30%
ASD	10%
Patent ductus arteriosus (PDA)	10%
Pulmonary stenosis	7%
Coarctation	7%
Aortic stenosis	6%
Tetralogy of Fallot	6%
Transposition	4%
Other	20%

Table 16.2 WHO classification of maternal cardiovascular risk

Risk Class	Risk of pregnancy
I	Increasing risk of mortality and morbidity requiring increased specialist input
II	
III	
IV	

Table 16.3 High-risk obstetric patients

Obstetric patients have an overall risk of >1%
Any cyanotic CHD
Pulmonary hypertension
Poor systemic ventricular function
Severe left heart obstruction – mitral and aortic stenosis
Marfan's with dilated root
Dacron patch repair of coarctation
Previous peripartum cardiomyopathy
Poor cardiac function

classification of maternal cardiovascular risk (Table 16.2). Risk Class IV is where pregnancy is relatively contraindicated and termination should be discussed, if the patient presents as pregnant. If pregnancy is to continue, treat the same as Risk Class III, with expert input for the duration of the peripartum period. High-risk groups are illustrated in Tables 16.3 and 16.4. Pregnancy is associated with a thrombotic tendency, which is exacerbated by the polycythaemia that occurs

Table 16.4 Comparison of complications with different conditions

Obstetric risk comparison	Percentage risk of complications
Healthy woman	0.005%
Average population	0.01%
Corrected Fallot's	0.1%
Severe stenosis	1.0%
Uncorrected Fallot's	10%
Pulmonary hypertension	33%
Eisenmenger's	50%

Table 16.5 Incidence of congenital heart defect in babies

Abnormality in parent	Incidence in child
Marfan's	50%
VSD	15%
ASD	10%
Aortic stenosis	10%
Tetralogy of Fallot	3%

Table 16.6 Main areas of focus during outpatient assessments

Clinical assessment of deterioration

Ventricular decompensation

Incipient pulmonary oedema

Pulmonary hypertension and exacerbation

Systemic desaturation

Onset of new arrhythmias

SABE (subacute bacterial endocarditis)

in patients with cyanotic heart disease. Congenital heart disease patients also have a higher incidence of pre-eclampsia, which is associated with high mortality in patients with Eisenmenger's. In addition, they also have a tendency to develop new arrhythmias.

In 50% of patients there will be intrauterine growth retardation (IUGR) with fetal indication of early delivery. The babies have an increased risk of heart defect, which is often similar to that of the parents (3–5%) (Table 16.5).

Assessment

The most import part of the assessment is to identify patients that have complete repair, palliative surgery or no repair. Those with complete correction should behave in a similar manner to normal patients. Palliative correction or no correction is likely to be associated with primary and secondary cardiac, pulmonary or systemic dysfunction.

These patients should be seen in clinic at fortnightly intervals in the first 24 weeks and then on a weekly basis, looking for specific signs of deterioration (Table 16.6).

History of shortness of breath and palpitations should be specifically sought and examination should focus on signs of failure. Periodic transthoracic ECHO may also be helpful in identifying deterioration and the need for early hospitalization and delivery. Pulse oximetry particularly before and after exertion can be helpful in identifying patients that are deteriorating.

Fetal scans at 20 weeks will pick up 80% of major cardiac defects and should be repeated at 24 weeks. Nuchal scans help indicate fetal cardiac disease (>4 mm = Down's and cardiac disease likely; <4 mm = 1:1000 risk of CHD).

In addition, many patients with CHD have other syndromes, which will have specific anaesthetic implications. Noonan's, Turner's and trisomy can be associated with problems with airway management as well as communication and consent. Di George syndrome, which is also called CATCH 22 (Cardiac defect, Abnormal facies, Thymic hypoplasia, Cleft palate, Hypocalcaemia due to chromosome 22), is associated with potential airway problems, electrolyte problems and immune deficiency requiring the use of irradiated blood products for transfusion.

Ventriculoseptal defects (VSD)

These are graded according to the flow through the defect and its site. Therefore, unrestricted defects, which are associated with high flow, will be associated with more problems. Small to moderate VSDs are usually well tolerated in pregnancy and generally behave as well as repaired defects. The main aim is to identify pulmonary hypertension or even Eisenmenger's, which will be associated with increased risk of complications.

Atrioseptal defects (ASD)

If previously undiagnosed, these patients present with an enlarged heart and murmurs in pregnancy, usually secundum ASDs. Primum ASDs are associated with other endocardial cushion defects with involvement of atrioventricular valves and earlier presentation. These patients may develop arrhythmias. Pregnancy is usually tolerated well in unoperated patients unless they have developed pulmonary hypertension.

Atrioventriculoseptal defects (AVSD)

Of complete AVSD, 75% occur in patients with Down's syndrome whilst 90% of partial AVSD occur in non-Down's patients. Patients with partial AVSD present in a manner similar to secundum VSD. Complete AVSD act essentially as univentricular hearts and are associated with heart failure.

These patients have a high risk during pregnancy due to the problems of cardiac failure risk, but particularly due to a tendency to pulmonary hypertension and Eisenmenger's.

Tetralogy of Fallot (TOF)

These patients are usually identified in infancy. Patients with complete repair will often behave in a similar manner to normal patients. In patients that have not been repaired completely, pulmonary hypertension and Eismenger's is a major complication. Patients with saturations <85% have a high incidence of IUGR and intrauterine death, in addition to a high incidence of maternal complications.

They can have right ventricular outflow tract obstruction (RVOTO), pulmonary regurgitation, tricuspid regurgitation, right ventricular failure and arrhythmias.

Ebstein's anomaly

These patients have apical displacement of the tricuspid valve. This is associated with an enlarged right atrium, tricuspid regurgitation and often right ventricular outflow obstruction and 50% will have a patent foramen ovale (PFO) or a secundum ASD. Accessory conduction pathways occur in 25% and are associated with atrial tachyarrhythmias.

Extreme forms are associated with *in-utero* death with hydrops fetalis. Severe forms present with failure to thrive. Patients with moderate and less severe defects present in adolescence or adulthood with dyspnoea, tachyarrhythmias, paradoxical emboli or cyanosis.

Pregnancy is usually well tolerated unless complicated by right heart failure, tachyarrhythmias and cyanosis.

Fontan's

These patients have had palliative surgery to improve pulmonary circulation and rely on passive flow from the venous system to the pulmonary artery and lungs. Examples of such patients include pulmonary and tricuspid atresia. Therefore, they normally have signs of elevated systemic venous pressure and venous congestion with hepatic congestion and even cirrhosis. They are often on multiple medications such as amiodarone, angiotensin converting enzyme (ACE) inhibitors and warfarin, which can affect the fetus.

These patients often have heart failure, atrioventricular (AV) valve dysfunction and arrhythmias. There is also tendency to bleeding as well as hypercoagulability.

Outcome of pregnancy can be good if they have good exercise tolerance and do not have signs of heart failure, tachyarrhythmias and embolism. Hypovolaemia is poorly tolerated in these patients. High intrathoracic pressure associated with assisted ventilation during general anaesthesia can reduce pulmonary venous flow and increases the risk of dysfunction and hypoxia.

Pulmonary hypertension

In historical series, there is a high (up to 50%) maternal mortality rate reported with pulmonary hypertension, but more recent data suggests lower mortality figures of 15–30%. Nevertheless the risks are still very high. Death generally occurs in the third trimester or during the first months after delivery due to worsening of the pulmonary hypertension, pulmonary thrombosis or right heart failure. Causes of pulmonary hypertension are shown in Table 16.7.

Most of the patients with shunts will develop cyanosis. Oxygen therapy (4–5 L/min) may improve oxygenation, reduce the risk of pulmonary hypertensive crisis and improve fetal growth. All these patients should be given anticoagulant prophylaxis. Ideally patients with significant pulmonary hypertension should be managed in pulmonary hypertension centres where all therapeutic options such as sildenafil, bosentan, prostacyclin and nitric oxide therapy are available.

Table 16.7 Commonest causes of pulmonary hypertension

Primary pulmonary hypertension

Collagen vascular disease

Congenital heart defects

Portal hypertension

HIV infection

Drugs/toxins/appetite suppressants

Table 16.8 Co-morbidities in patients with Eisenmenger's syndrome

Hepatic and renal dysfunction
Clotting dysfunction leading to bleeding tendency
DVT risk
Polycythaemia
Haemochromatosis
Arrhythmias
Gout
Haemoptysis
Risk of SABE

Table 16.9 Complications in patients with Eisenmenger's syndrome

IUGR	30%
Premature delivery	50%
Stillbirth incidence	20–40%
Thromboembolism	44%
Hypovolaemia	25%
Preeclampsia	18%

Eisenmenger's

This is invariably due to pulmonary hypertension with flow reversal and cyanosis as a consequence of another defect of flow. Atrio-ventricular septal defects (AVSD), and patent ductus arteriosus (PDA) and atrial septal defect (ASD) (often due to embolic phenomena) account for 70–80% of these patients. Other causes include truncus arteriosus, surgical aortopulmonary connections, complex pulmonary atresia and univentricular heart.

Of Eisenmenger's patients, 42% will survive to 25 years of age, with poor prognosis if they develop syncope, elevated right atrial pressures or severe resting hypoxaemia (<85%). They have many associated medical problems, as illustrated in Table 16.8.

Pregnancy is associated with 30–45% mortality and it should be discouraged (Table 16.9).

Worsening heart failure and progressive hypoxaemia are common. Therefore these patients need close monitoring and hospitalization by 25–30 weeks. They should be hospitalized for a further 1–3 weeks after delivery.

Anticoagulation should be considered after 20 weeks for these patients. Good hydration is vital throughout pregnancy and particularly during labour. Vaginal delivery is the best option for these patients.

Acquired heart disease

Acute coronary syndromes

As the average maternal age increases, the number of women at risk of an ischaemic event will also increase. Acute coronary syndromes (ACS) are estimated to occur at 3–6 per 100,000 deliveries and are related to the characteristic risk factors of smoking, hypertension, hyperlipidaemia, diabetes and a positive family history. Spontaneous coronary artery dissection is more common in pregnancy, usually occurring in the peripartum period. Maternal mortality after an ACS is estimated at 5–10%, which has improved with the increased availability of primary percutaneous coronary intervention (PCI).

The diagnostic criteria of an ACS are similar to those of non-pregnant patients. There must be a low threshold for further investigation of parturients and postpartum women that present with chest pain. A history of chest pain, ECG changes and troponin rise are the hallmarks, although inverted T waves may occur in pregnancy without underlying ischaemia. PCI is the preferred therapy of choice and stenting has been performed successfully during pregnancy. Tissue plasminogen activator does not cross the placenta, however, it may cause catastrophic bleeding around the placenta and should only be used in life-threatening ACS where PCI is not available. Low-dose aspirin and β-blockers are safe to use in pregnancy. If clopidogrel is indicated, it should be used for the shortest duration possible and stopped prior to delivery.

Valvular heart disease

Stenotic valvular disease carries a higher risk than regurgitant lesions during pregnancy. In mitral stenosis (MS), heart failure occurs frequently in those with valve areas less than 1.5 cm^2, even when previously asymptomatic. Pulmonary oedema may occur, particularly if atrial fibrillation occurs. The third stage of labour may also precipitate pulmonary oedema in these patients, which should be managed in the same way as for non-pregnant patients.

Those with moderate or severe MS should be advised to delay pregnancy until balloon dilatation or valve replacement is performed. In those already pregnant, β-blockers are used to control the heart rate and allow a longer diastolic phase, and diuretics can be used to manage fluid retention. In those who remain symptomatic, percutaneous balloon dilatation can be performed. Open surgery to the valve should be avoided if at all possible. Vaginal delivery is appropriate for most patients, however, those with NYHA class 3 or 4, or in those where balloon dilatation has failed, should be considered for caesarean section.

Aortic stenosis (AS) is primarily caused by a congenital bicuspid valve at this age and causes left ventricular outflow tract obstruction (LVOTO). LVOTO can also be sub-valvular or supra-valvular in origin. Supra-valvular obstruction is often associated with anomalies of other major vascular branches, such as the coronary arteries and pulmonary arteries.

This is often well tolerated if obstruction is mild or moderate. Patients with symptomatic AS and impaired LV function are at the greatest risk of heart failure and arrhythmias from the increase in cardiac output associated with pregnancy. These patients also have a greater risk of aortic dissection and rupture.

A general anaesthetic for caesarean section is often utilized for patients with severe AS in order to avoid the drop in systemic vascular resistance associated with a regional technique. However, combined spinal and epidural anaesthesia or intrathecal spinal catheters have been used successfully.

Mechanical heart valves and anticoagulation

Mechanical heart valves are generally avoided in young women, but in patients with an existing prosthesis, lifelong anticoagulation is required and there is additional concern of valve thrombosis during pregnancy. There is an increased maternal risk of bleeding, osteoporosis and thrombocytopenia. Maternal mortality risk is 2.9%, major bleeding is 2.9% and thrombus/embolus is 3.9%. The safest strategy for the mother is to continue warfarin, as this is associated with the lowest rate of valve thrombosis. However, warfarin is associated with a risk of embryopathy (up to 80%) and 70% incidence of poor fetal outcome, including middle trimester miscarriage, stillbirth, and fetal internal and intracerebral haemorrhage. Unfractionated heparin (UFH) and low-molecular-weight heparin (LMWH) are alternative methods of anticoagulation, but carry a higher risk of valve thrombosis. LMWH may be used throughout

pregnancy or in the 6–12-week period to avoid embryopathy associated with warfarin. Close monitoring of the anti-Xa levels, keeping peak levels at 0.8–1.2 U/mL, is essential, as increased volume of distribution and renal clearance often lead to an increase in the dose requirement. Choice of anticoagulation regimen depends on valve type, previous thrombosis, dose of warfarin, and maternal preference. It should be explained to the woman that the risk of embryopathy is low when the daily dose of warfarin is <5 mg. There is a 6.4% risk of fetal teratogenicity. However, she should also be given the option to replace it with LMWH during weeks 6–12. The use of LMWH throughout the entire pregnancy is not recommended, although warfarin should be switched to LMWH prior to delivery.

Endocarditis prophylaxis

The 2008 National Institute for Health and Care Excellence guideline on antibiotic prophylaxis for infective endocarditis has advised against routine antibiotic prophylaxis for women during childbirth. The American Heart Association suggests that those patients with conditions posing high risk for infective endocarditis, namely prosthetic valve, congenital heart disease, previous infective endocarditis and cardiac transplant, should receive a prophylactic antibiotic active against enterococci (such as ampicillin, vancomycin or piperacillin) during operative procedures or prior to urinary tract manipulation.

Aortic disease

Various conditions may predispose to aortic disease (Table 16.10) Recommendations include counselling about risk to the mother antenatally, imaging the aorta and close monitoring of aortic size during the pregnancy, particularly looking for rapid increase in size. Aorta diameter of <4.0 cm is relatively safe, whilst those with an aorta >4.5 cm are at high risk of

Table 16.10 Causation of aortic disease

Marfan's syndrome
Ehlers-Danlos syndrome
Turner's syndrome
Bicuspid aortic valve
Familial aortopathy
Associated with congenital heart disease – coarctation; sinus of valsalva aneurysm

rupture. History of a rapid increase in size is also associated with a high risk of rupture. Aortic dissection is a potential risk and there were seven deaths in the last UK maternal mortality report. Measures to minimize cardiovascular stress at the time of delivery are important in patients with a dilated aorta. These include good blood pressure control with β blockade and regional anaesthesia. Caesarean should be considered in these patients.

Patients with sinus of valsalva aneurysms should have surgical repair prior to pregnancy.

Acute pulmonary oedema

Acute pulmonary oedema is a significant cause of morbidity and mortality. It typically presents with sudden onset breathlessness +/− agitation, and has several associated conditions/risk factors (Table 16.11) with an incidence of up to 1 in 200 pregnancies. Acute pulmonary oedema during pregnancy can be divided into that occurring with hypertension and without hypertension. This distinction allows appropriate management and pharmacological therapy.

Pulmonary oedema associated with hypertension may be due to pregnancy-induced hypertension, essential hypertension or a combination of the two. Development of pulmonary oedema in these patients is often associated with excessive fluid administration and increasing disease severity. Pre-eclampsia predisposes to pulmonary oedema due to several factors, including elevated systemic vascular resistance, increased left ventricular end diastolic pressure, a reduction in colloid osmotic pressure and increased

Table 16.11 Causes of pulmonary oedema

Pre-existing conditions	Cardiac conditions
	Obesity
	Endocrine disorders
	Increased maternal age
Diseases in pregnancy	Pre-eclampsia
	Sepsis
	AFE
	Preterm labour
	PE
Drugs	β-agonists
	Steroids
	Magnesium
	Cocaine
Iatrogenic	IV fluid
Fetal conditions	Multiple gestation

endothelial permeability. The precipitating event is an increased fluid load, which may be due to sudden vasoconstriction through sympathetic nervous system activation or excessive fluid administration. The immediate management includes activation of an emergency medical team, support of the woman's ventilation through non-invasive/invasive means, introduction of pharmacological therapy and transfer to a high-dependency area when appropriate. Glyceryl trinitrate (GTN) is recommended as the drug of choice and can be given intravenously or sub-lingually. Furosemide can also be added to produce vasodilation and diuresis. If hypertension persists despite this therapy, nifedipine can be added. Early echocardiography to assess left ventricular function may be helpful in these patients and considered early.

Pulmonary oedema without hypertension has several causes (Table 16.11). Early identification of at risk patients and careful fluid management in the perinatal period are essential to prevent development of pulmonary oedema. The acute management is similar to that of non-pregnant patients and includes furosemide, vasodilators, inotropes and ventilation when required.

Cardiomyopathy

Hypertrophic cardiomyopathy

Patients with hypertrophic cardiomyopathy are often asymptomatic and may present during pregnancy. It is often well tolerated and symptoms, such as breathlessness, may be treated with β-blockers. A recognized complication is diastolic dysfunction, which may predispose to pulmonary oedema, so strict fluid balance is essential.

Peripartum cardiomyopathy

Peripartum cardiomyopathy (PPCM) is a form of dilated cardiomyopathy carrying a worldwide mortality of 30% in the past with more recent published mortality rates of 10%. It is a pregnancy-specific disease condition causing systolic dysfunction and a decrease in left ventricular ejection fraction. It can occur late in pregnancy in the last month or in the first 5 months postpartum. There is no identifiable cause or any pre-existing heart disease before the last month of pregnancy. Diagnosis should be suspected in a patient presenting with breathlessness, tachycardia and signs of heart failure, including pulmonary oedema. A dilated ventricle and sluggish circulation predisposes to mural thrombus formation, which may cause systemic emboli, making thromboprophylaxis essential in these patients.

Management includes treatment of heart failure (oxygen, diuretics, vasodilators, β-blockers and inotropic support), elective delivery if antenatal and (ACE) inhibitors if postnatal. Severe cases may require ventilation, balloon pumps, other cardiac assist devices and transplantation. Approximately 50% of women make a full recovery, however there is a risk of recurrence of PPCM in future pregnancies. Failure of the heart size to return to normal at six months is a poor prognostic indicator.

Arrhythmias

Palpitations are a common complaint during pregnancy, with atrial and ventricular ectopics the most common cause. The most frequently occurring arrhythmia during pregnancy is a supraventricular tachycardia, which can be terminated in the same fashion as non-pregnant patients by use of vagal manoeuvres and drugs (adenosine, verapamil or β-blockers). Drugs to be avoided if possible during pregnancy include amiodarone and atenolol in the first trimester. An underlying cause of an arrhythmia should be sought, such as sepsis, pulmonary embolism or underlying structural heart disease. Pacemakers, implantable defibrillators and DC cardioversion have been used successfully and are thought to be safe during pregnancy.

Anaesthetic management of labour and caesarean section

In patients with cardiac disease, vaginal delivery has half the risk of caesarean section. In particular, elective section is associated with a twofold increase in the risk of haemorrhage, threefold for DVT and tenfold for infection.

Mode and timing of delivery

Spontaneous labour is suitable for women with normal cardiac function, otherwise induction of labour is preferable in women with cardiac disease. The timing of this is based on maternal cardiac status and maternal or fetal reasons. There is no consensus agreement on absolute contraindication to vaginal delivery, so indication for caesarean section is again down to maternal reasons, cardiac status and obstetric reasons. Caesarean section is indicated in situations, for example, when control of the timing of delivery is important (mechanical heart valve and anticoagulation), cardiac dysfunction (overt heart failure), minimizing CVS stress (dilated aortopathies), significant cardiac disease (severe aortic stenosis or severe pulmonary hypertension).

The first and second stages of labour are usually well tolerated, particularly with good analgesia. Therefore epidurals are potentially beneficial. Bearing down can be associated with significant cardiovascular changes. Therefore, it is important to monitor this stage in order to avoid significant prolongation. A shortened time-limited active second stage and early assisted delivery should be considered.

During the third stage, placental delivery is associated with autotransfusion and the extra blood in the circulation can lead to circulatory overload. Conversely, failure to contract the uterus may lead to haemorrhage and circulatory instability due to blood loss. These two effects have to be balanced. Ergometrine is associated with a tendency to raise blood pressure due to peripheral vasoconstriction and can cause coronary spasm. Syntocinon can reduce blood pressure due to vasodilation and is followed with an associated increase in cardiac output due to the autotransfusion and a reflex tachycardia. In addition, oxytocin can have a direct effect on the heart, causing a reduction in contractility and heart rate. If used it should be given by very slow injection or by infusion. Additional infusion of syntocinon at 10 IU/h can be considered. Carboprost can cause bronchospasm, pulmonary oedema and tachycardia. Its use in active cardiac conditions is not recommended. Misoprostol does not appear to modify the cardiovascular system.

Monitoring during labour

Standard fetal monitoring is paramount. However, interpretation may be difficult when the mother is being treated with drugs controlling heart rate, particularly β-blockers. ECG, pulse oximetry and invasive monitoring with arterial and occasionally central line may be necessary. Patients may need ongoing higher levels of care in the obstetric HDU, critical care unit or cardiac unit after delivery. Multidisciplinary team input after delivery and regular review is essential.

Management of caesarean section

Generally vaginal delivery should be encouraged and caesarean section should be scheduled so that support services such as cardiac anaesthetist, cardiology and cardiac intensive care are available. Many of these patients will require postoperative monitoring and management in a higher-care area.

Regional anaesthesia with combined spinal epidural or spinal catheters is well tolerated, even in patients with restrictive cardiac and stenotic valve disease. It is particularly helpful in patients with pulmonary hypertension or Eisenmenger's. However, general anaesthesia is also well tolerated with a careful approach. The use of appropriate monitoring is essential, including the use of transoesophageal echocardiography if available. Patients occasionally may require inotropic support perioperatively.

Antibiotic prophylaxis is indicated for the prevention of surgical site infection. The current guidance regarding endocarditis prophylaxis should also be referred to if required.

Drugs including breastfeeding

Thromboprophylaxis should be continued after delivery, as should other cardiac medication. There must be an assessment and a balance of risk, benefit and urgency. There are different resources that can be used, including the US FDA resource that classifies drugs from A (safest) through B, C, D and X (do not use, known danger).

Warfarin, flecainide and digoxin are safe, but β-blockers are excreted into breast milk and can cause neonatal bradycardia.

Key points

1. Cardiac disease is a significant cause of maternal mortality and morbidity, with an incidence of heart disease in pregnancy of up to 4% in the western world.
2. Early assessment and risk stratification of parturients using a multidisciplinary team approach is paramount.
3. It is essential to have a low threshold for further investigations of cardiac symptoms during pregnancy and in the postpartum period.
4. Stenotic lesions carry more risk during pregnancy.
5. Mode and timing of delivery need careful planning. Vaginal delivery reduces maternal risk; however, caesarean section may be preferable for reasons of timing, cardiac dysfunction and disease, or to minimize CVS stress.

Further reading

Cardiac Disease in Pregnancy (CARPREG) Investigators (2001). Prospective multicenter study of pregnancy outcomes in women with heart disease. *Circulation*, **104**, 515–521.

Chan, W. S., Anand, S. and Ginsberg, J. S. (2000). Anticoagulation of pregnant women with mechanical heart valves: a systematic review of the literature. *Arch. Intern. Med.*, **160**, 191–196.

Dennis, A. T. and Solnordal, C. B. (2012). Acute pulmonary oedema in pregnant women. *Anaesthesia*, **67**, 646–659

Ginsberg, J. S., Greer, I. and Hirsh, J. (2001). Use of antithrombotic agents during pregnancy. *Chest*, **126**, 344s–370s

Hossenbaccus, E., Robinson, C., Wadsworth, R. and Vohra, A. (2007). Is there a role for enoximone in the management of pregnant women with dilated cardiomyopathy? *Int. J. Obstet. Anaesth.*, **16**, S34, P14.

Hossenbaccus, E., Robinson, C., Wadsworth, R. and Vohra, A. (2007). Severe mixed aortic valve disease and cardiomyopathy. *Int. J. Obstet. Anaesth.*, **16**, S34, P41.

Lewis, G. (2007). The confidential enquiry into maternal and child health (CEMACH). Saving mothers lives: reviewing maternal deaths to make motherhood safer – 2003–2005. *The Seventh report on Confidential Enquiries into Maternal Deaths in the United Kingdom*. London: CEMACH.

Steer, P., Gatzoulis, M. and Baker, P. (2006). *Heart Disease and Pregnancy*. London: RCOG.

Thaman, R. (2003). Pregnancy related complications in women with hypertrophic cardiomyopathy. *Heart*, **89**(7), 752–756.

The Task Force on the Management of Cardiovascular Diseases during Pregnancy of the European Society of Cardiology (ESC) (2011). ESC guidelines on the management of cardiovascular diseases during pregnancy. *Eur. Heart J.*, **32**(24), 3147–3197.

Yentis, S., May, A. and Malhotra, S. (2007). *Analgesia, Anaesthesia and Pregnancy*. Cambridge: Cambridge University Press.

Respiratory disease in pregnancy

Christopher Kelly, Simon Maguire and Craig Carroll

Introduction

A number of significant physiological changes occur within the maternal respiratory system throughout pregnancy, either as a result of hormonal or neonatal effects. Chapter 1 details these changes.

Asthma

Asthma is a common condition characterized by intermittent reversible airways obstruction, chronic inflammation of the airways and bronchospasm. It affects approximately 5% of the population in the UK and is more common in women than men.

Asthma may be affected by pregnancy. Meta-analysis has shown approximately one-third of women will have improved symptoms, one-third will worsen and one-third will see no changes. Any worsening of symptoms will typically peak at six months gestation. There is often an improvement of symptoms during labour, perhaps due to endogenous corticosteroid production, with acute asthma being very rare at this stage.

Well-controlled asthma is unlikely to have any impact on the pregnancy. Uncontrolled asthma is associated with a variety of complications, including hyperemesis, hypertension, pre-eclampsia, vaginal haemorrhage, complicated labour, fetal growth restriction, preterm birth, increased perinatal mortality and neonatal hypoxia. Large cohort studies have shown an increased caesarean section rate in those with moderate and severe asthma.

Treatment should be optimized during pregnancy. A large case-controlled study showed no increased risk of congenital malformations in mothers being treated for asthma. There is good evidence that the older therapies have no teratogenic effects and no evidence to show the newer agents cause any harm. The risk of uncontrolled asthma is far greater than the theoretical risk of therapy.

Acute asthma should be managed in the standard way. Poor management is associated with poor outcomes for mother and fetus; there is no known risk to the fetus with standard treatment.

Asthma is not a contraindication to any form of labour analgesia. Should caesarean section be required, regional anaesthesia is suitable, as those with asthma are less likely to tolerate mechanical ventilation well.

Postpartum haemorrhage can safely be managed with syntometrine and prostaglandin E2. Prostaglandin F2α may cause bronchospasm.

Breastfeeding is not a contraindication to any of the treatments given for asthma, none of which are found in dangerous levels in the milk. Oral steroids may also be given safely to the breastfeeding mother.

Pulmonary hypertension

Pulmonary artery hypertension (PAH) is defined as mean pulmonary artery pressures >25 mmHg at rest or >30 mmHg with exercise. This can arise from a wide variety of disease states leading to a common end pathway of plexogenic pulmonary arteriopathy. It can be sub-classified into:

- Idiopathic pulmonary arterial hypertension
- Associated with left heart disease/congenital heart disease (e.g. Eisenmenger's)
- Associated with lung disease/hypoxaemia
- Associated with chronic thrombotic/embolic disease
- Miscellaneous (e.g. histiocytosis, lymphangioleiomyomatosis, sarcoidosis).

Idiopathic pulmonary hypertension is a rare disease with prevalence in the region of 10 per million. It is three times more common in women than men. Much more commonly, PAH is associated with cardiac or respiratory disorders giving an overall prevalence of around 100 per million.

Core Topics in Obstetric Anaesthesia, ed. Kirsty MacLennan, Kate O'Brien and W. Ross Mcnab.
Published by Cambridge University Press. © Cambridge University Press 2015.

The pathophysiology is worsened by physiological changes of pregnancy. Cardiac output fails to rise in response to the normal reduction in systemic vascular resistance. The pulmonary vasculature also fails in its response to an increased circulating volume. Hypercoagulability can lead to thromboembolism and further rises in PA pressures. The situation worsens in labour with further stress and tachycardia. This can lead to fatal pulmonary hypertensive crisis.

Women are often counselled against pregnancy as maternal mortality is between 30% and 50%, depending on the aetiology of PAH. In the event of pregnancy a multidisciplinary team with knowledge of the condition should be consulted.

Parturients are often started on low-molecular-weight heparin during pregnancy. Oxygen and diuretics may reduce the burden on the pulmonary vasculature. Many pulmonary vasoactive compounds are teratogenic, although sildenafil may be safe. There is no consensus on optimum mode of delivery, but this should be with full invasive monitoring and the facility to administer nitric oxide in order to reduce PVR and therefore pulmonary arterial pressure.

Mothers should be monitored closely for at least two weeks, as many deaths are in the postpartum period.

Pulmonary embolism

Pulmonary embolism (PE) is an obstruction to the lung vasculature by a substance that has travelled from elsewhere in the circulation. This is most commonly thrombus, but can be fat, air or amniotic fluid.

The haemostatic changes during pregnancy include increased concentrations of factors I, II, V, VII, VIII, X and XII, as well as reduced effectiveness of activated protein C and reduced levels of protein S. This leads to a hypercoagulable state and increased risk of thromboembolism. Large studies have demonstrated PE in 1–2 of 7000 pregnancies, most of these occurring postpartum. In the 2006–2008 CEMACE report there were 0.79 deaths per 100,000 maternities; this was the lowest level since 1985. Obesity is an independent risk factor with 14 of the 16 women dying from PE having a BMI >25 kg/m^2. Other predictors of risk are pre-eclampsia, caesarean section and multiple births.

A high index of suspicion should be employed and the clinician alert for dyspnoea or tachypnoea with or without pleuritic chest pain and/or haemoptysis.

Investigations should be as for the non-pregnant population. Those with suspected PE should have CT pulmonary angiography performed. The potential benefits of accurate diagnosis and subsequent treatment should be weighed against an increased lifetime risk of maternal breast cancer and theoretical harm to the fetus.

Current practice is an extrapolation of treatment used in non-pregnant patients and observational studies. Low-molecular-weight heparins are the treatment of choice; warfarin is teratogenic and should be avoided, although can be taken while breastfeeding. Unfractionated heparin is often substituted close to delivery because of the potential for reversal in the event of haemorrhage. Treatment should continue for the longest duration, either three months after the initial diagnosis or six weeks post delivery.

Sarcoidosis

Sarcoidosis is a multisystem disorder, of unknown aetiology, characterized by granulomas, which can be found in most tissues of the body, but are most commonly found in the lungs.

The condition typically presents between the ages of 20 years and 40 years and will affect an estimated 1 in 2000 pregnancies. Although the condition usually has a benign course, fatalities are reported.

Knowledge of sarcoidosis and pregnancy comes primarily from observational studies and case reports. There is often a relapsing remitting course of sarcoidosis; those in remission or with stable disease typically see no changes to their condition during pregnancy. Expectant mothers with active sarcoidosis will often find their symptoms improve as they approach term; radiological improvements are also recorded. Unfortunately there is often rebound exacerbation, potentially with new manifestations, three to six months post delivery.

There does not seem to be a correlation between sarcoidosis and poor outcome from pregnancy. There have been individual reports of preterm labour and low birth weights, but this seems to be in keeping with the background rates.

The condition should be optimized prior to and during pregnancy. Pulmonary function tests may be of use when planning labour strategies. Corticosteroids are the first-line treatment and have not been shown to have major teratogenic effects in large studies of patients with asthma. If right heart hypertrophy and/or dilatation are present due to pulmonary hypertension women should be advised against pregnancy. The second-line agents methotrexate and cyclophosphamide are teratogenic and should be avoided, although some agents may be safe.

Women should be actively followed up post partum in anticipation of potential worsening of their condition.

Cystic fibrosis

Cystic fibrosis (CF) is an autosomal recessive condition affecting chloride channels found throughout the body. It is a multisystem disorder, but morbidity and mortality arise principally from the respiratory system. The resulting thickening of secretions causes blockages, chronic inflammation, recurrent infections and architectural damage to the lungs.

CF occurs in approximately 1 in 2500–3200 live births. The prevalence is ever increasing as median life expectancy is rising with improved care. There are more adults than children with CF in some European countries.

Although all pregnancies in CF patients should be considered high risk, a baseline FEV1 >60% predicted is associated with favourable outcomes. The normal physiological changes of pregnancy can present a significant challenge to these patients. Increasing minute ventilation with little functional reserve and raising cardiac output with existing right heart strain can be problematic. Indeed, as previously mentioned, pulmonary hypertension can present grave risk.

Predictors of increased risk are weight gain <4.5 kg, BMI <20 kg/m^2, colonization with *B. cepacia*, frequent infections, diabetes mellitus, pancreatic insufficiency and recurrent infections. These patients have increased frequency of preterm labour.

Treatment should be optimized during pregnancy and multidisciplinary input sought. Mildly impaired mothers may labour normally with epidural analgesia. Should caesarean section be deemed necessary, each patient must be assessed individually, as no robust evidence exists to guide treatment. Regional anaesthesia is often preferable to reduce impact on the respiratory system and avoid mechanical ventilation. High block should be avoided because of dependence on the accessory muscles. A CSE technique seems a reasonable approach to allow epidural analgesia post section and aid compliance with physiotherapy. These patients require meticulous attention to detail in the perioperative period, with senior input from the CF team, physiotherapy and microbiology, as well as obstetrics/midwifery/anaesthesia.

Musculoskeletal disease

Myopathies

The myopathies are a heterogenous group of diseases that affect skeletal muscle cell function. They can be divided into different groups:

1. The hereditary dystrophies (muscular dystrophies)
   These can have a dominant, recessive or sex-linked inheritance. They usually affect proximal muscles and have no sensory involvement.
2. The hereditary myotonic disorders
   Myotonic dystrophy (autosomal dominant) is the most common inherited myopathy with a prevalence of 5:100,000.
3. Metabolic myopathies
   These include the mitochondrial myopathies, as well as disorders of glycogen storage and lipid metabolism.
4. Myasthenic syndromes
   Predominantly myasthenia gravis (see below) but also Eaton–Lambert syndrome.
5. Others, e.g. inflammatory myopathies
   These are proximal myopathies associated with muscle pain, tenderness and markedly raised muscle enzymes and include dermatomyositis and polymyositis. Associated restrictive lung defects, conduction abnormalities and bulbar symptoms are a cause for anaesthetic concern. These myopathies are often steroid-responsive.

These all have in common a tendency to progression and deterioration over time with a reduction in muscle strength. The level of input from the multidisciplinary maternity team will therefore be dictated by the symptoms at presentation and progression over the course of the confinement.

Myotonic dystrophy

Myotonic dystrophy has two clinically and molecularly distinct forms, DM1 and DM2.

DM1 is the most common form and presents earlier with more progressive symptoms, including restrictive lung defects with carbon dioxide retention and a reduced response to hypoxia. Pulmonary function tests and arterial blood gas analysis should be considered. Bulbar involvement and oesophageal dysmotility increase the risk of aspiration. An ECG is essential to rule out any conduction defect and there is also an association with cardiomyopathy. These parturients should be screened for diabetes as they can have insulin resistance. DM2 is typically milder, with myotonia in 90%, muscle dysfunction in 82%, but less commonly cardiac conduction defects, cataract and diabetes.

Parturients with myotonic dystrophy suffer a higher incidence of obstetric complications, including premature labour. Providing there are no contraindications, regional anaesthesia is the preferred choice for labour analgesia or operative intervention. Points for consideration in myotonic dystrophy:

- Spinal anaesthesia may be contraindicated in those patients with severe respiratory involvement.
- Prevent myotonic crisis by keeping the patient warm, avoiding suxamethonium and gentle surgical technique. (Although case series have reported the use of suxamethonium without complications in this patient group.)
- Regional anaesthesia does not prevent a myotonic crisis.
- Myotonic crisis can be treated with intravenous dantrolene, phenytoin or procainamide.
- Use rocuronium and sugammadex to eliminate the possibility of postoperative residual neuromuscular blockade.

Myasthenia gravis

Myasthenia gravis is a chronic, autoimmune disorder resulting from autoantibodies to the postsynaptic acetylcholine receptors. It is more common in women and is characterized by muscle weakness and fatigability with repetitive use of the involved muscle. Over 80% of patients have detectable antibodies and those who do not tend to have a milder form of the illness. Treatment includes anticholinesterase medication, thymectomy, steroids, azathioprine and plasma exchange. Exacerbations may be provoked by stimuli, including pain, temperature fluxes, infection, stress and many drugs. The illness tends to progress from the head down, typically with early involvement of the eye and facial muscles, bulbar symptoms and progression to involvement of respiratory muscles and proximal muscles of the upper limbs. It has a variable peripartum course, but symptoms are reported to be exacerbated more frequently during the first trimester and post partum. One-third of patients will remain clinically unchanged, one-third will improve while one-third will have an exacerbation of their symptoms.

Anaesthetic considerations include:

- Antenatal assessment to discern the degree of bulbar and respiratory involvement/impairment.
- Baseline pulmonary function tests. FVC <2.6 L has been shown to be predictive of the need for postoperative ventilation.
- Anticholinesterase dosage may require alteration during pregnancy, especially if associated with emesis.
- Consider the possibility of both myasthenic and cholinergic crises if a patient presents with worsening weakness. Intravenous edrophonium will improve a myasthenic, but not a cholinergic, crisis.
- Use magnesium sulfate with caution as it will temporarily interfere with neuromuscular function and power.
- The preferred method of analgesia or anaesthesia is a regional technique, thus avoiding the respiratory depressive effects of opioids and the need for muscle relaxants.
- Progressive bulbar involvement or deteriorating respiratory function may result in the need for general anaesthesia and securing of the airway. Care must be taken in the use of muscle relaxants and monitoring of neuromuscular function. These parturients may require an increased dose of depolarizing muscle relaxant, but a significant reduction in the dose of non-depolarizing relaxants, with atracurium the drug of choice. Prolonged postoperative ventilation should be anticipated.

Scoliosis

Scoliosis is a major source of referral to obstetric anaesthetic assessment clinics. Mostly, these will be minor to moderate, surgically uncorrected scoliosis. Scoliosis is more common in women and most cases (90%) are idiopathic. There are, however, a large number of conditions associated with scoliosis, including spina bifida, neurological disorders (e.g. cerebral palsy), myopathies (e.g. muscular dystrophy), connective tissue disorders (e.g. Marfan's) and metabolic disorders (e.g. mucopolysaccharidosis).

Factors affecting morbidity include age of onset, cardiorespiratory involvement and other associated pathologies.

With patients in whom scoliosis has developed relatively late in childhood and puberty, cardiorespiratory function is usually well maintained.

Deformity from early childhood is associated with greater impact upon lung development and may adversely affect cardiac function. The resulting restrictive lung defect can potentially progress to chronic hypoxia and pulmonary hypertension. Investigations to detect cardiorespiratory defects should be considered as part of anaesthetic assessment.

Factors affecting choice of anaesthesia and analgesia are discussed below.

Uncorrected scoliosis

- The level of the vertebral deformity needs to be identified.
- More than one curve can exist (i.e. thoracic + lumbar curve). The curve may not be evident towards the lower region of the lumbar spine.
- The defect is three-dimensional, with vertebral rotation in conjunction with curvature.
- The spinal cord may not terminate at the usual level (i.e. T12–L1).
- The morphology of the epidural space may be altered, resulting in unpredictable passage of epidural catheters, with an increased risk of failed block and possibly inadvertent dural puncture.

Corrected scoliosis

Scoliosis corrective surgery consists of a number of steps that can compromise the ability to perform regional blockade safely and effectively.

Posterior scoliosis correction surgery results in tissues superficial to the ligamentum flavum being disrupted, posterior spinous processes are usually removed and laminae disrupted. Decortication of bone and addition of inert bone graft will obliterate the midline and paramedian access to the epidural space. The epidural space itself may be disrupted.

Attempts to perform epidural analgesia in the corrected scoliosis patient are therefore linked with an increase in both complications of insertion and sub-optimal/inconsistent analgesic outcome.

The literature suggests that continuous spinal analgesia is used with increased frequency in this patient group (either as a planned procedure or possibly as a result of inadvertent dural puncture).

Practical suggestions when contemplating regional anaesthesia in the scoliosis patient include:

- Consider avoiding epidural analgesia, using spinal catheters instead.
- Consent for an increased risk of failure and complications of neuraxial technique (failed access, prolonged procedure, neuropraxia, inadvertent dural puncture, failure to thread epidural catheter, blood in catheter, inconsistent block, unpredictable height of block, spinal cord trauma.
- Perform the technique low in the lumbar spine (L4–5, L5–S1), where the pelvis tends to limit the rotational element of deformity.
- Avoid attempting regional analgesia through areas of surgical scarring.
- Restrict the number of needling attempts; be prepared for failure.
- Consider the risk of infecting metalwork with needling of the instrumented surgical area.

Lumbar spine disease

Mechanical lumbar back pain and nerve root pain are common causes for antenatal anaesthetic consultation.

It is important to distinguish the pathology causing the symptoms so that the patient can be appropriately consented for risks of regional anaesthesia.

Assessment and documentation of neurological function prior to performing a regional procedure is important for both clinical and medicolegal reasons.

Nerve compression in the lumbar region can be caused by disc disease, alignment abnormalities, tumour or osteophytes.

Alignment abnormalities

Either by anatomical or progressive traumatic/degenerative. Spondylisthesis of the lumbar vertebrae (usually L5 on S1) results in a slip and malalignment of the vertebrae with resulting narrowing of the exit foramen and spinal nerve compression. The listhesis itself is thought to contribute to mechanical back pain.

True disc disease

The intervertebral disc consists of an outer annulus fibrosus and inner soft nucleus pulposus. Pathologies include:

- The annulus remains intact, but bulges, compressing the cauda and spinal nerve root.
- The annulus ruptures and pulposus tissue exudes into the spinal canal causing compression and chemically mediated irritation.

Disc prolapse can be posterolaterally or from the true posterior position (central disc prolapse). Compression of the entire thecal sac in the latter scenario can result in *cauda equina syndrome*, which consists of back or leg pain, saddle anaesthesia with loss of bladder and bowel continence – these are red flag signs and represent a neurosurgical urgency.

Lumbar spine decompression surgery

In order to understand the risks of regional anaesthesia, it is important to understand which operation has been performed and at what level.

- Laminectomy: the lamina and possibly posterior spinous process will have been removed. The ligamentum may have been obliterated and removed at this level. The epidural space may not exist. An epidural cannot be performed at this level. Epidural anaesthesia performed at another level may be ineffective, as the spread of local anaesthetic past the operative level may be impeded. Spread of spinal anaesthesia is unaffected.
- Lateral approach with fenestration: The midline structures are left intact and a fenestration made in the ligamentum at an interlaminar level (similar to the site of a paramedian approach to the epidural space). Spread of epidural anaesthesia may be affected.

When considering regional anaesthesia do not attempt needling though the scar. (NB: surgery may have been performed beyond the limit of the scar.)

A recent study demonstrated similar LA use for labour analgesia in women with previous lumbar discectomy compared to controls. The only difference between the groups was the number of interspaces attempted.

Patients with untreated thecal or spinal nerve compression may have a flattened or deviated thecal sac. This may result in a decreased thecal target, with possible deviation from the midline and obliteration of epidural fat, reducing the size of the epidural space.

There have been historical links between labour epidurals and long-term back pain, but all recent studies have failed to demonstrate any link. A Cochrane Database Systematic Review in 2011 comparing epidural vs. non-epidural or no analgesia in labour found no link between labour epidural analgesia and long-term backache.

Anaesthetic considerations:

- Document existing neurology
- Obtain information relating to previous diagnosis, level of disease and surgery
- Counsel the patient and obtain consent before attempting neuraxial blockade

- Avoid needling at the level of or close to any surgical scar
- Be aware of red flag signs of back pain and features of cauda equina syndrome.

Neural tube defects

Spina bifida encompasses a range of neural tube defects from spinal bifida occulta (SBO), which occurs incidentally in up to 25% of the population, to spina bifida cystica, a more severe form, which occurs in 1 in 2000 live births.

SBO is often an incidental finding on X-ray and occurs when two halves of a vertebral arch (usually at level L5–S1) fail to fuse. The overlying skin is intact, but can have cutaneous angiomata, pigmented areas, lipoma, a tuft of hair or simple dimple. It is not associated with neurological symptoms.

Spinal bifida cystica is defined as failed closure of the neural arch with herniation of the meninges (meningocoele) or the meninges and neural elements (meningomyelocoele). Tethering of the spinal cord is a well-recognized association and neurological defects can occur below the level of lesion.

Occult spinal dysraphism, sometimes confused with SBO, is a condition where bony defects of the spine are associated with spinal cord anomalies, including tethering (in 35–87% cases), intraspinous lipomas, dermoid cysts, fibrous bands and split cord.

Issues complicating regional anaesthesia (RA) include:

- Increased risk of neural/dural injury, especially at the level of defect
- Abnormal spread of local anaesthetic, either excessive cranial or inadequate caudal
- Performance of RA in presence of pre-existing neurology.

Recommendations:

- In patients with SBO always consider occult spinal dysraphism. Patients with neurological abnormalities, cutaneous manifestations or involvement of more than one lamina should have MRI imaging to determine the extent of spinal involvement
- Careful documentation of pre-existing neurology
- Consent patient for risks of failure and complications
- Perform neuraxial procedure above the level of defect.

Malignant hyperthermia

This inherited disorder (mainly autosomal dominant) results in an error in skeletal muscle calcium control. There is a loss of control of calcium flux and an increase in the calcium concentration in the cytosol of skeletal muscle. The proposed site of action is the Ryanodine receptor, which spans the calcium-releasing channels on the sarcoplasmic reticulum and T-tubule.

The increase in intracellular free calcium results in the clinical picture of:

- Increased skeletal muscle contraction
- Increased skeletal muscle metabolism
- Glycolysis
- Rhabdomyolysis
- Uncoupling of oxidative phosphorylation.

The triggers for this condition are volatile anaesthetic agents and suxamethonium. The majority of UK cases are in patients with a known family history and therefore preparations can be made during pregnancy. The two main presentations are therefore acute presentation in patients previously undiagnosed and known cases presenting in the antenatal clinic.

Known cases should be seen antenatally in order to discuss the benefits of an early labour epidural, which can safely provide intrapartum and intraoperative analgesia and anaesthesia.

Delivery suite and theatres should be prepared, ensuring the availability of a vapour-free anaesthetic machine, TIVA equipment, dantrolene, rocuronium and sugammadex.

Algorithms for recognition and treatment of malignant hyperthermia should be readily available.

Key points

1 Respiratory disease can improve, remain stable or deteriorate during the antenatal and postpartum period.

2 Evaluation of respiratory function outside of pregnancy can guide preconceptual counselling.

3 MDT management, with regular antenatal review and appropriate peripartum and postpartum plans are essential.

4 Knowledge of pre-existing musculoskeletal disease is essential to guide intrapartum analgesic and anaesthetic options.

Further reading

Anim-Somuah, M., Smyth, R. M. and Jones, L. (2011). Epidural versus non-epidural or no analgesia in labour. *Cochrane Database Syst Rev.*, **12**, CD000331.

Bauchat, J. R., McCarthy, R. J., Koski, T. R. *et al.* (2012). Prior lumbar discectomy surgery does not alter the efficacy of neuraxial labor analgesia. *Anesth. Anal.*, **115**(2), 348–353.

British Thoracic Society. (2014). British guideline on the management of asthma. London: The British Thoracic Society.

British Thoracic Society Standards of Care Committee Pulmonary Embolism Guideline Development Group. (2003). British Thoracic Society guidelines for the management of suspected acute pulmonary embolism. *Thorax*, **58**, 470–484.

Crochetiere, C. (2008). *Myopathies: Musculoskeletal Disorders: Obstetric Anesthesia and Uncommon Disorders.* Cambridge. Cambridge University Press.

Huffmyer, J., Littlewood, K. and Nemergut, E. (2009). Perioperative management of the adult with cystic fibrosis. *Anaesth. Analg.*, **6**, 1949–1961.

Imison, A. R. (2001). Anaesthesia and myotonia: an Australian experience. *Anaesth. Intens. Care*, **29**, 34–37.

Madden B. P. (2009). Pulmonary hypertension and pregnancy. *Int. J. Obstet. Anaesth.*, **2**, 156–164.

Vahid, B., Mushlin, N. and Weibel, S. (2007) Sarcoidosis in pregnancy and postpartum period. *Curr. Respir. Med. Rev.*, **3**, 79–83.

Chapter 18

Obesity and ultrasonography for central neuraxial blocks

Sophie Bishop and Preye Zuokumor

Obesity is a global health pandemic with increasing prevalence, and is arguably one of the biggest challenges facing maternity services today.

Obesity is defined as a condition of abnormal or excessive fat accumulation in adipose tissue to the extent that health may be impaired. Obesity is often expressed with reference to body mass index (BMI). This is calculated by the person's weight in kilograms (kg) /divided by the square of their height in meters (m^2). The World Health Organization (WHO) defines obesity as a BMI of at least 30 kg/m^2, which is further divided into five classes (Table 18.1).

In 2011, an estimated 26% of women in the UK aged 16 years or over were obese (*cf*. 16% in 1993). The UK prevalence of women with a known BMI ≥35 kg/m^2 at any point in pregnancy is ~5% (approximately 38,478 maternities/year). The prevalence of women with a BMI ≥ 40 kg/m^2 in the UK is 2%, whilst a BMI ≥ 50 kg/m^2 affects 0.19% of all parturients.

Maternal obesity is associated with a substantial increase in both obstetric and fetal morbidity, as well as being a significant risk factor for maternal mortality (see Table 18.2).

Pregnant women with obesity are at higher risk of anaesthesia-related complications. Obesity has been identified as a significant risk factor for anaesthesia-related maternal mortality. Prepregnancy BMI >40 kg/m^2 and a delivery BMI >45 kg/m^2 have been found to be predictive of a higher incidence of anaesthetic complications, including: failure to establish neuraxial anaesthesia, inadequate neuraxial anaesthesia requiring conversion to general anaesthesia and other anaesthesia-related morbidity and mortality.

The Confidential Enquiry into Maternal and Child Health (CEMACH) report on maternal deaths in the 2003–2005 triennium showed that 28% of mothers that died were obese, whereas the prevalence of obesity in the general maternity population within the same time period was 16–19%. Six maternal deaths were directly related to anaesthesia, of which four patients were obese and two were morbidly obese. As a result in 2008 the Centre for Maternal and Child Health Enquires (CMACE) conducted a 3-year UK-wide Obesity in Pregnancy project and with the Royal College of Obstetricians and Gynaecologists (RCOG) have published clinical guidelines on the

Table 18.1 WHO classification of obesity

WHO Classification	Popular description	BMI (kg/m^2)	Risk of co-morbidity
Underweight	Thin	< 18.5	Low
Normal	Normal	18.5–24.9	Average
Overweight	Overweight	25–29.9	Mildly increased
Obese Class 1	Obese	30–34.9	Moderately increased
Obese Class 2	Obese	35–39.9	Severely increased
Obese Class 3	Morbidly obese	> 40	Very severely increased
Super Obese		> 50	Very severely increased
Super Super Obese		> 60	Very severely increased

Core Topics in Obstetric Anaesthesia, ed. Kirsty MacLennan, Kate O'Brien and W. Ross Mcnab.
Published by Cambridge University Press. © Cambridge University Press 2015.

Table 18.2 Risks related to obesity in pregnancy

Maternal	Spontaneous first trimester and recurrent miscarriage Maternal death Left ventricular hypertrophy/dysfunction/failure, cardiomyopathy, ischaemic heart disease Obstructive sleep apnoea, asthma Gestational diabetes (GDM) Hypertension, pre-eclampsia Thromboembolism Dysfunctional labour Lower success rate of vaginal birth after caesarean section Shoulder dystocia Operative vaginal delivery (increases with increasing BMI) Higher caesarean section rate Postcaesarean wound infection Postpartum haemorrhage Low breastfeeding rates
Fetal	Stillbirth and perinatal mortality Congenital anomalies, birth injuries Macrosomia (birth weights >4000 g) Neonatal intensive care admission Possible long-term obesity problems for child

management of women with obesity in pregnancy (see Further reading). The CMACE report (2006–2008) noted obesity was still a major contributor to maternal mortality, with 27% of mothers who died being obese.

Physiological changes in obesity

Pregnancy induces a number of physiological changes to support the uteroplacental unit, as discussed in Chapter 1. Obesity also results in a number of significant physiological changes (additive with increasing BMI). The further physiological impact of obesity on pregnancy leads to significant functional impairment and decreased physiological reserve. The most important physiological changes are listed in Table 18.3. These effects need to be taken into consideration when planning regional and general anaesthesia for these patients.

Airway

Obesity and pregnancy each increase the risk of difficult intubation and pulmonary aspiration during anaesthesia. Careful assessment, planning and management of

the airway are important. Poor head positioning, a short neck, an increased fat pad at the back of neck, airway oedema and increased breast tissue make laryngoscopy and tracheal intubation technically challenging. The incidence of difficult intubation may be as high as 15%. The combination of Mallampati score and thyromental distance are useful to predict difficult laryngoscopy. Mallampati class III–IV has been found to be an independent risk factor for difficult intubation in obese patients.

Positioning before induction of general anaesthesia remains critical for the morbidly obese parturient, and time should be taken to do this even in an emergency situation. The optimal position is the 'ramped' position, where the head and neck are elevated until the external auditory meatus is in a horizontal plane with the sternal notch, when assessing the patient from the side view. This can be accomplished by using either a stack of blankets or a commercially available pillow such as the Oxford Head Elevating Laryngoscopy Pillow (HELP) (Alma Medical, Oxford, UK).

Patients with a known difficult airway may require an awake oral fibre optic intubation (FOI). (Nasal FOI is not recommended on account of mucosal congestion and risk of bleeding).

Thromboprophylaxis

Venous thromboembolic (VTE) disease is a major cause of maternal mortality in developed countries and both caesarean delivery and obesity are major risk factors. Obese parturients are at significantly higher risk of thromboembolic events throughout pregnancy and puerperium. Low-molecular-weight heparin (LMWH) is recommended for antenatal and postnatal thromboprophylaxis (see Table 18.4). This highlights the importance of documentation of the patients' recent weight for appropriate dosing. In addition mechanical methods such as graduated compression stockings and sequential calf compression devices should be used and mobilization encouraged. Clear guidelines should be provided regarding safe timing of neuraxial anaesthesia and analgesia following thromboprophylaxis administration.

Equipment

Maternal weight should be re-measured in the third trimester to allow appropriate plans to be made for specialist equipment and personnel required during

Table 18.3 Physiological changes in obesity

Respiratory system

- Reduced functional residual capacity (FRC) with risk of hypoxia
- FRC below closing capacity resulting in shunting
- Increased work of breathing due to reduced chest wall compliance (sometimes up to 30%) secondary to increased chest wall weight and impaired diaphragm function. Increased oxygen consumption and CO_2 production
- Restrictive respiratory defect resulting in a rapid, shallow breathing pattern
- Obstructive sleep apnoea with risk of pulmonary hypertension and cor pulmonale
- Obese hypoventilation syndrome 5–10% of morbidly obese

Cardiovascular system

- Increase in blood volume
- Increase in cardiac output proportional to degree of obesity
- (30–50 mL/min for every 100 g of adipose tissue)
- Presence of endothelial dysfunction with increased peripheral resistance
- Hypertension
- Left ventricular hypertrophy with subsequent systolic and diastolic dysfunction, leading to heart failure
- Increased risk of fatal gestational and peripartum arrhythmias
- Peripartum cardiomyopathy (difficult to diagnose as symptoms masked and technical difficulties in performing echocardiography)
- Obese supine hypotensive syndrome due to aortocaval compression

Gastrointestinal

- Raised intragastric pressure, relaxed lower oesphageal sphincter
- Increased gastric acidity and volume
- Increased incidence of gastro-oesphageal reflux and hiatus hernia. The volume and acidity of gastric contents may be 5 × greater

Endocrine

- Type II diabetes mellitus (DM) (+/− complications of DM)
- Nutritional status – may be malnourished

Musculoskeletal

- Difficulty in positioning patient, including left lateral tilt
- Risk of rhabdomyolysis with prolonged surgery e.g. buttock ischaemia

Coagulation

- Increased risk of thromboembolic disease

Table 18.4 RCOG guidelines for thromboprophylactic doses of LMWH

Weight	Enoxaparin	Dalteparin	Tinzaparin
< 50 kg	20 mg daily	2500 units daily	3500 units daily
50–90 kg	40 mg daily	5000 units daily	4500 units daily*
91–130 kg	60 mg daily*	7500 units daily*	7000 units daily*
131–170 kg	80 mg daily*	10000 units daily*	9000 units daily*
> 170 kg	0.6 mg/kg/day*	75 units/kg/day*	75 units/kg/day*

"Reproduced from: Royal College of Obstetricians and Gynaecologists. *Thrombosis and Embolism during Pregnancy and the Puerperium.* Green-top Guideline No. 37A. London: RCOG; 2009, with the permission of the Royal College of Obstetricians and Gynaecologists."

Table 18.5 Equipment list

- Maximum weight that operating table can support must be known (minimum of 160 kg)
- Lateral extensions for operating table and arm boards
- Weighing scales
- Wide wheelchairs
- Bariatric hover mattress
- Slide sheets
- HELP pillow or pillows to allow for ramping
- Electric beds
- Large gowns
- Large compression stockings/mechanical calf compressors
- Large blood pressure cuff
- Ultrasound for IV cannulae/epidural insertion

Table 18.6 CAVE assessment

C	Co-morbidities
A	Airway assessment
V	Venous access
E	Epidural (including U/S back)/Equipment required

labour and delivery (Table 18.5). Familiarity with specialist beds for the morbidly obese is necessary in case a woman needs to be laid flat for resuscitation.

Anaesthetic antenatal assessment

It is recommended that all women with a BMI ≥ 40 kg/m^2 have an antenatal consultation with an obstetric anaesthetist, so that potential difficulties can be identified and an anaesthetic management plan for labour and delivery can be documented. Obstetric units may decide to use a lower BMI threshold, taking into consideration the local prevalence of maternal obesity. Women with a BMI <40 kg/m^2 with anticipated problems related to co-morbidities, airway management, vascular access and regional anaesthetic techniques will also require an antenatal anaesthetic consultation. All other obese parturients should be assessed as soon as possible after arrival on delivery suite.

The CAVE assessment (Table 18.6) is a useful mnemonic for assessment of these patients, which includes a physical and ultrasound examination of the patient's back. Tactful discussion with the patient should include both the increased risk of difficult labour analgesia initiation and potential failure and the goals for comfort and safety. Surveys suggest that this type of discussion rarely occurs, possibly because of concerns of offending the patient. Lack of discussion may contribute to unrealistic patient expectations or incomplete informed consent. The Obstetric Anaesthetists' Association (OAA) have published a leaflet 'Information for pregnant women with a high

body mass index', which is helpful to give to women, and also for those women not referred to the anaesthetic antenatal clinic.

Anaesthetic management for labour

Delivery of the morbidly obese parturient should take place on a consultant-led delivery suite with the senior obstetrician and anaesthetist aware. On admission, the antenatal anaesthetic plan should be reviewed, or a CAVE assessment performed. Oral intake should be limited to clear fluids, and an H$_2$ antagonist commenced and continued 6 hourly whilst in labour. A large-bore intravenous cannula should be inserted early in labour (ultrasound guidance may be needed), by those with expertise, as multiple failed attempts may make it more difficult.

The provision of regional analgesia for labour reduces the need for entonox or systemic opioid analgesia, which have been proven to lead to maternal drowsiness, airway obstruction and hypoxaemia. Intramuscular diamorphine in obese patients is unreliable due to variable absorption and effect. Increasingly, remifentanil patient-controlled analgesia (PCA) is used as a labour analgesic. Extreme care should be taken to ensure obese women using PCA are well monitored and have continuous one-to-one midwifery care until delivery.

As the obese parturient is more likely to require operative delivery and general anaesthesia is associated with greater morbidity, central neuraxial block is the most effective form of analgesia in labour. Due to the technical challenges of siting an epidural in these patients, placement of an epidural early in labour is recommended as patient position can be optimized more easily. As landmarks are more difficult to palpate and back flexion is limited (both factors predictive of difficult neuraxial placement) the epidural failure rate is high and multiple attempts are not uncommon.

The sitting position is best as the midline may be identified more easily than in the lateral position, and

133

it reduces the distance from the skin to the epidural space. Interestingly, despite an increased depth of epidural space with increasing weight and BMI, very few patients actually have an epidural space that is deeper than 8 cm. However, it may be necessary to use a longer epidural needle. Techniques to facilitate epidural insertion include the use of the patient's light touch discrimination to determine the midline, tilting of the table towards the operator to open the lumbar interspaces and the use of a seeker needle to identify a spinous process. Ultrasound visualization is discussed below.

In obese patients, successfully placed epidural catheters can easily be dislodged by the drag of the back fat pad, so it is advisable to leave extra catheter length in the space i.e. 5–6 cm; also tunnelling the epidural catheter may help. The catheter site should be protected whilst repositioning in bed. Catheter position and sensory levels should be checked regularly during labour to ensure adequate position and function. Epidural re-sites have been reported to increase with increasing BMI and the epidural catheter should be replaced early if the block is ineffective.

There is evidence that after accidental dural puncture, the incidence of post dural puncture headache is less in obese parturients compared with non-obese parturients. This may be due to increased pressure in the epidural space. This effect may also result in higher than expected sensory and motor block levels. Careful titration of local anaesthetic should be used to avoid a high block.

Anaesthesia for caesarean section

Anaesthetic challenges may lead to increased decision-to-delivery time if emergency operative delivery is required and may increase anaesthetic morbidity. Advanced warning of such challenges may influence the planned mode of delivery and allow appropriate staff to be made available.

General considerations for delivery in theatre

- Appropriate equipment available
- Surgery is technically more difficult with reduced surgical access and bleeding
- Retraction of the panniculus may worsen aortocaval compression
- Adequate left lateral tilt is required
- Operating times are often longer
- Increased risk of PPH.

Monitoring

Reliable monitoring of obese obstetric patients is essential. Measure the mid-arm circumference to assess the appropriate size of non-invasive blood pressure (NIBP) cuff. If >33 cm (13 inches) use large or adult thigh cuff size. Note that normal-size cuffs can be applied to the forearm to monitor BP if larger cuffs are unavailable.

Invasive arterial pressure monitoring may be required. Central venous access may also be necessary.

Regional anaesthesia

Extending labour epidural analgesia avoids general anaesthesia and allows a titratable level of anaesthesia and dose, with the ability to extend the block for prolonged surgery and slower and more controllable haemodynamic changes. For elective caesarean section, single-shot spinal is probably the most practiced technique. However combined spinal-epidural techniques is an attractive alternative technique, combining the advantages of rapid onset and dense block with the ability to prolong regional anaesthesia if required. In addition, reducing the intrathecal dose may help to control the haemodynamic effects of the block, which are compounded by aortocaval compression in this group.

General anaesthesia

General anaesthesia can be slightly quicker than regional anaesthesia and is indicated when there is an immediate threat to life of mother or fetus, and where central neuraxial block is contraindicated or has failed – i.e. only done when absolutely necessary. General anaesthesia for caesarean section is associated with a much higher risk of maternal mortality than regional anaesthesia, with failed intubation and aspiration as contributing factors. A senior anaesthetist should be present, to assist with airway management. Standard aspiration prophylaxis must be given. Optimal patient positioning, in the ramped position as previously discussed are and good preoxygenation vital, as rapid desaturation is common. Careful attention to left lateral tilt even during general anaesthesia is mandatory. A relatively high inspired-oxygen concentration may be necessary compared to non-obese parturients and the use of pressure-controlled ventilation and positive end-expiratory pressure to maintain adequate oxygenation. Awake extubation with adequate reversal of neuromuscular blockade, with a

45° head-up tilt is a more favourable position than supine in the obese population.

Postpartum care

Postoperatively women with a BMI >40 kg/m^2 should be assessed individually to determine if they need an extended recovery period on the delivery suite or the high-dependency unit (likely if BMI ≥50 kg/m^2) for the first 24 hours. If there is respiratory or cardiovascular compromise, early referral to ITU should be considered. Common postoperative complications include hypoxia, pulmonary atelectasis and pneumonia, so humidified oxygen supplementation should be maintained. Early postnatal and postoperative mobilization is vital, with adequate pain control, VTE prophylaxis and chest physiotherapy.

Ultrasonography for central neuraxial blocks in obstetrics

Ultrasonography for obstetric regional anaesthesia is a novel way of identifying the structures within and around the lumbar vertebrae. Conventionally, siting epidurals and spinals relies on the anaesthetist's skills and ability to correctly identify the bony landmarks of the spine and pelvis, and to introduce the needle blindly into the epidural or intrathecal space. Not surprisingly, the landmark-based technique is associated with difficulties and failures, particularly amongst inexperienced anaesthetists, obese patients and patients with scoliosis or previous back surgery. With the introduction of high-resolution portable ultrasound machines, the lumbar spine can be imaged with some degree of accuracy. When appropriately utilized, ultrasonography increases the success rate of central neuraxial blocks, while minimizing the risks to the patient. The use of ultrasound imaging has been shown to improve the efficacy of epidural analgesia and reduce technical difficulties.

In 2008, guidance from NICE reported that although evidence of U/S guided catheterization of the epidural space was limited, it is safe and may be helpful in achieving correct placement.

Spinal ultrasound can be challenging, as the structures imaged are protected by an articulated encasement of bones, limiting the acoustic windows for the ultrasound beam. The structures of interest are located deeper than expected. Accordingly, spinal ultrasonography requires a probe that is curved and of low frequency (2–5 Hz), with the ability for deep penetration. However, with deeper penetration of the ultrasound beam there is some loss of image resolution.

There are two ways of facilitating epidural catheterization under ultrasound guidance. The first is the most common and is referred to as prepuncture ultrasound. It is used as a guide to the conventional technique of central neuraxial block and involves an initial ultrasound scan of the vertebral spines to determine the midline, vertebral interspaces and depth of the space. The interspaces can be marked on the skin to facilitate actual needle placement. The second, which is still at its infancy in terms of development, is real-time ultrasound imaging, and this approach allows observation of the epidural needle as it passes towards the epidural space. Subsequent discussions will be limited to the first approach.

Sonoanatomy of the lumbar spine

The aim of ultrasound imaging of the lumbar spine is to encourage pattern recognition, which is essential to the interpretation of images:

- Patient should be placed in the position the block is to be performed, which is sitting in most obstetric patients.
- A curved array, low frequency (2–5 MHz) probe gives the best image quality.
- The initial depth is set to 7–10 cm (the depth may be fixed with some devices)
- For the sake of simplicity, there are two main orientations of the probe: paramedian sagittal (PS) and transverse views. Information from each scanning plane compliments the other.
- With the probe in a PS orientation 3–4 cm from the midline (PS transverse process view), the 'Trident sign' is the main feature and it represents finger-like shadows of the transverse process. If the probe is tilted towards the midline, the 'sawtooth' appearance of the laminae is seen. Also, the posterior complex (ligamentum flavum, epidural space and posterior dura) and anterior complex (anterior dura, posterior longitudinal ligament and vertebral body) will be discernable (Figure 18.1).
- With the probe still in the PS orientation, slide the probe caudally until the L5–S1 interspace is at the centre of the screen. The horizontal hyperechoic line of the sacrum is used to identify the L5–S1 interspace, and its location can be used to mark intervertebral levels (Figure 18.2).

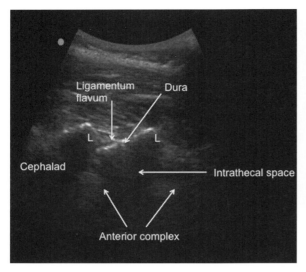

Figure 18.1 Parasagittal (oblique) view. The laminae (L) form a 'saw-tooth' pattern.

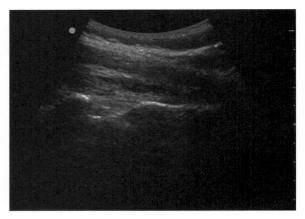

Figure 18.2 Parasagittal (oblique) view of L5–S1 junction.

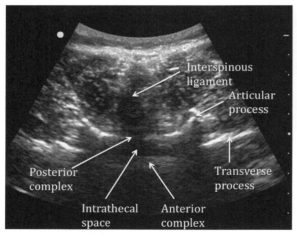

Figure 18.3 Transverse (interlaminar) view of the lumbar spine.

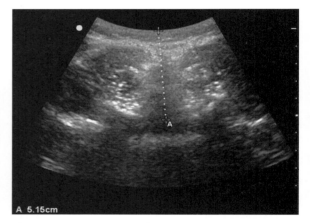

Figure 18.4 Transverse view showing the depth to the posterior complex.

- Rotate the probe transversely to obtain a transverse interlaminar view of the desired interspace. Optimal views may be obtained by tilting the probe cephalad or caudad. The depth from skin surface to the posterior complex may be measured using the inbuilt electronic calipers (Figures 18.3 and 18.4).

Indications for ultrasound imaging of the spine:

- As part of preoperative assessment of obstetric patients at the antenatal anaesthetic assessment clinic, in delivery suite or theatre

- Facilitates insertion of central neuraxial block, especially in patients with difficult surface anatomy, e.g. morbidly obese, scoliosis or previous back surgery
- Previous problematic central neuraxial blocks
- Previous post dural puncture headaches.

The perceived advantages of imaging of the spine include:

- Prediction of depth of epidural and intrathecal spaces
- Aids identification of intervertebral levels
- Assists in locating important landmarks such as the midline and interlaminar spaces
- Fewer puncture attempts
- Higher first time success rate
- Less time required to catheterize epidural space

- Higher patient satisfaction
- Improves teaching of regional techniques to anaesthetic trainees.

Limitations of the ultrasound spinal imaging technique:

- Poor image quality in certain patient populations. In obese patients images are less distinct because of attenuation of ultrasound waves. Patients with metal implants may distort the image quality.
- Inaccuracies of skin marking due to patient movement
- Operator inexperience
- May lead to delays (if an urgent caesarean section is needed).

Key points

1. Maternal obesity significantly increases both obstetric and fetal morbidity and is an independent risk factor for maternal mortality.
2. Prepregnancy BMI >40 kg/m^2 and a delivery BMI >45 kg/m^2 are predictive of a higher incidence of anaesthetic complications.
3. Antenatal anaesthetic assessment is recommended for parturients with BMI >40 kg/m^2 at booking.
4. Early epidural placement is recommended during labour. Timing in relation to administration of LMWH may be required.
5. Spinal ultrasound may be helpful in achieving correct placement of central neuroaxial blocks.
6. Prepare for difficult laryngoscopy in the obese parturient with optimal patient positioning and an appropriate airway plan.
7. Meticulous care is required to reduce significant postoperative risks, including respiratory complications, thromboembolism and infections.

Further reading

Association of Anaesthetists of Great Britain and Ireland (2007). *Peri-Operative Management of the Morbidly Obese Patient.* London: AAGBI.

Centre for Maternal and Child Enquires (CMACE) (2010). *Maternal Obesity in the UK: Findings from a national project.* London: CMACE.

Centre for Maternal and Child Enquires (CMACE) (2011). Saving Mothers' Lives: reviewing maternal deaths to make motherhood safer: 2006–2008. The Eighth Report on Confidential Enquires into Maternal Deaths in the United Kingdom. *BJOG*, **118**(1), 1–203.

Chin, K. J., Karmakar, M. K. and Peng, P. (2011). Ultrasonography of the adult thoracic and lumbar spine for central neuraxial blockade. *Anesthesiology*, **114**(6), 1459–1485.

Grau, T., Bartusseck, E., Conradi, R., Martin, E. and Motsch, J. (2003). Ultrasound imaging improves learning curves in obstetric epidural: a preliminary study. *Can. J. Anaesth.*, **50**, 1047–1050.

Grau, T., Leopold, R. W., Fatehi, S., Martin, E. and Motsch, J. (2004). Real time ultrasonic observation of combined spinal-epidural anaesthesia. *Eur. J. Anaesthesiol.*, **21**, 25–31.

Knight, M., Kurinczuk, J. J., Spark, P. and Brocklehurst, P. (2010). Extreme obesity in pregnancy in the United Kingdom. *Obstet. Gynaecol.*, **115**, 989–997.

Labor, E. E. (2012). Analgesia for the obese parturient. *Anaesth. Analg.*, **115**, 889–903.

National Institute for Health and Clinical Excellence (2008). *Ultrasound Guided Catheterization of the Epidural Space.* London: NICE.

Obstetric Anaesthetists' Association. (2013). Information for pregnant women with a high body mass index (BMI). Available on www.oaa-anaes.ac.uk (accessed May 2015).

Endocrine disease in pregnancy, including diabetes mellitus, thyroid and adrenal disease

Jenny Myers and Dan Mallaber

Diabetes

Introduction

Diabetes mellitus (DM) is a common and growing problem, affecting approximately 650,000 pregnancies in England and Wales each year (representing 2–5% of the obstetric population). Women with diabetes have an increased risk of both fetal and maternal complications, and of requiring anaesthetic intervention. Close monitoring and treatment during pregnancy, and careful anaesthetic management during labour and delivery, can reduce these risks and improve outcomes for both mother and baby.

Classification

DM is a multisystem disorder of carbohydrate metabolism, which can result from a number of distinct pathophysiological processes. Around 7.5% of pregnancies complicated by diabetes are due to type 1 and 5% due to type 2 diabetes. Gestational diabetes (GDM) accounts for the remaining 87.5%.

Type 1

Type 1 DM is attributable to an absolute lack of insulin production and secretion by the pancreatic β cells of the Islets of Langerhans. It is primarily an autoimmune disorder, although genetic and environmental factors also play a role. It accounts for around 10% of all DM. There is an association with other autoimmune conditions, including hypothyroidism.

Type 2

Type 2 DM is caused by a combination of both relative lack of insulin secretion and insulin resistance in target tissues. It accounts for 90% of all DM cases

and is primarily associated with obesity. As such, its prevalence in both obstetric and non-obstetric populations is increasing and this is particularly so amongst several ethnic groups (including people of African, black Caribbean, South Asian, Middle Eastern and Chinese family origin).

Gestational diabetes mellitus

Gestational diabetes (GDM) is defined as glucose intolerance, which is first identified during pregnancy. Insulin resistance is known to increase progressively during the second and third trimesters of pregnancy due to an increase in counter-regulatory hormones (including placental lactogen, placental growth hormone, cortisol and progesterone). GDM may therefore be thought of as a preclinical state of glucose intolerance unmasked by the physiological changes in pregnancy. For most mothers glucose levels return to normal, but there is an increased risk of subsequent type 2 diabetes in women diagnosed with GDM.

Diagnosis and screening

The diagnosis of type 1 DM is usually made in adolescence or early adulthood. It is confirmed by a fasting glucose greater than 7 mmol/L, random glucose greater than 11.1 mmol/L or greater than 11.1 mmol/L 2 hours following a 75 g oral glucose tolerance test, and accompanying classical symptoms such as thirst, weight loss, fatigue and polyuria.

Patients with type 2 DM are rarely symptomatic and the diagnosis is usually made during routine screening. The threshold values are the same as for type 1 DM. A glycated haemoglobin (HbA1c) level of greater than 48 mmol/mol is also considered strongly suggestive of DM.

Core Topics in Obstetric Anaesthesia, ed. Kirsty MacLennan, Kate O'Brien and W. Ross Mcnab.
Published by Cambridge University Press. © Cambridge University Press 2015.

Table 19.1 Risk factors for GDM

Previous GDM

BMI > 30 kg/m^2

Previous large baby (>4.5 kg or >95th centile on customized chart)

Parent, brother or sister with diabetes

Family origin (South Asian, Black Caribbean, Middle Eastern)

Screening criteria taken from NICE guidelines 2008

Diagnosis of GDM can be more challenging because of the changes in carbohydrate metabolism that occur normally during pregnancy, and the lack of international consensus on the diagnostic criteria. Universal screening is not currently recommended and screening is currently targeted at women who have risk factors for GDM (see Table 19.1). It is worth noting, however, that one or more of these risk factors is found in 30–50% of the pregnant population in the UK. Screening of high-risk patients currently takes place at between 16 and 18 weeks' gestation for those with previous GDM, and 24–28 weeks for those with other risk factors.

Management

The treatment of women with diabetes begins before pregnancy and includes optimization of glycaemic control and cessation of medications contraindicated in pregnancy (e.g. *angiotensin converting enzyme* (ACE) inhibitors, angiotensin receptor blockers (ARBs), statins) with conversion to alternative antihypertensive medication if required (calcium-channel blockers, β-blockers). High-dose folate (5 mg daily) is recommended preconceptually to reduce the risk of congenital abnormalities, particularly neural tube defects. Early pregnancy assessment of women with pre-existing diabetes should include an assessment of renal function (creatinine and urine protein:creatinine ratio) and referral for retinopathy screening, which should be conducted each trimester. Recent NICE guidelines also recommend low-dose aspirin (75 mg daily) from 12 weeks' gestation to reduce the risk of pre-eclampsia, which is more common in women with diabetes. Low-molecular-weight heparin should be considered in women at increased risk of thrombosis (BMI >40 kg/m^2 and diabetic nephropathy with >3 g proteinuria).

For women with DM, rigorous glycaemic control and close monitoring during pregnancy is associated with improved outcomes for both the woman and her baby. Preconception care and advice should be offered to all women with pre-existing DM. Women with HbA1C >85 mmol/mol should be advised to avoid pregnancy until glycaemic control is improved.

Women with type I diabetes are ideally managed in a joint antenatal diabetes clinic, combining obstetric, diabetic and specialist midwifery care. If safely achievable, then fasting blood glucose levels should be kept between 3.5 and 5.9 mmol/L and 1-hour postprandial blood glucose levels below 7.8 mmol/L during pregnancy. Women should be warned of the significant risk of hypoglycaemia, which may be complicated by reduced hypoglycaemia symptom awareness. Glucagon kits should be made available and insulin therapy adjusted if hypoglycaemia is occurring frequently. Increasingly women with type 1 diabetes are being offered continuous sub-cutaneous insulin infusion (CSII) therapy. To date there is little evidence that use of pumps improves pregnancy outcomes, but it may reduce the frequency of hypoglycaemic episodes. Insulin requirements increase in pregnancy, but may decline in the last few weeks of pregnancy and during labour. Insulin doses should be reduced by approximately 50% following delivery or adjusted to the prepregnancy regime.

Women with type 2 diabetes who have previously been treated with oral hypoglycaemic agents (e.g. metformin, glibenclamide) are usually advised to continue these during their pregnancy, although many women require additional insulin treatment to achieve the rigorous glycaemic control required in pregnancy.

Women with GDM are often able to achieve adequate glycaemic control with dietary adjustments, but 20–30% will require treatment with either metformin or insulin.

Complications

Maternal complications
Acute

Diabetic ketoacidosis (DKA) occurs mainly in patients with Type I DM and is due to either failure to administer sufficient insulin or to the development of a new source of insulin resistance (e.g. infection, trauma, stress). Emesis, steroid and β-blocker use are also important triggers during pregnancy. The lack of insulin favours lipolysis, the β-oxidation of free fatty acids and the formation of acetoacetate. These biochemical events result in metabolic acidosis, hyperglycaemia and an osmotic diuresis. Signs and symptoms of DKA include tachycardia, tachypnoea, hypotension, nausea and vomiting.

The incidence of DKA in pregnancy is between 1% and 2% and occurs most commonly in the second and third trimesters. As with the non-obstetric population, the management of DKA in pregnant patients involves rehydration, control of glucose with an intravenous sliding scale insulin regime and removal/treatment of any precipitating factors. All pregnant patients with DKA should be cared for in a level 2 critical-care facility with input from both medical and obstetric teams.

The hyperosmolar hyperglycaemic state (HHS) occurs predominantly in patients with type 2 DM and is characterized by very high blood glucose levels (frequently >40 mmol/L) without accompanying ketosis. It is rare in pregnancy.

Hypoglycaemia poses a significant risk for pregnant women, occurring in up to two-thirds of patients with pre-existing type 1 DM – a rate up to 15 times higher than in the non-pregnant population. It is most common before 20 weeks' gestation. The intensification of treatment to achieve tight glycaemic control and impairment of the counter-regulatory hormonal responses that accompany insulin therapy are the main causes. Symptoms of hypoglycaemia are non-specific and include abdominal pain, vomiting, weakness, dizziness and drowsiness. These may be absent or reduced in pregnant women who are at an increased risk of hypoglycaemic unawareness. Hypoglycaemia is much less common in women with type 2 DM or GDM.

Chronic

The prevalence of chronic complications generally correlates to the duration of DM and the adequacy of glycaemic control. Atherosclerotic macrovascular complications include disease of the coronary, cerebral and peripheral vasculature. Although rare, myocardial infarction is a potential risk and suspected cardiovascular disease should be thoroughly investigated.

Microvascular complications include diabetic retinopathy and nephropathy. Pregnancy may accelerate the rate of progression of both retinopathy and nephropathy.

Diabetic neuropathy can lead to autonomic cardiovascular dysfunction and gastroparesis. This may be difficult to assess, but in the non-pregnant diabetic patient, prolongation of the QT interval on the ECG correlates with the severity of autonomic dysfunction.

The diabetic stiff joint syndrome (also known as diabetic scleroderma) occurs in patients with long-standing type I DM and is associated with short stature, joint contractures and tight skin.

Obstetric

Rates of gestational hypertension, pre-eclampsia, fetal macrosomia, preterm delivery, induction of labour and caesarean section are all higher in diabetic obstetric patients. Recent studies have suggested that the risk of pre-eclampsia and gestational hypertension can be reduced by optimal glycaemic control during pregnancy.

Pre-existing DM, but not GDM, is associated with a 36% risk of preterm labour and delivery – approximately two to three times the non-diabetic rate. The incidence of early fetal loss, miscarriage and still birth is also higher.

Fetal macrosomia (birth weight >4 kg) complicates up to 50% pregnancies in women with pre-existing diabetes. There is a corresponding increase in the risk of birth trauma and shoulder dystocia. The high rates of macrosomia, along with other obstetric complications such as pre-eclampsia, mean that up to two-thirds of women with diabetes will be delivered by caesarean section. Shoulder dystocia is also more common in women with both pre-existing and gestational diabetes. Warning signs such as slow progress in labour, particularly in the second stage, should be heeded with early recourse to operative delivery where significant fetal macrosomia is suspected.

Neonatal hypoglycaemia is more common, occurring in 5% and 12% of cases of pre-existing DM and GDM, respectively. An increase in fetal insulin production in response to sustained intrauterine fetal hyperglycaemia is thought to be the cause.

Anaesthetic management

Meticulous glycaemic control is the cornerstone of management of women with diabetes. Local multidisciplinary protocols should be developed to cover the treatment of both pre-existing DM and GDM in the intra- and postpartum periods. Ideally, an individualized management plan should be drawn up in advance of delivery.

In labour or prior to caesarean delivery, an intravenous sliding scale insulin regime will be necessary for the majority of women with pre-existing diabetes and for some women with gestational diabetes. Tight glycaemic control in labour can reduce risk and severity of neonatal hypoglycaemia. Insulin requirements may fall dramatically during labour and should be reduced by at least 50% after delivery. Frequent blood glucose measurements (every 30–60 minutes) should be performed to avoid severe maternal hypoglycaemia or hyperglycaemia. Women who require fluid restriction because of severe pre-eclampsia will require a modified regime to reduce infusion volumes.

The anaesthetist should be alert to the possibility of complications related to diabetes, and history and examination should be directed accordingly. For women with long-standing diabetes with known complications, antenatal anaesthetic review is desirable.

Autonomic cardiovascular dysfunction increases the possibility of hypotension during neuraxial blockade. More frequent blood pressure measurement, judicious use of vasopressors and vigorous IV hydration may be required. In severe cases, use of continuous intra-arterial blood pressure measurement should be considered. Gastroparesis increases the risk of regurgitation and aspiration. Antacid prophylaxis should be prescribed regularly during labour.

Women with type 1 diabetes and the diabetic stiff joint syndrome may suffer from limited movement of the atlanto-occipital joint. Direct laryngoscopy and tracheal intubation may be more difficult. This is in addition to the increased incidence of difficult intubation present in the non-pregnant type 1 diabetic population. The 'prayer sign' (an inability to approximate the palmar surfaces of the phalangeal joints when the hands are bought together as if praying and despite maximum effort) has been suggested as a screening test for difficult intubation. The stiff joint syndrome is also associated with a reduction in compliance of the epidural space. Smaller volumes of local anaesthetic may be required to avoid an unexpectedly high block.

With the above in mind, epidural or combined spinal-epidural (CSE) anaesthesia may be preferred over single-shot spinal technique because of the slower onset of sympathetic blockade and the greater degree of control that it affords.

Finally, diabetic patients are at an increased risk of infection. Strict aseptic technique must be used during all procedures and surgical antibiotic prophylaxis as dictated by local guidelines given in theatre.

Thyroid disease

Thyroid disease is common in women of childbearing age and hypo- and hyperthyroidism complicate up to 4% of pregnancies. Its presence has implications for the mother and the developing fetus. An understanding of the diagnosis, treatment, and the metabolic and anatomical changes that may accompany thyroid disease are important to allow safe management in the puerperium.

Thyroid gland and pregnancy

During pregnancy there is an oestrogen-mediated increase in the plasma binding protein thyroxine-binding globulin (TBG). This occurs up to around 20 weeks' gestation, after which levels plateau. TBG binds most circulating tri-iodothyronine (T3) and thyroxine (T4), and total levels of these show a corresponding increase during pregnancy. It is the unbound ('free') T4, however, that generally determines thyroid activity in target tissues, and this remains unchanged, or falls slightly, during pregnancy. Normal pregnancy is, therefore, a clinically euthyroid state.

T3 and T4 are synthesized in the follicular cells of the thyroid gland from dietary iodine. The amount of iodine available falls in pregnancy due to a combination of fetal iodine uptake and enhanced maternal renal clearance. Iodine deficiency may ensue in areas where intake is low and lead to a reactive hyperplasia of the thyroid gland (goitre).

Hyperthyroidism

Hyperthyroidism is diagnosed by finding a raised serum concentration of free T4. Causes are shown in Table 19.2. Measurement of thyroid stimulating hormone (TSH), TSH receptor antibodies (TSH-RAb), ultrasound examination and fine needle aspiration may be needed to help differentiate the exact pathophysiology.

Symptoms are related to the increase in basal metabolic rate and include a hyperdynamic circulation, tachyarrhythmias, nervousness, sweating, tremor, weakness, diarrhoea and changes in appetite.

In pregnancy, direct stimulation of the thyroid gland by human chorionic gonadotrophin (hCG) can result in transient gestational thyrotoxicosis.

Table 19.2 Causes of hyperthyroidism

Overstimulation:
- Graves' disease
- TSH secreting pituitary tumour
- Gestational trophoblastic neoplasia

Intrinsic thyroid over-activity:
- Toxic adenoma
- Toxic multinodular goitre

Inflammation:
- Sub-acute thyroiditis

Other:
- Ectopic thyroid tissue
- Thyroxine ingestion

In the absence of symptoms, mild biochemical hyperthyroidism should be monitored with repeat thyroid function tests (TFTs) and referral to an endocrinologist made only if the derangement persists beyond 4–6 weeks.

Graves' disease accounts for 70% to 90% of cases of overt hyperthyroidism in pregnancy, followed by toxic multinodular goitre and toxic adenoma. Graves' disease is an autoimmune disorder with a multifactorial aetiology. Autoantibodies are directed against the TSH receptor and usually augment (although may inhibit) its action. Some patients may also develop Graves' eye disease with exopthalmus, proptosis and irritation. Graves' disease has an association with other autoimmune conditions.

Thyroid nodules are common amongst the general population and may increase in size and number during pregnancy.

Treatment of hyperthyroidism may be medical, surgical or a combination, and aims to keep free T4 normal or in the upper range of normal throughout pregnancy. The drug of choice for most women in pregnancy is propythiouracil, although carbimazole can also be used. Propythiouracil interferes with synthesis of T3 and T4 in the thyroid gland and inhibits peripheral conversion of T3 to the more active T4. Both can cross the placenta and potentially impair fetal thyroid function and cause fetal goitre, so the lowest effective dose should be used. The dose may be reduced after the first trimester and often discontinued in the third trimester.

Surgery, in the form of total or sub-total thyroidectomy, is usually reserved for patients who have failed medical therapy. It is generally considered safe

from the second trimester onwards. Radioiodine therapy is contraindicated in pregnancy.

Uncontrolled hyperthyroidism is associated with a number of maternal and fetal complications. Pre-eclampsia, preterm labour, miscarriage and placental abruption are all more common. TSH-RAbs are able to cross the placenta and may lead to fetal tachycardia, growth retardation, low birth and congenital malformations. Very high titres of TSH-RAbs are associated with an increased risk of fetal intrauterine or neonatal thyrotoxicosis.

Severe cases of untreated or under-treated hyperthyroidism may result in a thyroid storm. This is a life-threatening exacerbation of hyperthyroidism, which can lead to hyperpyrexia, cardiac failure, coma and death.

Anaesthetic management

The management of patients with hyperthyroidism involves giving careful consideration to both the metabolic effects of the disease and the possibility of partial airway obstruction secondary to an enlarged thyroid gland.

Surgery in the presence of uncontrolled hyperthyroidism carries a risk of precipitating a thyroid storm and a high mortality. If time allows, the goal should be to render the patient euthyroid. In the emergency situation, treatment involves supportive measures (cooling, oxygen, fluid and electrolyte replacement), reduction of synthesis and peripheral conversion of thyroid hormones (propothiouracil, glucocorticoids, sodium iodide) and amelioration of the metabolic effects (β-blockers). Drugs associated with tachycardia should be avoided.

Both general and neuraxial anaesthesia have been used safely. The decision must be made on an individual patient basis, taking into account such factors as the presence and severity of any airway compromise, cardiac involvement and electrolyte disturbance.

Patients with hyperthyroidism have a relative deficiency of glucocorticoids and should be given supplementation. Care should be taken to protect the eyes and prevent corneal abrasions during general anaesthesia in those with Graves' eye disease and exophthalmus.

Hypothyroidism

Hypothyroidism is diagnosed by finding a low level of free T4. The causes can be split into primary and secondary and are shown in Table 19.3. Hashimoto's

Table 19.3 Causes of hypothyroidism

Primary

Autoimmune:

- Hashimoto's thyroiditis
- Atrophic thyroiditis

Iatrogenic:

- Thyroid surgery
- Radio-iodine therapy

Drug-induced:

- Antithyroid drugs (propothiouracil, methimazole)
- Amiodarone
- Lithium

Congenital:

- Dyshormonogenesis
- Thyroid dysgenesis or agenesis

Other:

- Iodine deficiency

Secondary

Pituitary dysfunction:

- Radiotherapy
- Surgery
- Neoplasm
- Sheehan's syndrome

Hypothalamic dysfunction:

- Radiotherapy
- Neoplasm
- Granulomatous disease

disease (autoimmune thyroiditis) is the most common cause in women of childbearing age.

Symptoms can be vague and include fatigue, weight gain, muscle cramps, constipation and memory problems. Women with hypothyroidism also have lower fertility rates. Sub-clinical hypothyroidism is relatively common in the pregnant population and may be picked up by antenatal screening programmes.

During pregnancy, untreated hypothyroidism is associated with an increased risk of anaemia, pre-eclampsia, abruption, miscarriage, low birth weight and postpartum haemorrhage. The growing fetus is dependent on maternal thyroxine, particularly during the first half of the pregnancy, and hypothyroidism at this stage can adversely affect neuropsychological development. Outcomes for both mother and fetus are improved with treatment.

Medical management is with oral thyroxine replacement until the patient is clinically and biochemically

euthyroid. Requirements may change during pregnancy and regular TSH measurements are needed to allow appropriate dose titration.

Anaesthetic management

As with hyperthyroidism, the patient should ideally be clinically and biochemically euthyroid before any anaesthetic intervention. History, examination and investigations should focus on identifying the potentially more serious consequences of prolonged or untreated hypothyroidism. These can include myocardial dysfunction, coronary artery disease and obstructive sleep apnoea. In the emergency situation, glucocorticoid supplementation should be given to the untreated patient as, like those with hyperthyroidism, there is a decrease in glucocorticoid reserves and hyponatraemia. Intravenous thyroxine is rarely indicated and its use carries a risk of precipitating myocardial ischaemia.

Hypothyroidism is a rare cause of acquired von Willebrand's disease and untreated hypothyroidism can result in abnormal platelet function, despite normal platelet levels. Laboratory and/or near-patient testing of coagulation should therefore be performed before administering neuraxial anaesthesia. Patients may show a blunted response to phenylephrine.

Any patient with a goitre requires careful assessment of the airway and neck to check for retrosternal spread or evidence of tracheal deviation. A chest radiograph may be helpful. The history should include the duration of swelling (long-standing goitre is associated with tracheomalacia) and symptoms such as stridor or breathlessness, which may indicate dynamic tracheal compression. Patients who have had previous thyroid surgery, or who have malignant disease may suffer from vocal cord palsy.

Adrenal disease

Adrenal disorders (including congenital adrenal hyperplasia, Addison's disaease, pheochromocytoma and Cushing's disease) frequently have a negative impact on fertility and so are relatively uncommon in pregnancy. Undiagnosed and untreated disease can have serious consequences for maternal and fetal health with maternal mortality rates historically approaching 50% for untreated Addison's disease or pheochromocytoma.

Proper diagnosis and treatment of adrenal dysfunction with steroid therapy or surgery can dramatically improve outcomes and lead to successful pregnancy and delivery. As always, patients are best managed in joint obstetric endocrine clinics by those with experience in their management.

Addison's disease

Addison's disease, or primary adrenal insufficiency, is most commonly caused by autoimmune adrenalitis, but can also be the result of infection, haemorrhage, metastases or genetic causes. New onset disease in pregnancy is rare. Symptoms are vague and include weight loss, weakness, fatigue, nausea, diarrhoea and postural hypotension. These can easily be mistaken for symptoms of pregnancy itself or associated conditions such as hyperemesis gravidum.

Patients with known disease are initially maintained on their preconception doses of gluco- and mineralocorticoids with regular electrolyte monitoring throughout the antenatal period. In normal pregnancy, cortisol levels rise due to increased levels of corticosteroid-binding globulin and decreased clearance. Doses of glucocorticoids may therefore need to be increased in the third trimester for some patients. Intravenous steroids and hydration should be considered in any patient suffering from nausea and vomiting. Mineralocorticoids should be stopped if the patient develops pre-eclampsia.

Severe adrenal insufficiency is known as an Addisonian crisis and is a potentially life-threatening medical emergency. It may be the result of previously undiagnosed Addison's or due to an intercurrent stress (e.g. infection, trauma, labour) in someone with known disease. Signs include hypotension, hyponatraemia, hypoglycaemia, hyperkalaemia, hypercalaemia, psychosis and convulsions. Treatment is with IV steroids, IV hydration with saline and dextrose and correction of the underlying cause (if any). Hyperkalaemia should be treated with dextrose and insulin.

Patients with well-controlled Addison's should receive an increased dose of parenteral steroids for labour or caesarean delivery (e.g. 100 mg hydrocortisone IV QDS) and IV saline. After delivery, doses can be tapered back to maintenance over 3 days.

Congenital adrenal hyperplasia

Congenital adrenal hyperplasia (CAH) refers to a heterogenous group of autosomal recessive disorders that affect the enzymes controlling the synthesis of cortisol from cholesterol. The majority (90%) of cases are due to 21-hydroxlase deficiency with 11-β-hydroxylase deficiency accounting for a further 5–8%. Clinical features can include precocious puberty, virilization and ambiguous genitalia in some females.

The treatment of choice for pregnant women with CAH is steroid replacement with glucocorticoids, which can be inactivated by the placenta (hydrocortisone, prednisone, methylprednisolone) to minimize the risk of fetal adrenal suppression. If the fetus is at risk from CAH, then dexamethasone, which easily crosses the placenta, may be used to prevent masculinization of the genitalia of female infants. Mineralocorticoids (fludrocortisone) can be added in those patients with the salt-wasting form of the disease.

High-dose glucocorticoid therapy (e.g. hydrocortisone 50–100 mg IV QDS) should be initiated at the start of active labour, continued until after delivery and then tapered back down to the patient's normal maintenance dose. Elective caesarean delivery should be considered for patients who have undergone previous reconstructive genital surgery. Electrolytes should be measured prior to anaesthesia and disturbances corrected. Good hydration should be maintained, if necessary with 0.9% saline IV.

Pheochromocytoma

Pheochromocytomas are rare catecholamine-secreting neuroendocrine tumours of chromaffin cells; 90% occur within the adrenal medulla, the other 10% arising from extra-adrenal chromaffin tissue. It is thought to complicate only around 1 in 50,000 pregnancies.

The classical presentation is with paroxysms of headache, sweating, palpitations and anxiety associated with severe hypertension. Patients may have postural hypotension and dizziness on standing due to a contracted intravascular volume. Hypertension is common in pregnancy and so it is possible for the diagnosis to be overlooked.

Raised levels of catecholamines in a 24-hour urine sample confirm the condition with a high level of sensitivity and specificity. Catecholamine levels do not change in pregnancy and so the biochemical diagnosis is no different from a women who is not pregnant. Once confirmed, the tumour is localized using MRI or ultrasound examination if pregnant, to avoid ionizing radiation.

Surgical removal is the definitive treatment for pheochromocytoma and should ideally take place prior to 24 weeks' gestation. After this time the gravid uterus may make surgical exploration of the abdomen and tumour removal difficult. The choice may then be to defer surgery until the fetus is mature and consider adrenalectomy immediately after caesarean delivery.

Whatever the timing of surgery, preoperative management aims to control blood pressure, correct volume depletion and prevent intraoperative hypertensive crises. This is usually achieved using α-adrenergic blockade (e.g. with phenoxybenzamine or doxazocin, both of which are safe in pregnancy) for 10–14 days prior to surgery to allow time for volume expansion. β-Blockade should not be used without adequate α-blockade to avoid the risk of unopposed α-adrenergic activity leading to a hypertensive crisis. Expert help should be sought in the obstetric, surgical and anaesthetic management of the pregnant patient diagnosed with pheochromocytoma.

The condition still carries a significant risk to mother and fetus. Maternal mortality is around 2% if the condition is diagnosed antenatally, but rises to between 4% and 17% if diagnosed during pregnancy, with a fetal mortality of up to 26%. Unrecognized pheochromocytoma carries a significantly higher mortality and the diagnosis may not be made until post mortem.

Cushing's syndrome

Cushing's syndrome occurs very rarely in pregnancy because of the impact on fertility caused by hypercortisolism. The spectrum of disease changes, with adrenal adenomas more commonly the cause rather than the pituitary-dependent disease that predominates in the general population. Diagnosis is made difficult because of the previously mentioned changes in cortisol levels during pregnancy. The low dose dexamethasone suppression test is also inaccurate in the presence of high levels of oestrogens.

GDM occurs in up to a third of patients with Cushing's disease and rates of pregnancy-induced hypertension are increased. Severe hypertension and congestive cardiac failure may occur in up to 10% of patients. Premature delivery occurs in two-thirds of cases, with a neonatal mortality rate of around 15%.

Both adrenalectomy (usually early in the second trimester) and trans-sphenoidal hypophysectomy have been successfully reported in pregnant patients. Steroid replacement should be started immediately after surgery and the mother and neonate monitored for signs of cortisol withdrawal.

Anaesthetic management may be complicated by obesity, poor venous access, an increased risk of difficult intubation and of impaired respiratory muscle function in the postoperative period due to proximal myopathy.

Vaginal delivery is preferable to caesarean delivery because of the increased incidence of poor wound healing and wound breakdown in patients with Cushing's.

Key points

1. Diabetes is associated with higher rates of gestational hypertension, pre-eclampsia, polyhydramnios, shoulder dystocia, caesarean section and increased risk of fetal anomalies.

2. Insulin resistance increases progressively through the second and third trimester, largely due to an increase in hormones like human placental lactogen, cortisol and progesterone.

3. Gestational diabetes is defined by glucose intolerance, which is first identified during pregnancy.

4. In pregnancy, direct stimulation of the thyroid gland by human chorionic gonadotrophin can result in transient thyrotoxicosis.

5 Thyroid surgery during pregnancy is usually reserved for patients who have had failed medical therapy.

6. Undiagnosed and untreated adrenal disease can have serious consequences for maternal and fetal health. Correct and early diagnosis, appropriate treatment of adrenal dysfunction, steroid therapy or surgery can significantly improve outcomes.

Further reading

Wissner, R. N. (2014). Endocrine disorders. In D. H. Chestnut (ed.), *Obstetric Anaesthesia, Principles and Practice*, 5th edn. Elsevier, 1003–1032.

National Institute for Health and Clinical Excellence (2008). *Diabetes in Pregnancy: Management of Diabetes and its Complications from Pre-conception to the Postnatal Period.* CG63. London: NICE.

Centre for Maternal and Child Enquires (2010). *The CEMACH/OAA Diabetes Project: A national audit of anaesthetic records and care for women with type 1 or type 2 diabetes undergoing caesarean section.* London: CMACE.

Royal College of Obstetricians and Gynaecologists (2011). *Diagnosis and Treatment of Gestational Diabetes.* Scientific Impact Paper No. 23. London: RCOG.

Chapter 20

Renal disease

Jessica Longbottom and W. Ross Macnab

Introduction

Chronic renal insufficiency occurs in 0.03–0.2% of all pregnancies. Although rare, these parturients have a significantly increased maternal and fetal morbidity and mortality and can present a significant challenge to the anaesthetist. The management of this high-risk group of patients is often complicated and is supported by little evidence. It requires an understanding of the physiological changes of pregnancy, the optimization of existing management, close monitoring of both mother and fetus, and early involvement of obstetricians, nephrologists, neonatologists and anaesthetists, with early intervention as required.

Renal insufficiency in pregnancy may be classified into three categories. These include known pre-existing renal disease diagnosed prior to the pregnancy, sub-clinical chronic renal disease unveiled by the pregnancy or new-onset disease that develops during the pregnancy. Although general principles can be applied to the management of these patients, the causes, associated co-morbidities and prognosis of these patients may differ greatly.

It is important to consider both the impact of renal insufficiency upon maternal and fetal outcome, and the impact of a pregnancy upon the short- and long-term course of chronic kidney disease. These patients have an increased risk of pregnancy-induced hypertension, pre-eclampsia, preterm delivery, intrauterine growth restriction and perinatal mortality. The demands of pregnancy may result in a transient, and sometimes a permanent decline in renal function.

The assessment of renal function in pregnancy

Pregnancy itself results in anatomical and physiological changes in the renal system (See Chapter 1).

Changes in water metabolism, extracellular fluid volume regulation, acid–base regulation and the renal handling of electrolytes, protein and glucose result in altered 'normal ranges' of typical laboratory values. These values continue to change from the first to the second and third trimesters. This complicates the diagnosis, assessment and surveillance of renal insufficiency. The gold standard for measuring and therefore monitoring renal function remains inulin clearance, but it is difficult to perform. Creatinine clearance measured with a 24-hour urine collection is the most well-validated method for approximating glomerular filtration rate (GFR). Formulaic estimations of GFR lack validity in pregnancy.

GFR and creatinine clearance typically increase by 40–65% and serum creatinine concentrations fall. It has been suggested that the upper limit of serum creatinine concentration should approximate 85, 80 and 90 mol/L in the first, second and third trimesters, respectively. A blood urea nitrogen concentration of >13 mg/dL may also indicate renal insufficiency in pregnancy.

The associated increase in urinary protein excretion also results in an altered definition of proteinuria during pregnancy of greater than 300 mg/day (correlating to 1+ on urine dipstick) compared to a nonpregnant value of 150 mg/day.

For these reasons the usual prepregnancy NICE classification of the stages of chronic kidney disease (Table 20.1) is difficult to apply during pregnancy, yet it remains a useful tool when considering a patient's prepregnancy values. Traditionally parturients have been stratified into mild impairment serum creatinine <125 μmol/L, moderate 125–250 μmol/L and severe >250 μmol/L.

Core Topics in Obstetric Anaesthesia, ed. Kirsty MacLennan, Kate O'Brien and W. Ross Mcnab.
Published by Cambridge University Press. © Cambridge University Press 2015.

Table 20.1 Stages of chronic kidney disease

Stage[a]	GFR (mL/min/1.73 m^2)	Description
1	≥ 90	Normal or increased GFR with other evidence of kidney damage
2	60–89	Slight decrease in GFR with other evidence of kidney damage
3a	45–59	Moderate decrease in GFR with or without other evidence of kidney
3b	30–44	damage
4	15–29	Severe decrease in GFR with or without other evidence of kidney damage
5	<15	Established renal failure

[a] Use suffix (p) to denote presence of proteinuria (protein creatinine ratio ≥ 50 mg/mmol)

Chronic kidney disease in pregnancy

There are many causes of CKD in women of child-bearing age, all of which will be seen in pregnancy. The most common include diabetic nephropathy, hypertensive nephropathy, chronic glomerulonephritis, systemic lupus nephritis, polycystic kidney disease and chronic pyelonephritis among many rarer causes. The underlying pathology and its associated systemic co-morbidities, as well as the systemic manifestations of chronic renal impairment itself provide significant challenges to the anaesthetist. The risk of adverse outcome to either mother or fetus does not appear to be related to the specific underlying disorder, but to the degree of renal impairment and the presence or absence of hypertension.

The effect of pregnancy on kidney disease

Pregnancy can exacerbate pre-existing renal disease and, in some cases, can cause irreversible deterioration in renal function. Adverse outcomes tend to relate to the degree of maternal renal function and blood pressure control. The pathogenesis is not clearly evident, but altered immune function, increased inflammation, endothelial dysfunction and platelet aggregation resulting in microvascular thrombi have all been implicated.

Proteinuria and associated peripheral oedema worsens in approximately 50% of cases and hypertension may develop or worsen in 25% of cases. These features frequently resolve post partum.

Evidence suggests that patients with a normal or only mildly reduced GFR and a serum creatinine concentration less than 132 µmol/L have a less than 10% risk of a permanent decline in renal function as a consequence of pregnancy. The presence of hypertension in this group of patients gives a poorer prognosis. Patients with moderate renal insufficiency, a serum creatinine concentration between 132 and 255 µmol/L, are likely to experience an initial fall in serum creatinine concentration as GFR increases, but this will continue to rise up to and beyond the baseline by the third trimester. These patients have approximately a 50% risk of a permanent reduction in GFR and a 10% risk of developing end-stage renal disease within 12 months of delivery. This figure may increase to 50% if there is associated uncontrolled hypertension. In severe renal failure the likelihood of conception and carrying a fetus to term is very low. Up to 40% of these patients will require dialysis. It is important to note that pregnancy may result in immune sensitization and potential difficulties for future donor matching should renal transplant be indicated. CKD also increases the risk of urinary tract infection, which in turn may cause a rapid deterioration in renal function. Co-existing pre-eclampsia is also associated with subsequent progression to end-stage renal disease.

The prevention of deterioration of renal function in these patients relies upon close surveillance by a multidisciplinary team, monthly serial monitoring of maternal renal function, early detection and treatment of asymptomatic bacteriuria and aggressive treatment of maternal hypertension. Although the management of hypertension is important, many antihypertensives are contraindicated in pregnancy. Labetalol, α-methyldopa and nifedipine are considered safe. Preterm delivery may be necessary to preserve long-term kidney function.

The effect of kidney disease on pregnancy outcomes

A large systematic review demonstrated a fivefold higher incidence of maternal morbidity and twofold higher incidence of fetal morbidity in the presence of maternal CKD.

Patients with CKD are more likely to develop gestational hypertension, pre-eclampsia and eclampsia. Preterm deliveries are around twice as common and there is a recognized association with intrauterine growth restriction and still birth. Again the risks of maternal and fetal complications seem to be directly proportional to the degree of renal impairment and are further increased by the presence of uncontrolled hypertension. Patients with mildly reduced GFR and well-controlled blood pressure have very favourable outcomes. However, there may be as high as a 20–30% and 40% increased risk of pre-eclampsia in patients with moderate and severe renal insufficiency, respectively. In this situation, the diagnosis of pre-eclampsia is often difficult. The presence of hypertension at the time of conception increases the risk of fetal loss by up to tenfold. Significant proteinuria is also associated with an increased risk of preterm delivery.

These patients may require weekly antenatal reviews, with close monitoring of blood pressure to allow the early diagnosis and treatment of co-existing pre-eclampsia, in addition to aggressive management of pre-existing hypertension. Fetal growth and well-being should be monitored.

The systemic manifestations of chronic kidney disease

Chronic kidney disease is a multisystem disorder with far-reaching systemic manifestations. These may occur irrespective of the underlying pathology and have implications in the antenatal, intrapartum and peri-operative anaesthetic management of these patients (Table 20.2).

Common underlying chronic renal disorders

Diabetic nephropathy

Diabetes, gestational or otherwise, is one of the most common diseases occurring in pregnancy. Diabetic nephropathy most frequently occurs in those in whom type 1 diabetes has been present for over 10 years and is characterized by proteinuria,

Table 20.2 The systemic manifestations of CKD

Cardiovascular system	Hypertension, ischaemic heart disease, peripheral vascular disease, aortic calcification, calcific valvular heart lesions, uraemic pericarditis, cardiomyopathy
Respiratory system	Potential difficult airway, pulmonary oedema, atelectasis and infection
Haematological system	Normochromic normocytic anaemia, platelet dysfunction Low/normal platelet count
Immune system	Immunosuppression, risk of hepatitis B and C
Gastrointestinal system	Delayed gastric emptying, reduced gastric pH, malnutrition
Neurological system	Myoclonus, encephalopathy, convulsions, autonomic neuropathy, peripheral neuropathies
Endocrine system	Impaired glucose tolerance, tendency towards hypothermia, reduced fertility
Fluid and electrolytes	Hyperkalaemia, hyponatraemia, hypocalcaemia, renal osteodystrophy, hypermagnesaemia
Acid–base regulation	Chronic metabolic acidosis, poor buffering capability
Pharmacokinetic changes	Reduced protein binding Accumulation of renally excreted drugs

hypertension and a reduced GFR. Patients with good glycaemic control, microalbuminuria, well-preserved renal function and well-controlled blood pressure are likely to have a successful outcome. However, patients with overt nephropathy preconception are at increased risk of pre-eclampsia, fetal growth restriction, preterm delivery and irreversible deterioration in renal function.

The principles of management include preconception assessment of nephropathy, patient counselling and optimization of glycaemic control. Hypertension should be controlled with labetalol, α-methyldopa or calcium-channel blockers such as nifedipine. Close monitoring should continue throughout pregnancy. Good intrapartum glycaemic control and fluid balance are important.

Systemic lupus nephritis

Systemic lupus erythematosus (SLE) is a common autoimmune disorder in women of childbearing age. The associated nephritis presents unique challenges in pregnancy.

Lupus nephritis may have spontaneous exacerbations during pregnancy, which are associated with a 75% chance of fetal loss. The presence of active disease at the time or within six months of conception and the duration of disease significantly increase the risk of an exacerbation during pregnancy. It remains unclear whether pregnancy itself is a risk factor for lupus flares.

A lupus flare is characterized by deteriorating renal function, hypertension, worsening proteinuria and thrombocytopenia, making it difficult to distinguish from pre-eclampsia, a condition which may also co-exist. Presentation prior to 20 weeks' gestation or the presence of hypocomplementaemia, urinary red blood cell casts, a typical rash, arthritis or serositis make lupus nephritis more likely. The mainstay of the management is general supportive care and immunosuppression with steroids and azathioprine, which may exacerbate pre-eclampsia. When stabilization is not achieved, delivery may be indicated.

SLE is associated with the presence of antiphospholipid antibodies, which increase the risk of both lupus flares and thrombotic events such as deep vein thrombosis, pulmonary embolism, myocardial infarction and stroke. Patients should undergo preconception antibody screening. When antibodies are present patients should receive aspirin prophylaxis with additional heparin if there is a history of thrombotic events.

Chronic glomerulonephritis

None of the histological sub-types of glomerulonephritis appear to be associated with a particularly good or poor prognosis. The severity of renal impairment and presence of hypertension are useful prognostic factors.

Polycystic kidney disease

Autosomal dominant polycystic kidney disease (ADPKD) is often asymptomatic, with renal function preserved until well after childbearing age. However, there is an increased risk of urinary tract infection, hypertension, oedema and pre-eclampsia. Associated liver cysts may enlarge during pregnancy, but liver function is usually preserved. Due to the association of ADPKD with cerebral aneurysms antenatal screening should be considered.

Chronic pyelonephritis

Chronic pyelonephritis often worsens during pregnancy. Urinary tract abnormalities such as vesicoureteric reflux are a common feature. Prophylactic antibiotics, high fluid intake and regular screening for bacteruria minimize deterioration.

New diagnosis of chronic kidney disease in pregnancy

The increased monitoring of the pregnant patient combined with the anatomical and physiological changes that occur in pregnancy may lead sub-clinical renal impairment to become clinically detectable for the first time. Superimposed obstetric disorders such as pre-eclampsia may unveil underlying renal disease.

Renal diseases most commonly diagnosed in this way include immunoglobulin A nephropathy, focal and segmental glomerulosclerosis, polycystic kidney disease and reflux nephropathy. Investigations that may aid diagnosis include ultrasonography and renal biopsy. Renal biopsy is often deferred to the postnatal period due to the increased risk of complications secondary to increased renal blood flow and difficult patient positioning. However, a sudden unexplained deterioration in function or marked nephrotic syndrome prior to 32 weeks' gestation may warrant a biopsy. Once the diagnosis has been made, close monitoring by the multidisciplinary team, including regular assessment of blood indices, proteinuria and protein:creatinine ratio is essential.

Acute kidney injury in pregnancy

Acute kidney injury requiring dialysis occurs in 1 in 20,000 pregnancies in Europe and North America. In the developing world, 20% of AKI cases are pregnancy related and there is an incidence of AKI of up to 1 in 50 pregnancies. AKI is a significant cause of maternal mortality, with little overall change of the mortality figures in the developed world quoted between 0 and 30% and a figure of up to 50% in the developing world. It is suggested by an acute deterioration in renal function, reduced GFR, rise in serum creatinine, symptoms of uraemia, hyperkalaemia, hyponatraemia and metabolic acidosis often, but not always, associated with oliguria. In the general population the RIFLE criteria have been used to define three stages

Table 20.3 RIFLE criteria for AKI

Grade	GFR criteria	Urine output
Risk	Creatinine ×1.5; GFR reduced >25%	UO <0.5 mL/kg/h for 6 h
Injury	Creatinine ×2; GFR reduced >50%	UO <0.5 mL/kg/h for 12 h
Failure	Creatinine ×3; GFR reduced >75%	UO <0.3 mL/kg/h for 24 h or anuria for 12 h
Loss	Loss of function >4 weeks	
End stage	Loss of function >3 months	

of severity of acute renal dysfunction and two potential outcomes (Table 20.3).

Any cause of AKI that occurs in the non-pregnant population may also cause AKI in the pregnant population. There are, however, specific pregnancy-related conditions, occurring in both early and late pregnancy, which may result in AKI. AKI in early pregnancy is most commonly due to hyperemesis gravidarum or septic abortion. Most cases of AKI occur after 35 weeks' gestation and may be caused by severe pre-eclampsia or HELLP syndrome, major obstetric haemorrhage, acute fatty liver of pregnancy, urinary tract obstruction, acute pyelonephritis or exposure to nephrotoxins. The principles of management are to identify and correct any reversible cause, careful fluid management and the early use of renal replacement therapy although this may necessitate delivery. Outcome of AKI will depend on cause and supportive treatments provided. When causes are reversible function often recovers in 3–4 weeks. However, if bilateral cortical necrosis has occurred, recovery will be limited. Full renal recovery is reported in up to 60–90% of obstetric cases.

Thrombotic microangiopathy

Although rare, thrombotic microangiopathies (TMA), such as thombotic thrombocytopaenic purpura (TTP) and haemolytic uraemic syndrome (HUS), are associated with significant morbidity and are difficult to distinguish from severe pre-eclampsia, HELLP syndrome and acute fatty liver of pregnancy. TMA is defined by the occurrence of thrombi of fibrin and/or platelets in the microvasculature of various organs, mainly the kidney and brain. Other pathological features can affect endothelial cells and basement membranes. In more recent times there has been a better understanding of different mechanisms of causation and the chance for improved management strategies.

TTP and HUS are characterized by unexplained thrombocytopaenia, microangiopathic anaemia and renal failure. Associated hypertension, proteinuria, elevated liver enzymes or disseminated intravascular coagulation (DIC) indicate a probable alternative diagnosis. The dominance of either neurological features or renal failure suggests a diagnosis of TTP and HUS, respectively. The timing of onset is also an important distinguishing factor, with TTP occurring in the second and third trimester, HUS usually occurring post partum and severe pre-eclampsia and HELLP occurring after 20 weeks' gestation. Renal failure associated with severe pre-eclampsia will most likely resolve spontaneously, unlike in TTP-HUS where renal replacement therapy and resultant end-stage renal disease are common. The mainstay of treatment is plasma exchange.

Acute tubular necrosis

Can occur due to hypotension, prolonged volume depletion and vasoconstriction and can be secondary to other pathologies: PET, HELLP syndrome, sepsis. Exposure to nephrotoxins or ischaemic injury secondary to prerenal failure may result in acute tubular necrosis. In severe obstetric haemorrhage, acute cortical necrosis with DIC may occur, which can require renal replacement therapy.

Acute fatty liver of pregnancy

This rare cause of acute kidney injury occurs in late pregnancy and is associated with rapidly progressive liver failure, elevated liver enzymes, elevated bilirubin, hypofibrinogenaemia, anaemia, thrombocytopaenia and deranged coagulation, and up to 40% of patients can develop AKI. Delivery is often indicated and renal function usually recovers.

Urinary tract obstruction

It is important to exclude any potential postrenal cause of AKI. Relaxation of smooth muscle and ureteric obstruction by the gravid uterus frequently results in a functional hydronephrosis, particularly affecting the right side, but rarely results in renal

Table 20.4 Dialysis in pregnancy

	Method of delivery	Potential complications
Haemodialysis	5–7 sessions per week, total 20 h per week Slow ultrafiltration rate to avoid hypotension Minimal heparinization	Risk of cardiovascular instability and reduced uteroplacental perfusion Continuous fetal heart rate monitoring required Difficult to establish target weight
Peritoneal dialysis	Increased frequency with reduced exchange volumes	Abdominal fullness and discomfort Catheter problems Polyhydramnios and placental abruption

failure. The presence of large uterine fibroids or renal calculi may result in obstructive renal impairment. Most calculi will pass spontaneously, but cystoscopy and stent insertion may be required.

The dialysis patient

Dialysis patients have a reduced fertility. Over 85% of women deliver before 36 weeks' gestation and the frequency of live births is reduced to only 30–60%. Associated pre-eclampsia is the greatest risk factor for an adverse perinatal outcome. Other poor prognostic factors include maternal age >35 years and more than 5 years on dialysis.

The management of these patients requires a multidisciplinary approach with close maternal and fetal surveillance. The intensification of peritoneal dialysis (PD) and haemodialysis (HD) must be significantly increased during pregnancy to maintain a predialysis serum urea concentration below 20 mmol/L and avoid metabolic acidosis. Both PD and HD have comparable perinatal outcomes; however, there are complications associated with both (Table 20.4).

Careful attention must be paid to nutrition, particularly increasing daily protein intake (1.2 g per kg body weight), calcium and vitamin D supplementation. Concurrent anaemia requires iron and folic acid supplementation and erythropoietin. Hypertension should be aggressively managed. Antihypertensives contraindicated in pregnancy must be stopped (e.g. ACE inhibitors, angiotensin receptor blockers) and replaced with labetalol, metoprolol, nifedipine or methyldopa.

Specific anaesthetic considerations when caring for the dialysis parturient are similar to that in the general population. Arteriovenous fistulas must be protected with appropriate positioning and padding, and avoidance of intravenous access and blood pressure monitoring on that arm. Peripartum blood loss on a background of anaemia should be anticipated and cross-matched blood products and cell salvage be available as necessary. The increased frequency of dialysis in pregnancy usually means the patient has undergone dialysis within the previous 24–48 hours. Patients on haemodialysis may have residual heparin that prohibits a neuraxial technique. Thromboelastography in combination with routine tests of coagulation may be reassuring and support a neuraxial technique. It is important to assess the intravascular volume of these patients prior to any anaesthetic intervention as this may significantly fluctuate between dialysis. Patient weight compared to dry weight, heart rate, the presence of postural hypotension and urine output (if not usually anuric) are useful indicators of hypovolaemia. Hypovolaemia in the presence of autonomic neuropathy may result in profound hypotension and poor uteroplacental perfusion, with the onset of sympathetic blockade. Euvolaemia and a slow induction of CSE anaesthesia will minimize hypotension. Vasopressors should be used to manage hypotension in the euvolaemic individual to avoid fluid overload. The altered pharmacokinetics of the dialysis patient dictates the prudent use of highly protein bound or renally excreted drugs. Patients on magnesium must have their loading dose and infusion rate modified and levels monitored.

The renal transplant recipient

Compared to the dialysis patient, renal transplant recipients have a greater frequency of a successful perinatal outcome, with live births occurring in up to 80% of occasions. However, hypertension occurs in 50% and pre-eclampsia in 30% of these patients. Intrauterine growth restriction and low birth weight is common and 50% of deliveries occur prior to 36 weeks' gestation.

The effect of pregnancy on the renal allograft varies. If renal function is stable, pregnancy does not have long-term adverse effects on allograft function. Severe proteinuria or a serum creatinine concentration greater than 130 μmol/L significantly increases the risk of graft loss. The incidence of rejection is not increased, although it is advised to avoid pregnancy for 1–2 years post transplantation. The diagnosis of rejection may require renal biopsy.

Care should be provided by a multidisciplinary team of nephrologists and obstetricians familiar with these patients. Careful and regular monitoring of mother and fetus is necessary. Vaginal delivery should be possible in most patients with a renal allograft. However, the precise location should be assessed by ultrasound. It is particularly important to know the allograft's exact location and involve the transplant surgery team should the patient require caesarean section.

Immunosuppressants and corticosteroids have potential maternal and fetal side effects and may interact with anaesthetic drugs and techniques. The adverse effects of chronic steroid use should be evaluated particularly with respect to cardiovascular disease and altered glucose metabolism. Although immunosuppressants are never entirely risk-free in pregnancy, azathioprine is considered safe. However, potential adverse effects include life-threatening bone marrow suppression and associated coagulopathy. Tacrolimus and cyclosporin are also used; however, they require an altered dosing regime and close monitoring. Mycophenalate mofentil is generally contraindicated in pregnancy. An increased risk of infection is associated with all immunosuppressant therapy, necessitating the appropriate use of prophylactic antibiotics covering all surgical procedures and use of a meticulous aseptic technique at all times.

The anaesthetic management of the parturient with chronic kidney disease

Assessment and optimization

Preoperative evaluation must include the assessment of the degree of renal impairment, the systemic manifestations of chronic renal disease and the co-morbidities and pathologies associated with the underlying cause of renal failure. These patients will have been closely monitored in the antenatal period and care plans may already be in place for intrapartum management.

Full blood count, urea and electrolytes and a coagulation screen are essential investigations on admission to the delivery unit. Anaemia may require correction with iron, folic acid, erythropoietin and a red cell transfusion. Patients with CKD often display a bleeding tendency. Conversely, the increase in coagulation factors may also increase the risk of thrombosis. Thrombocytopenia and platelet dysfunction in the presence of a normal platelet count are common. These patients may give a history of easy bruising, bleeding from oral mucosa, melaena or excessive haemorrhage following invasive procedures. Thromboelastography may be useful in evaluating global coagulation status. There is no obvious correlation between excessive bleeding and severity of renal dysfunction. Heparin-free haemodialysis, peritoneal dialysis, arginine vasopressin (DDAVP) and cryoprecipitate have all been used to improve coagulation. Intravenous arginine vasopressin (usually 300 μg) increases von Willebrand factor (vWF) release for up to 8 hours. Repeated doses are less effective.

During the peripartum period, it is important to ensure the patient is euvolaemic, has electrolytes that are stable and any metabolic acidosis is minimized. This requires careful fluid balance, close monitoring of electrolytes, knowledge of daily diuretic doses, daily urine output and potentially dialysis.

Left ventricular dysfunction and pulmonary oedema due to chronic fluid overload, ischaemic heart disease or uraemic cardiomyopathy may all result in poor cardiorespiratory reserve. Patients with severe disease of long duration or anaemia are particularly at risk. ECHO cardiography may be useful in evaluating function. Hypertension in renal patients is very common. These patients require screening for pre-eclampsia and aggressive management aiming for a diastolic pressure of less than 80–90 mmHg.

Delayed gastric emptying and reduced gastric pH increases the risk of aspiration pneumonitis. Premedication with ranitidine, metoclopramide and sodium citrate is advised.

Peripartum monitoring

In mild or moderate disease, standard non-invasive monitoring will usually suffice. In patients at risk of ischaemic heart disease S-T segment monitoring may be useful. Temperature must be monitored, as these patients possess a tendency towards hypothermia. Neuromuscular function following muscle relaxants is unpredictable, especially after magnesium infusion, and monitoring is essential. Invasive monitoring is indicated in the presence of uncontrolled hypertension, severe cardiorespiratory disease or a rapidly fluctuating volume status.

Neuraxial analgesia and anaesthesia

The presence of thrombocytopenia may contraindicate neuraxial techniques for analgesia or anaesthesia. More frequently, altered arachidonic acid metabolism, increased nitric oxide production and defective endothelial release of vWF results in platelet dysfunction in the presence of a normal platelet count. Normal values derived by thromboelastography in the presence of a normal coagulation screen can support the use of a neuraxial technique. Residual heparin following dialysis and the prolonged effect of low-molecular-weight heparin may also prohibit neuraxial techniques. The use of low-dose epidural solutions and close monitoring of sensory and motor function will aid early diagnosis of epidural haematomas.

Hypovolaemia, especially in the presence of autonomic dysfunction, may result in severe hypotension with sympathetic blockade following epidural or spinal anaesthetic. It is important to ensure euvolaemia, particularly prior to a spinal anaesthetic, and slowly load epidurals to prevent precipitous drops in blood pressure. Excessive intravenous fluids may cause pulmonary oedema, therefore once euvolaemic, vasopressors should be used to maintain normotension.

The pharmacokinetics of bupivacaine and ropivacaine are relatively unaffected and similar doses produce the expected clinical response. Remifentanil patient-controlled analgesia (PCA) is useful for labour analgesia where neuraxial analgesic techniques are contraindicated.

General anaesthesia

Patients with stable mild to moderate renal impairment may require little adaptation of general anaesthetic technique. Severe disease, particularly in the presence of uncontrolled hypertension or cardiorespiratory complications, may present a significant challenge to the anaesthetist.

Knowledge of preoperative fluid and electrolyte status and the patient's ability to handle fluids is extremely important for intraoperative fluid management. Invasive monitoring may be indicated. Postoperatively, insensible loss in addition to the previous hour's urine output is a common regimen.

Induction of anaesthesia is complicated by the increased risk of a difficult airway and aspiration. Decreased protein binding, greater blood–brain barrier penetration, uraemia and prolonged elimination half-lives potentiate anaesthetic agents. The pharmacokinetics of propofol are unchanged. Thiopentone, etomidate and benzodiazepine all require a reduction in dose. Suxamethonium is best avoided if the serum potassium is unknown or greater than 5.5 mEq/L. Rocuronium will produce acceptable intubating conditions within 90 s but duration of action will be significantly longer. Suggamadex is safe to use in the presence of renal insufficiency. Atracurium and cisatracurium produce predictable results, due to Hofmann degradation. Isoflurane and desflurane preserve renal blood flow better than sevoflurane. Enflurane should be avoided. Patients on magnesium may require a reduced infusion rate and monitoring of magnesium levels.

The active metabolite of morphine, morphine-6-glucuronide, accumulates in renal failure and careful titration is advised. Alfentanil, fentanyl or remifentanil can provide useful, reliable analgesia without accumulation although prolonged infusions of fentanyl may still accumulate. Regional anaesthesia such as transverse abdominal plane block or a rectus sheath block may be a useful analgesic adjunct. Paracetamol is safe in renal failure, however non-steroidal anti-inflammatories should be avoided.

Many intraoperative renal protective strategies, including dopamine, furosemide, mannitol, calcium-channel blockers or excessive intravenous fluids, have been explored, yet there is very little evidence supporting any of them. It is important to avoid nephrotoxic drugs and hypovolaemia.

The anaesthetic management of the parturient with acute kidney injury

The anaesthetic management of the patient with AKI is similar to that with chronic disease. The systemic manifestations of chronic kidney disease will be absent and the underlying pathology is different and sometimes unknown. Particular attention should be paid to assessment of fluid and electrolyte status, blood pressure, severity and symptoms of uraemia, metabolic acidosis and urine output as these patients may have unstable physiology. Renal replacement therapy and invasive monitoring may be indicated. General and neuraxial anaesthetic techniques require similar considerations to those with chronic impairment.

Key points

1. Renal disease significantly increases maternal and fetal morbidity and mortality.
2. Parturients with CKD are more likely to develop gestational hypertension, pre-eclampsia and eclampsia.
3. Kidney disease during pregnancy may become apparent for the first time. This can be due to the physiological and anatomical changes of pregnancy, increased levels of monitoring or diseases associated with pregnancy e.g. pre-eclampsia.
4. Dialysis patients require a multidisciplinary approach, modification of their renal replacement regimes and close surveillance of the mother and fetus.
5. Although in renal transplant patients a successful obstetric outcome is common, a multidisciplinary approach is essential. Particular attention should

be paid to close and regular monitoring of mother and fetus, immunosuppression regimes and knowledge of the precise location of the allograft. Ideally, transplant surgeons should be available if caesarean section is required.

Further reading

August, P. and George, J. N. (2013). Acute kidney injury (acute renal failure) in pregnancy. *UpToDate* (online). Available at http://www.uptodate.com (Accessed May 2015).

August, P. and Vella, J. (2013). Pregnancy in women with underlying renal disease. *UpToDate* (online). Available at http://www.uptodate.com (Accessed May 2015).

Chinnappa, V., Ankichetty, S., Angle, P. and Halpern, S. H. (2013). Chronic kidney disease in pregnancy. *Int. J. Obstet. Anesth.*, 22(3), 223–230.

Podymow, T., August, P. and Akbari, A. (2010). Management of renal disease in pregnancy. *Obstet. Gynecol. Clin. North Am.*, 37(2), 195–210.

Haematologic disease in pregnancy

Pavan Kochhar, Andrew Heck and Clare Tower

Introduction

The haematological system undergoes significant changes during pregnancy. A knowledge of these changes is essential to enable clinicians to determine what is within normal parameters and what is pathological. The recognized haematological changes during pregnancy are detailed in Chapter 1.

Anaemia of pregnancy

A measure of haemoglobin (Hb) levels should be made at booking and at 28 weeks' gestation.

Anaemia during pregnancy may result from dilutional physiological changes, iron deficiency, folate deficiency, new-onset pernicious anaemia, or pre-existing diseases, including haemoglobinopathies or hereditary spherocytosis. Establishing the cause is paramount and early treatment will minimize the harmful effects.

The 2011 UK guidelines for the management of iron deficiency in pregnancy defined anaemia as:

- <110 g/L in the first trimester
- <105 g/L in the second and third trimesters
- <100 g/L postpartum.

Anaemia impairs oxygen delivery and results in an increase in cardiac output and oxygen demand, with a loss of functional reserve and an increased risk of maternal and fetal ischaemia. Remember, blood loss is expected at an uncomplicated normal delivery (500 mL) and at caesarean section (1000 mL).

Iron deficiency is the leading cause of anaemia; this may be due to pre-existing low iron levels secondary to menorrhagia, inadequate diet, pregnancy within the last year or due to increased iron demands (such as multiple pregnancy). It is associated with low birth weight, preterm delivery and increased blood loss at delivery.

Iron deficiency can be diagnosed using serum ferritin and total iron binding capacity saturation more reliably than mean corpuscular volume or mean corpuscular haemoglobin concentration. Without the presence of inflammatory disease, serum ferritin is the best indicator of iron stores in pregnancy. The 2011 UK guidelines for the management of iron deficiency in pregnancy advise iron replacement therapy for women with serum ferritin levels less than 30 µg/L, as this represents early iron depletion that will deteriorate with increasing gestation. A serum ferritin <15 µg/L is diagnostic of iron deficiency. Treatment is with 100–200 mg elemental iron per day. Inhibitors to iron uptake in the intestine, such as phytic acid and tannins, should be avoided. Parenteral iron may be indicated when oral therapy is not tolerated, absorbed or compliance is in doubt. The World Health Organization (WHO) recommends iron supplementation for all women. However, analysis of studies in the Cochrane database have not provided sufficient evidence to support this.

Folate deficiency most often results from dietary deficiency, but can occur secondary to haemoglobinopathies, anticonvulsants or specific folate antagonists.

Recombinant human erythropoietin is not recommended for use, other than in patients with end-stage renal failure.

In women found to be markedly anaemic at the onset of labour, a careful assessment should be made. Transfusion may be necessary for symptomatic women or those with Hb < 70 g/L. Active management of the third stage is necessary to minimize blood loss.

Core Topics in Obstetric Anaesthesia, ed. Kirsty MacLennan, Kate O'Brien and W. Ross Mcnab.
Published by Cambridge University Press. © Cambridge University Press 2015.

Haemoglobinopathies

Sickle cell disease (SCD)

SCD describes a group of inherited single-gene auto-somal recessive disorders caused by a 'sickle gene'. This includes HbSS (the most common homozygous form) and heterozygotes of haemoglobin S and another abnormal haemoglobin such as haemoglobin C, D, E or β-thalassaemia. About 300 newborns are diagnosed with SCD each year in the UK. Patients rarely live to their sixth decade.

Haemoglobin S results from a mutation on chromosome 11, causing a valine for glutamic acid substitution on the β-globin sub-unit. This formation is biochemically unstable and prone to precipitating out of solution, markedly so when PO_2 <6 kPa. The agglutinated masses cause vaso-occlusive problems and the sickled red cells have a shorter life of 12 days compared to the normal 120 days.

Untreated, the consequences of sickle cell disease occur due to anaemia or occlusive end-organ damage:

- Cardiomegaly secondary to an anaemia-induced high-output state, pulmonary artery hypertension and pulmonary infarction.
- Pulmonary infarctions can lead to an 'acute chest syndrome' with haemoptysis, dyspnoea and pleuritic pain, which can ultimately lead to pulmonary failure.
- Marrow hyperplasia causes frontal bossing and maxilla enlargement.
- Lymphoid tissue enlargement may cause obstructive sleep apnoea.
- Renal impairment begins in childhood.
- Sequestration of red blood cells (RBCs) within the spleen can lead to severe life-threatening anaemia.
- Hyposplenism results from autoinfarction, rendering the patient immunocompromised.
- Repeated microvascular occlusion causes retinopathy and aseptic necrosis of susceptible tissues, including the femoral head.
- Transient ischaemic attacks and strokes are more prevalent.

In parturients, SCD is associated with increased perinatal mortality (up to 20%), maternal death (<1%), preterm labour, fetal growth restriction and acute painful crises. An increased risk of infection, spontaneous miscarriage, thrombotic events and antepartum haemorrhage may also occur.

The RCOG Guidelines for the Management of SCD in Pregnancy (2011) make the following recommendations:

1. Management should involve a multidisciplinary team comprising a haematologist and an obstetrician with an interest in this area.
2. Preconception counselling is recommended to allow optimization of disease control and medication adjustments. Medications contraindicated during pregnancy include ACE-inhibitors, angiotensin receptor blockers and hydroxycarbamide (used to reduce the incidence of sickle crisis). Folic acid supplementation (5 mg per day) is recommended to commence preconception and vitamin D status should be optimized.
3. Evidence of end-organ damage should be sought, including echocardiography to assess pulmonary hypertension.
4. The partner's carrier status should be ascertained enabling counselling and antenatal screening to occur if the couple wish.
5. Blood pressure and urine should be screened regularly. Multiple transfusions can result in alloimmunization and iron overload. Serum iron should be measured.
6. All vaccinations should be up to date. Low-dose aspirin (75 mg) should be taken to reduce the risk of pre-eclampsia.
7. The risk of venous thromboembolism should be assessed in order to guide the need for thromboprophylaxis.
8. Ultrasound scanning to assess fetal growth is required throughout the third trimester.
9. Prophylactic top-up transfusions are contentious due to the risks of iron overload, delayed transfusion reaction and the possible risk of precipitating a crisis. These should be administered only on the advice of a specialist haematologist. Women with recurrent crisis managed with regular exchange transfusions outside pregnancy should usually continue this programme throughout pregnancy with the involvement of the specialist haematologist.

Anaesthetic management may be in the provision of aggressive treatment of a sickle crisis or facilitating early analgesia as part of planned labour to minimize the risk of a crisis. On the labour ward the patient should be monitored in a high-risk room, receive continuous saturation monitoring and aim to keep saturations greater than 95%. Invasive monitoring may be required. Regional anaesthesia should be provided when safe to do so (note timing of anticoagulants). These patients are often opioid tolerant and pethidine should be avoided. Blood products should be at the discretion of the joint haematology and obstetric team. In the event of a general anaesthetic, meticulous attention to oxygenation, analgesia, temperature control, minimizing stasis and maintaining hydration is essential. Postpartum care should be in an obstetric high-dependency unit and a high index of suspicion for subsequent sickle crisis.

Thalassaemias

These are divided into two main groups: the α-thalassaemias, where one to four of the α-genes are deleted, and the β-thalassaemias, where one or two of the β-genes are absent.

α-Thalassaemia major is incompatible with life, with the fetus becoming severely hydropic; α- and β-thalassaemia traits are usually asymptomatic, but individuals are prone to anaemia and should be managed accordingly.

β-Thalassaemia major sufferers have a defective β-globin gene from each parent. Untreated, this condition is fatal, with markedly ineffective erythropoiesis and severe haemolysis. Outcome has improved to beyond the fourth decade now with repeated, regular transfusions. The clinical features of this condition are the consequence of iron overload following repeated transfusion. This includes hepatic, endocrine and cardiac dysfunction. Death occurs secondary to myocardial haemochromatosis. Where transfusions have not been regular, the effects of marrow hyperplasia are evident with bone deformities. Women with this disorder are usually sub-fertile without the use of reproductive technologies. Care for these women should be in specialist joint clinics with careful screening for the sequelae of iron overload. Preconception counselling is paramount, with optimization of medication prior to fertility treatment and pregnancy. Chelating agents are contraindicated during pregnancy. Closely supervised transfusion regimes may reduce the risk of prematurity and intrauterine growth restriction. Women should be screened for Hep B+C, diabetes, thyroid disease and cardiac insufficiency. Exclude spinal abnormalities, including osteoporosis and scoliosis.

Thrombocytopenia

A platelet count of $<150 \times 10^9/L$ may occur during pregnancy due to gestational thrombocytopenia, laboratory error (EDTA can cause Ca^{2+} and platelet agglutination, artificially reducing platelet count), platelet autoantibodies (immune thrombocytopenia, ITP) or widespread activation (e.g. TTP/haemolytic uraemic syndrome and pre-eclampsia/HELLP). Other causes of impaired platelet production include bone marrow suppression, folate deficiency, platelet destruction (such as disseminated intravascular coagulation) and drugs (unfractionated heparin, thiazides, hydralazine, digoxin, H_2 blockers). Diagnosis and correction of thrombocytopenia is vital to reduce the risk of haemorrhage at the time of delivery.

The timing and placement of neuraxial blocks in the presence of thrombocytopenia can be challenging. The nature of the thrombocytopenia and trend of platelet count is important, and the decision must be made on an individual basis. Discussion with senior doctors is important and consideration must be made for the most experienced operator to perform the block.

Gestational thrombocytopenia

This accounts for 70% of all cases and is probably caused by accelerated platelet destruction. Platelet count rarely falls below $75 \times 10^9/L$ and most authors regard them as needing no particularly special management other than platelet count monitoring. Regional anaesthesia is generally considered safe when the platelet count is stable around $80 \times 10^9/L$, but this should be decided on an individual basis, taking into account the absolute platelet count and the trend. An urgent full blood count should be sent on admission in labour. Diagnostic difficulty can occur when thrombocytopenia is identified for the first time during pregnancy, as confirmation of the cause can only be determined with a platelet count postnatally.

Autoimmune thrombocytopenic purpura (ITP/ATP)

This condition stems from IgG destruction of platelets and was previously known as *immune thrombocytopenic purpura* or *idiopathic thrombocytopenic purpura*. The incidence is around 0.1% and diagnosis is essentially one of exclusion, with platelets $< 100 \times 10^9/L$ usually occurring early in the antenatal period with normal coagulation profiles. High-dose oral corticosteroid therapy is initiated when the count is found to be falling in the third trimester, with the aim of achieving a platelet count of more than 50×10^9/L for delivery. If corticosteroids are ineffective, oral cyclosporin can be used. Those failing to achieve a satisfactory platelet count using oral therapy can be treated with intravenous IgG to transiently increase platelet count. Platelet transfusions are occasionally required to cover the delivery.

Maternal IgG can cross the placenta and in around 5% of cases can cause neonatal thrombocytopenia, theoretically increasing the risk of neonatal haemorrhage. As yet no study has conclusively demonstrated a link between fetal platelet count and intrapartum risk. The occurrence of neonatal intraventricular haemorrhage is rare and does not seem to correlate with the method of delivery. A care plan should be put in place to reduce the theoretical risk to the fetus, including potential avoidance of ventouse delivery.

The same principles regarding the appropriateness of regional anaesthesia should be applied as for gestational thrombocytopenia.

Thrombotic thrombocytopenic purpura (TTP) and haemolytic uraemic syndrome (HUS)

TTP is a rare condition usually presenting in the second trimester. Intravascular clot formation leads to platelet consumption and vascular occlusion. A classical pentad exists of:

1. Fever
2. Thrombocytopenia
3. Microangiopathic haemolytic anaemia
4. Focal neurology
5. Renal failure.

HUS presentation is similar, but with more pronounced renal failure and absence of neurological sequelae. Microscopic differences in the number and cluster of von Willebrand factor deposits help differentiate between the two conditions. Effective treatments include plasma exchange and plasmapheresis, intravenous IgG, prednisolone and prostacyclin. Renal replacement therapy may be required. Due to the coagulopathy present, neuraxial anaesthesia is not recommended.

Pre-eclampsia/HELLP

Pre-eclampsia is accompanied by a low platelet count in approximately 20% of cases, often with a coagulopathy on a continuum with the more severe HELLP variant (Haemolysis, Elevated Liver enzymes, Low Platelets). More extensive information is provided in Chapter 14. These patients require regular monitoring of their platelet and coagulation status, with any fall indicating a worsening of their condition. Any consideration of regional anaesthesia will be guided by this and point-of-care testing of coagulopathy.

Congenital coagulopathies

von Willebrand's disease (vWD)

vWD is a heterogenous group of mainly autosomal dominant disorders (types 1,2,3) in which there is reduced or abnormal circulating von Willebrand factor (vWF). vWF has two functions:

1. It combines with factor VIII to produce a procoagulant complex (VIIIc) that protects factor VIII from premature destruction.
2. It mediates platelet adhesion by binding to platelets (a reaction enhanced by ristocetin) and collagen.

The incidence of von Willebrand's disease is 1:100 to 1:2500 for the mild form and 1:200,000 to 1:2,000,000 for the severe homozygous form. Patients may present with a history of epistaxis, menorrhagia and bleeding after dental extractions. The bleeding risk associated with delivery and the immediate puerperal period can be significant. Women should be managed in close liaison with an obstetric haematology team. Consideration for the fact that the fetus may also be affected is necessary.

Type 1 disease results from a partial quantitative vWF deficit. Increase in vWF and factor VIII levels in pregnancy result in correction of this deficit by the third trimester in 80–90% of cases. When haematological abnormalities are corrected, management of labour and delivery should be as normal, and regional anaesthesia is acceptable. Following delivery, levels typically fall rapidly to those recorded prepregnancy. These women are at risk of primary and secondary postpartum haemorrhage.

In a minority of women, the disease does not correct, but some women will be responsive to desmopressin (DDAVP) to increase vWF levels.

Type 2 disease (9–15% of cases) is a qualitative defect; the vWF is abnormal and may not respond to DDAVP.

In Type 3 disease (<1% of cases) vWF is undetectable and factor VIII very low. Some women will require factor replacement (fresh frozen plasma (FFP), cryoprecipitate or vWF/factor VIII concentrates) to cover delivery of the fetus, and a detailed haematological care plan should be in place.

Types 2 and 3 patients are more complex and should be managed on an individual basis with the involvement of specialist haematologists. Regional anaesthesia is generally contraindicated, but has been described after clotting correction.

Treatment is usually started when factor VIII levels reach less than 25% of normal. Levels should be 50% for labour, and treatment should be instituted to raise this to 80% for caesarean delivery. Factor VIII levels should be checked daily post partum and treatment instituted if levels fall below 25% or significant bleeding occurs. There may be a role for oral tranexamic acid to reduce blood loss in the puerperal period.

Haemophilia

Haemophilia A (factor VIII deficiency) and haemophilia B (factor IX deficiency) are X-linked traits that classically do not affect women. Some female carriers (up to 10%) can be symptomatic and have clinically significant clotting deficiency.

Factor VIII or IX levels of 30% or more are considered satisfactory for vaginal delivery. For planned operative delivery, levels are increased to normal. Specialist haematology teams will guide administration of FFP, cryoprecipitate, DDAVP, tranexamic acid or purified clotting factors. Regional anaesthesia is generally contraindicated, but may be considered after specialist advice following factor correction and a risk–benefit assessment of individual cases.

Half of all male children of heterozygous carriers for haemophilia A or B will have haemophilia. These infants have an increased risk of bleeding and certain procedures should be used only where careful balance of risks and benefits has been assessed: fetal scalp electrode; fetal scalp pH sampling; vacuum extraction and difficult forceps delivery.

Acquired coagulopathies

Disseminated intravascular coagulation

DIC results from abnormal activation of the coagulation system. Procoagulant substances, including thromboplastin, phospholipid and those resulting from endothelial injury are released into the circulation. Stimulation of coagulation activity results in excess thrombin, consumption of clotting factors and platelets, with concomitant activation of the fibrinolytic pathway.

Common obstetric causes of DIC include:
- Placental abruption
- Sepsis
- Intrauterine death
- Pre-eclampsia
- HELLP syndrome
- Acute fatty liver of pregnancy
- Amniotic fluid embolus (AFE).

Diagnosis of DIC depends on the clinical presentation and laboratory tests. Patients may present with cardiovascular, respiratory or renal failure. There may be bleeding from venepuncture sites, gums, gastrointestinal and urogenital tracts, and also from the uteroplacental bed.

Laboratory tests can show a variable prolongation of the prothrombin time (PT) and activated partial thromboplastin time (aPTT), decreased platelet count, decreased fibrinogen and an increase in fibrin degradation products (FDPs) and D-dimers. The use of thromboelastography may allow rapid assessment of the coagulation disruption and monitoring of correction.

Acute fulminant DIC should be treated aggressively, with the emphasis on maternal resuscitation. Onset of DIC may be more insidious, e.g. pre-eclampsia and fetal demise. Removal of the underlying triggering is paramount, which usually requires delivery of the fetus and placenta.

Management of massive obstetric haemorrhage should be by a senior team, according to local protocols (see Chapter 25).

The management of DIC requires blood and blood products:
- Packed red cells to replace ongoing losses
- Fresh frozen plasma (FFP) to replace coagulation products
- Platelet concentrates
- Cryoprecipitate (contains more fibrinogen than FFP and should be considered if there is haemorrhage and the fibrinogen level is <1 g/L).

The other considerations for patients in DIC are:
- Regional anaesthesia is contraindicated
- Removal of previously sited epidural catheter should be delayed until correction of coagulopathy

- Arterial line for monitoring and blood sampling
- Central line for inotrope/vasopressor administration and for further monitoring
- Remain vigilant for complications of massive transfusion, including transfusion-related acute lung injury (TRALI)
- Utilization of cell salvage is advised in massive haemorrhage
- Surgical haemostasis may be difficult and may necessitate hysterectomy
- Internal iliac artery balloon catheterization can be considered if some degree of coagulation correction has been achieved and further surgical intervention is needed
- Use of recombinant factor VII and prothrombin complex concentrates (PCC) has been described
- Metabolic acidosis may take a few hours to correct
- Postoperative management in a high-dependency or critical care unit.

Thrombophilia/hypercoagulable states

Thrombophilia is a familial or acquired abnormality of haemostasis likely to predispose to thrombosis. A congenital deficiency in anticoagulant activity occurs in approximately 30–50% of patients with a history of venous thromboembolism (VTE). Pregnancy is a hypercoagulable state, and pre-existing thrombophilia increases the risk of thrombosis further, especially in the postpartum period. Some thrombophilias have been associated with recurrent miscarriage and an increased risk of pregnancy complications such as abruption, fetal growth restriction and pre-eclampsia. Antenatal management should be personalized and involve assessment of VTE risk and the risk of pregnancy complications. Management typically comprises low-dose aspirin and prophylactic subcutaneous low-molecular-weight heparin (LMWH). This has implications for the anaesthetist with regard to timing for regional techniques.

Congenital thrombophilias

Hereditary thombophilia is found in 20–50% of women with pregnancy-related VTE. These factor deficiencies can be quantitative and/or qualitative, hence specialist haematology input is required.

Protein C deficiency

Protein C inhibits activated factors V and VIII. The incidence of protein C deficiency is 1 in 15,000. Protein C levels typically rise by 30% in pregnancy, but this rise does not occur in patients with deficiency. These patients are greatly predisposed to VTE. In the absence of anticoagulation, VTE rates of up to 25% have been reported, mostly in the postpartum period.

Protein S deficiency

Protein S is a co-factor for protein C. Protein S levels typically fall during pregnancy, thus assessment of protein S levels must occur outside pregnancy. There may be an association with arterial thrombosis. Treatment is as for Protein C deficiency.

Antithrombin III (AT) deficiency

AT inactivates thrombin and coagulation factors IXa, Xa, XIa and XIIa.

AT deficiency occurs in around 1 in 5,000 pregnancies, accounting for 15% of thromboembolic events. Left untreated, the rate of VTE can be 55–70%. Deficiencies can be quantitative (type 1) or qualitative (type 2). Heparins may not be as effective in AT deficiency, as their mode of action is antithrombin-dependent, thus effectiveness of heparin prophylaxis should be monitored using anti-Xa levels. Different sub-types of AT deficiency are associated with different levels of VTE risk and therefore expert advice should be sought. Treatment should start in early pregnancy and continue for 6 weeks postpartum. The use of antithrombin III concentrate has been described in women at particular risk.

Factor V Leiden mutation

Factor V is a co-factor that allows factor Xa to activate thrombin, which cleaves fibrin from fibrinogen.

This common hereditary thrombophilic tendency results from a mutation in a single amino acid in the factor V gene. The mutant factor V Leiden persists for longer in the circulation. It is degraded more slowly by activated protein C, hence leading to a hypercoagulable state. Heterozygous factor V Leiden has an incidence of 3–5% and has a fivefold increase in VTE risk. Homozygous factor V Leiden status is associated with higher VTE risk. LMWH timing will guide safety for regional anaesthesia.

Acquired thrombophilias

Antiphospholipid syndrome is the most common cause of acquired thrombophilia. Recognized antibodies include lupus anticoagulant and anticardiolipin antibodies. A preceding history of arterial or venous thrombosis or adverse pregnancy outcome (defined as three or more unexplained miscarriages before 10 weeks of gestation, a fetal death after 10 weeks of gestation or a premature birth (before 35 weeks) due to pre-eclampsia or intrauterine growth restriction) is common. Antiphospholipid syndrome is associated with a 5% incidence of VTE or cerebrovascular accident in pregnancy.

Women with previous thromboses and antiphospholipid syndrome should be offered both antenatal and 6 weeks of postpartum thromboprophylaxis. Women with persistent antiphospholipid antibodies with no previous VTE and no other risk factors or fetal indications for LMWH may be managed with close surveillance antenatally, but should be considered for LMWH for 7–42 days post partum.

Assessment of coagulation

Assessment of coagulation begins with clinical examination of the patient and an index of suspicion over causes of coagulopathies. Excessive bleeding or bleeding from unusual sites, e.g. gums or venepuncture sites, can alert to the presence of a coagulopathy. Laboratory tests aid clinical evaluation, but unfortunately there is no single blood test that will give an overall study of haemostasis and blood coagulation.

Platelet count, PT and aPTT are measured. In normal pregnancy, an increase in coagulation factors results in a reduction in PT and aPTT. Fibrinogen assays are also useful in massive haemorrhage or sepsis. Gestational thrombocytopenia may lead to lower platelet counts at the end of pregnancy. A limitation of the platelet assay is that it measures platelet numbers, but not function. A summary of tests in clinical use is given in Table 21.1.

During a rapidly changing scenario such as haemorrhage, receipt of laboratory coagulation results often lags behind the current haematological picture. Coagulation products are often instituted empirically. Thromboelastography (TEG) and rotational thromboelastometry (ROTEM) evaluate real-time measurement of whole blood coagulation. They evaluate the viscoelastic properties of the sample, as well as coagulation factor and platelet activity. They can help with

Table 21.1 Laboratory tests used in the assessment of coagulation

Study	Measures	Normal values
Bleeding time	Platelets and vascular integrity	1–5 min
Platelet count	Number of platelets	140–440 × 10^9/L
aPTT	Extrinsic pathway (factors II, V, VIII, IX, X, XI)	24–36 s
PT	Intrinsic pathway (factors II, V, VII, X)	11–12 s
Thrombin time	Factors I, II, circulating split products, heparin	16–20 s

haemostatic decision-making and blood product use during surgery and severe haemorrhage.

The TEG analyzer has a sample cup into which 360 µL of whole blood sample is pipetted. This cup constantly oscillates at a set speed through an arc of 4°45'. A stationary pin attached to a torsion wire is immersed in the blood. Each oscillation lasts 10 s. When fibrin first forms, it begins to bind the cup and pin, causing the pin to oscillate in phase with the cup. The torque of the rotating cup is transmitted to the immersed pin only after fibrin or fibrin-platelet bonding has linked the cup and pin together. The degree of pin movement is converted into a graph (Figure 21.1) that represents the kinetics of clot development.

The reaction time (R-time) depicts the time for fibrin strands to form. It is decreased in hypercoagulable states such as pregnancy. A prolonged R-time may reflect decreased or dysfunctional coagulation factors leading to a delay in the formation of thrombin or fibrin. Consideration should be given to administer FFP for correction. A prolonged R-time may also reflect heparin activity, and this may be further evaluated using a heparinase cup that will remove the heparin effect on the sample.

The maximum amplitude (MA) represents clot strength with the amplitude of pin oscillation increasing with clot strength (Figure 21.1). The major contributors to clot strength are platelets (80–90%) and fibrinogen (10–20%), which binds the platelets together. Therefore, MA gives an indication as to the function of platelets present in the sample. A low MA value is indicative of insufficient platelet–fibrin clot

161

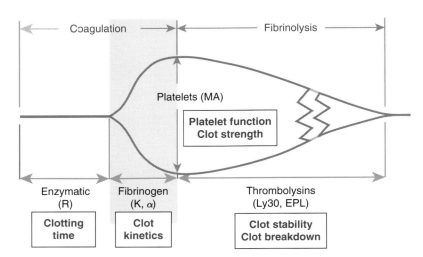

Figure 21.1 TEG graph and annotation.

formation due to poor platelet function, low platelet count, or low fibrinogen levels or function. The most common treatment of a low MA in a bleeding patient is transfusion of platelets. The amount of platelets required to reverse bleeding depends on the magnitude of the abnormality and on the patient's overall status.

Accepted non-pregnant reference ranges for R-time are 4–8 minutes and for MA, 55–73 mm. Studies on pregnant women reflect the hypercoagulable state of pregnancy; R-time values are shorter and MA values are higher, but further work is needed to define pregnancy values.

A platelet function analyzer (PFA-100) can also measure platelet function. This tests platelet activation and aggregation. Experience in obstetrics is limited and expert advice in the use and interpretation of samples is essential.

Clinical example of the use of TEG

A 24-year-old primigravida presented to labour ward with PV bleeding at 24 weeks' gestation. Her blood pressure was 150/110 and scans revealed fetal demise. Bleeding from venepuncture sites raised the clinical suspicion of DIC. TEG (Figure 21.2) was used as a rapid laboratory assessment and confirmed the presence of DIC. A prolonged R-time indicated a decrease in coagulation factors. A markedly reduced MA indicated reduced platelet activity. The concurrent blood tests revealed a PT of 24, aPTT of 42.7 and fibrinogen < 0.6 g/L. Renal function was impaired, with creatinine 182 μmol/L.

Four units of red cell concentrate, four units of FFP, three units of cryoprecipitate and two adult doses of platelets were infused. A repeat TEG (Figure 21.3) showed a marked improvement in the haemostatic profile. Blood tests confirmed the improvement with a PT of 14, aPTT of 35 and fibrinogen of 35 g/L.

The patient proceeded to caesarean section under general anaesthesia.

Key points

1. Pregnancy is a hypercoagulable state that develops in order to reduce blood loss at delivery.
2. Clear guidelines exist for the diagnosis and management of anaemia during pregnancy, including UK Guidelines on the Management of Iron Deficiency in Pregnancy by the British Committee for Standards in Haematology.
3. Women with sickle cell disease should be managed by an MDT, including specialist haematologists and obstetricians. RCOG guidelines should be consulted.
4. Thrombocytopenia can occur during pregnancy for a variety of reasons. Identification of cause, trend in platelet count and knowledge of platelet function all guide timing and appropriateness of regional anaesthesia.
5. Hypercoagulable states are typically managed antenatally with low-dose aspirin and low-molecular-weight heparin. Care must be taken when timing regional anaesthesia.
6. Point-of-care assessment of coagulation is becoming more widespread and is of particular benefit in rapidly changing scenarios such as haemorrhage.

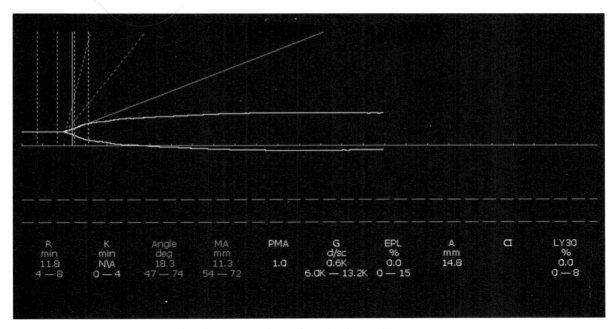

R min	K min	Angle deg	MA mm	PMA	G d/sc	EPL %	A mm	CI	LY30 %
11.8	N\A	18.3	11.3	1.0	0.6K	0.0	14.8		0.0
4 — 8	0 — 4	47 — 74	54 — 72		6.0K — 13.2K	0 — 15			0 — 8

Figure 21.2 TEG at presentation. For the colour version, please refer to the plate section.

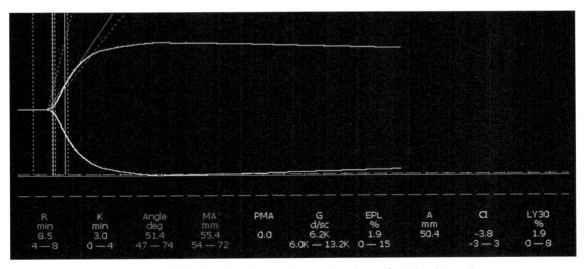

R min	K min	Angle deg	MA mm	PMA	G d/sc	EPL %	A mm	CI	LY30 %
8.5	3.0	51.4	55.4	0.0	6.2K	1.9	50.4	-3.8	1.9
4 — 8	0 — 4	47 — 74	54 — 72		6.0K — 13.2K	0 — 15		-3 — 3	0 — 8

Figure 21.3 TEG after correction with blood products. For the colour version, please refer to the plate section.

Further reading

Association of Anaesthetists of Great Britain and Ireland, Obstetric Anaesthetists Association and Regional Anaesthesia UK (2013). Regional Anaesthesia and Patients with Abnormalities of Coagulation. http://www. aagbi.org/sites/default/files/rapac_2013_web.pdf (accessed May 2015).

British Committee for Standards in Haematology (2011). UK guidelines on the management of iron deficiency in pregnancy. http://www.bcshguidelines.com/documents/ UK_Guidelines_iron_deficiency_in_pregnancy.pdf (accessed May 2015).

Chestnut, D.H., Polley, L.S., Tsen, L.C. and Wong, C.A. (2008). *Chestnut's Obstetric Anesthesia: Principles and Practice*, 4th edn. Philadelphia: Mosby/Elsevier.

Nelson-Piercy, C. (2010). *Handbook of Obstetric Medicine, 4th edn*. New York: Informa Healthcare.

Royal College of Obstetrics and Gynaecology (2007). Green-top Guideline No. 47: Blood Transfusions in Obstetrics. http://www.rcog.org.uk/womens-health/clinical-guidance/blood-transfusions-obstetrics-green-top-47 (accessed May 2015).

Royal College of Obstetrics and Gynaecology (2011). Green-top Guideline No. 61: Management of Sickle Cell Disease in Pregnancy. http://www.rcog.org.uk/womens-health/ clinical-guidance/sickle-cell-disease-pregnancy-management-green-top-61 (accessed May 2015).

Stoltzfus, R. J. and Dreyfuss, M. L. (1998). *Guidelines for the Use of Iron Supplements to Prevent and Treat Iron Deficiency Anemia*. Washington, DC: International Nutritional Anemia Consultative Group, International Life Sciences Institute.

Yentis, S., May, A. and Malhotra, S. (2007). *Analgesia, Anaesthesia and Pregnancy: A Practical Guide, 2nd edn*. Cambridge: Cambridge University Press.

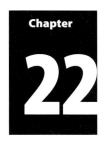

Neurosurgical and neurological disease in pregnancy

Kirsty MacLennan and Craig Carroll

Neurological disease in parturient prompts the anaesthetic and obstetric team to consider many aspects of care delivery. Pre-existing conditions may progress to cause significant compromise and the onset of new neurological symptoms may mimic more commonly encountered conditions, such as PET.

Even the presence of stable neurological conditions, of the spinal cord, neuro-axial skeleton or intracranium, may require careful consideration with respect to analgesia, anaesthesia and mode of delivery.

Quantification of anaesthetic risk is essential. A major anaesthetic concern relates to the safety of performing neuraxial blockade. The following questions arise:

- Is there risk of 'coning?' If a CSF leak results in a discrepancy in pressure within the cranium and infra foramen magnum (cranial: spinal CSF pressure gradient $CSF_{Cr}:CSF_{Sp}$), cerebellar tonsillar herniation can occur caudally with brain stem compression (coning).
- Is there risk of local trauma and neurological injury? Abnormal anatomy can result in spinal cord, cauda equina or spinal nerve trauma following needling of the perispinal region.
- Is there risk of spinal haemorrhage? Neuraxial vascular abnormalities can increase the risk of bleeding as a result of needling the spinal canal.
- Will the block work? Anatomical abnormalities can impede local anaesthetic spread.

General anaesthesia in parturients with neurosurgical pathologies is not without risks. Cardiovascular fluctuations during induction of anaesthesia can precipitate brain swelling or intracranial haemorrhage. Optimization of intracranial pressure (ICP), cerebral perfusion pressure (CPP) and cerebral blood flow (CBF) is essential. It is important, when evaluating known or perceived risk of complications of neuraxial blockade, to consider the risks of *not* performing the block or proceeding to general anaesthesia (see Chapter 11).

Neurosurgical issues relevant to pregnancy

See Chapter 17 for spinal abnormalities.

Intracranial mass lesions

Mass lesions can be caused by infection, tumour, vascular abnormalities, inflammation (e.g. MS), cystic lesions or haemorrhage. Presentation depends upon lesion size, rate of enlargement, aetiology and location, and includes:

- Asymptomatic; identified during investigation of other pathology
- Focal neurological deficit
- Ataxia
- Global reduction in cerebral function
- Headache classically worse when supine
- Nausea and vomiting
- Seizures.

Mass effect can cause disruption of neurological function by compression or destruction of brain tissue, causing oedema within the brain, causing hydrocephalus by obstructing CSF flow and by reducing cerebral compliance, thus increasing ICP and reducing CBF.

Posterior fossa lesions typically cause:

- Headache (usually with nausea and vomiting)
- Obstructed hydrocephalus (see later)
- Ataxia and co-ordination issues
- Lower cranial nerve dysfunction.

Core Topics in Obstetric Anaesthesia, ed. Kirsty MacLennan, Kate O'Brien and W. Ross Mcnab.
Published by Cambridge University Press. © Cambridge University Press 2015.

Table 22.1 Neurosurgical issues relevant to pregnancy

Category	Sub-category	Relevance
Mass lesions of the cranial vault	Intrinsic brain tumour Metastasis Infective lesions	ICP issue Altered neurology Seizure Influence on analgesia, mode of delivery, peripartum observation
Pituitary lesions	Functional/non-functional lesions	Mass effect CSF drainage Endocrine concerns Acute visual events Apoplexy
Posterior fossa abnormalities	Tumours Arnold Chiari malformations	CSF drainage Brainstem compression CSF gradient
Issues of CSF drainage	Hydrocephalus Benign intracranial hypertension (BIH) Shunting and diversion of CSF flow Consequences of low CSF pressure CSF pressure differential	CSF gradient Impact of indwelling shunts Acute pregnancy deterioration in vision Sub-dural haematoma
Vascular lesions of the central nervous system	Aneurysmal, non-aneurysmal SAH 'stroke' Cerebral venous thrombosis AVM Vascular tumours	Intracranial haemorrhage with altered cerebral blood flow Raised ICP Mass effects Venous hypertension Cerebral infarction
The vertebral column and related surgery	Disc abnormalities Previous lumbar surgery Scoliosis	Neurological trauma Failed regional analgesia
Head injury in pregnancy	Traumatic head injury	Immediate resuscitation Transfer Prioritization of therapeutic intervention Anaesthesia for delivery

Meningiomata and vestibular schwannomata (benign tumours of the VIII cranial nerve arising in the cerebropontine angle in the posterior fossa) are prone to marked expansion during pregnancy; this may reflect the alterations in hormonal secretion during pregnancy. They require close monitoring.

Investigation

If an intracranial mass lesion is suspected, discussion with neurosurgeons should ensue to decide upon the optimal imaging procedure (CT or MRI).

Treatment

Initial therapy may be medical (e.g. dexamethasone) to reduce brain swelling or reduce tumour volume. Surgical intervention may be initial control of CSF volume (with externalized ventricular drain). Craniotomy or craniectomy may be required for excision, debulking and tissue diagnosis. The timing of surgery will require a multidisciplinary approach, and will be influenced by the stage of pregnancy or puerperium. Immediate management of mass-related intracranial hypertension may require neurocritical care involvement.

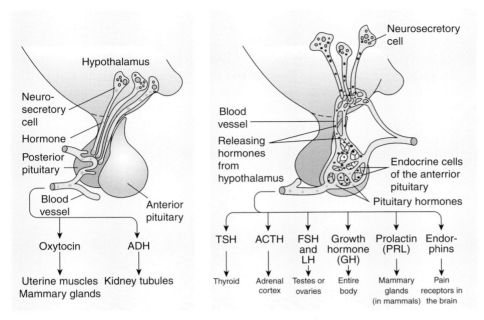

Figure 22.1 The pituitary. For the colour version, please refer to the plate section.

The pituitary

The pituitary gland consists of the anterior pituitary gland (adenohypophysis) and posterior pituitary gland (neurohypophysis). Connection to the hypothalamus is by the pituitary stalk. It receives its blood supply from the internal carotid artery, in addition to portal circulation linked to the hypothalamus.

The function of the anterior gland is endocrine and the posterior gland is a neurosecretory extension of the hypothalamus (see Figure 22.1).

Lesions of the pituitary

Mass lesions are usually primary adenomas of the anterior pituitary and stalk that may be secretory or non-secretory, and are either large enough to cause a mass effect, or small and only significant on account of their secretory activity. Patients with pituitary tumours may therefore have: hyposecretion of one of more hormones, disease resulting from isolated pituitary hormone over-secretion, hypersecretion of one hormone with deficient secretion of others, mass effect (compression of the optic chiasm), headache, possibly accompanied by hydrocephalus (rare), with or without hormonal pathology.

All anterior pituitary hormones except prolactin are under positive feedback control from the hypothalamus.

Compression of the pituitary stalk may reduce dopamine transit to the anterior pituitary gland and results in mild hyperprolactinaemia (<2000 mIU/L).

Disruption of the posterior pituitary may result in diabetes insipidus, due to the lack of ADH and reduced water resorption in the distal tubule and collecting ducts, characterized by hypernatraemia, with inappropriately dilute urine.

Apoplexy (haemorrhagic infarction) is a rare event resulting from bleeding into the pituitary fossa, in the presence of a pre-existing adenoma, causing sudden onset of mass effect and hormonal dysfunction.

Classical presentation is with acute severe retro-orbital headache. Pituitary swelling can cause compression of adjacent structures, resulting in visual field lesions, opthalmoplegia and cerebral hypoperfusion. It is a serious condition and if left untreated may be fatal.

Risk factors include anticoagulation, coagulopathy, treatment with dopamine agonists (e.g. bromocriptine) and pregnancy. Differential diagnoses include: sub-arachnoid haemorrhage, acute ischaemic stroke (AIS), Sheehan's syndrome or reversible cerebral vasoconstriction syndrome (RCVS), a rare condition presenting with recurrent severe headaches that can progress to intracranial haemorrhage or ischaemic stroke. It is more common post partum.

Investigation: CT Head is more easily organized in the emergency setting and requires the use of iodine-based contrast. MRI is more detailed than CT and requires the use of gadolinium contrast.

Treatment: Any patient with suspected apoplexy requires emergency neurosurgical referral and specialist endocrinology advice. Co-located obstetrics/neurosurgery care will be essential. Urgent hormonal replacement will be necessary (initially hydrocortisone).

Sheehan's syndrome results from haemorrhage into the pituitary gland in the peripartum period. It may present with headache, but classically presents with insidious onset of panhypopituitarism some weeks following delivery. Mass effect is uncommon. It is more common in parturients with delivery blood loss >2000 mL. Incidence is reported as 1–2% following large postpartum haemorrhage.

Investigation and management: Brain imaging by CT/MR is necessary. Involvement of an endocrinologist is necessary when the diagnosis is suspected.

Lymphocytic hypophysitis is a benign self-limiting autoimmune inflammatory disease, usually related to pregnancy. Treatment (under the guidance of endocrinology) is usually with steroids alone.

Cerebrospinal fluid

Hydrocephalus

Hydrocephalus is due to an increase in CSF volume within the cranial ventricular system, resulting in ventriculomegaly and (usually) raised intracranial pressure (ICP). See Figure 22.2.

Presentation is dependent upon the rate of CSF build up. Chronic impairment of flow results in headache, visual disturbance, confusion and ataxia with progression to decreased level of consciousness. Nausea and vomiting may exist. Acute cessation of CSF drainage results in rapid deterioration in conscious level. Those dependent upon non-anatomical drainage (shunts) are at risk of shunt blockage and acute hydrocephalus.

Non-communicating hydrocephalus occurs if CSF produced within the lateral ventricles fails to reach the sub-arachnoid space via drainage from the fourth ventricle. There is a $CSF_{brain}:CSF_{spinal}$ pressure gradient; lumbar drainage of CSF must be avoided as this can precipitate coning. Regional neuraxial anaesthesia is contraindicated. Causes include space-occupying lesions, haemorrhage (SAH, ICH) or CSF infection.

Communicating hydrocephalus occurs if CSF production exceeds reabsorption in the presence of normal anatomy. Causes include infection (meningitis, ventriculitis), haemorrhage, venous sinus thrombosis, following head injury or increased CSF protein content due to CNS tumour. Anatomically, neuraxial anaesthesia is not contraindicated.

Investigations

CT head confirms the diagnosis and may give indication as to the cause. See Figure 22.3. MRI will demonstrate increased ventricular size. T2-weighted images demonstrate periventricular oedema.

The presence of intracranial ventriculomegaly does not necessarily signify raised ICP; however, in symptomatic patients with headache and/or decreased level of consciousness, CSF flow obstruction must be assumed. Neurosurgical input is obligatory.

Treatment

Communicating hydrocephalus can be treated by CSF removal at lumbar puncture. For prolonged CSF pressure control, shunting of CSF is required (ventriculoperitoneal (VP)/atrial or lumboperitoneal (LP) shunt).

The standard emergency treatment of non-communicating hydrocephalus is with an externalized ventricular drain (EVD). Endoscopic third ventriculostomy (ETV) may be appropriate in some cases, with the aim to circumvent the aqueduct and VI ventricle by generating a fistula in the base of the III ventricle. See Figure 22.4. CSF flows directly to the basal cisterns. When successful, no additional CSF drainage procedure is necessary.

Ventriculoperitoneal/atrial shunt creates a conduit from the ventricular system to either peritoneum or right atrium. The system contains a valve, both preventing back flow and also dictating the CSF drainage pressure. This provides a permanent artificial route for CSF drainage.

Key points regarding CSF shunts in pregnancy:

- Parturients have a higher incidence of complicated pregnancy and worse fetal outcomes.
- Shunt malfunction can occur during pregnancy, though is more likely in the peridelivery period.
- Shunt blockage in a shunt-dependent parturient is a neurosurgical emergency.
- CSF infection risk is increased. If suspected, neurosurgical guidance is necessary and investigation is classically diagnostic LP after CT head to confirm shunt function.

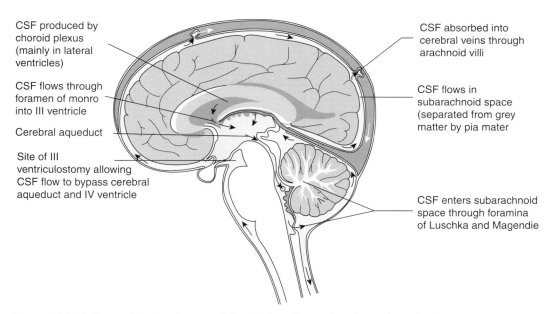

CSF produced by choroid plexus (mainly in lateral ventricles)

CSF flows through foramen of monro into III ventricle

Cerebral aqueduct

Site of III ventriculostomy allowing CSF flow to bypass cerebral aqueduct and IV ventricle

CSF absorbed into cerebral veins through arachnoid villi

CSF flows in subarachnoid space (separated from grey matter by pia mater

CSF enters subarachnoid space through foramina of Luschka and Magendie

Figure 22.2 Cerebrospinal fluid production and flow. For the colour version, please refer to the plate section.

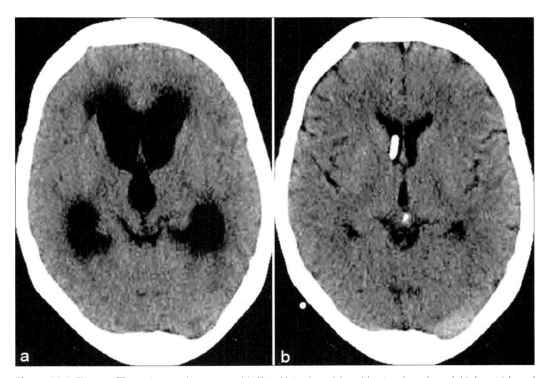

Figure 22.3 The two CT scan images demonstrate (a) dilated lateral venticles with a teardrop-shaped third ventricle and periventricular oedema. (b) An image of treated hydrocephalus with a ventricular drain *in situ* (this may be an EVD or ventriculo- shunt). For the colour version, please refer to the plate section.

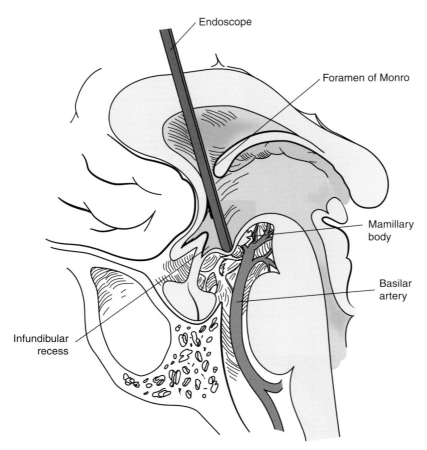

Figure 22.4 Endoscopic third ventriculostomy via a frontal burr hole through the base of the third ventricle.

- LP shunts are a relative contraindication for lumbar neuraxial blockade.
- Parturients with functioning ETVs and no hydrocephalus can be treated as normal.

Benign intracranial hypertension (BIH)

BIH occurs mainly in women of childbearing age and is associated with raised BMI. It is thought to result from an abnormality in central venous sinus pressure. CSF pressure is raised, with normal-sized ventricles. It causes chronic headache and is associated with papilloedema. Acute deterioration may occur, threatening ocular function. Pregnancy and labour may precipitate deterioration. Signs and symptoms can mimic cerebral venous thrombosis (CVT). Exclusion of this diagnosis must be made in BIH patients with worsening headache or neurological signs.

Investigation

CT brain and orbit will demonstrate small ventricles. MR venogram is needed to exclude CVT. Visual fields

need charting. CSF pressure monitoring is required (LP or parenchymal pressure monitor).

Treatment

- Neurology/neurosurgery input is essential.
- Therapeutic lumbar puncture can treat acute crises.
- BIH is occasionally treated with lumboperitoneal shunt.
- Labour and delivery have been successfully performed with epidural analgesia, lumbar puncture/sub-arachnoid anaesthesia. Specialist neurosurgical advice should be sought regarding anaesthetic management.
- Combined ICP management and regional anaesthesia has been reported using a lumbar drain.

Chiari malformation

The (Arnold) Chiari (type 1) malformation (ACM) consists of descent of the cerebellar tonsils and medulla through the foramen magnum (with or without syringomyelia). It has an incidence of ~0.7% in females, being completely asymptomatic in many cases. Classical presentation is with headache and neck pain, both worse on coughing and on neck extension. Issues of co-ordination, with nausea and vomiting, may occur. In the presence of syringomyelia, the loss of function in the central cord region can result in upper limb weakness and dissociative sensory loss with characteristic loss of pain sensation.

Key points

- Dural puncture in a symptomatic, untreated ACM may cause acute tonsillar descent and coning.
- CSF_{Brain}:CSF_{spinal} gradient is unlikely in the asymptomatic patient. Patients who have had corrective surgery may still have abnormal CSF flow.
- Surgical treatment is foramen magnum decompression, with the aim of improving CSF drainage. The full benefits of surgery may not be achieved for 12 months following surgery.
- Successful surgery results in lack of strain-related, or neck extension-related headache.
- Syringomyelia is associated with sensitivity to non-depolarizing muscle relaxants and hyperkalaemia with suxamethonium.

NAP3 did not identify any cases where neurological complications could have been attributed to undiagnosed ACM Type 1 or 2 in either the obstetric or general population.

Neurovascular pathology

Cerebral aneurysm

Arising from the cerebral arterial vessels, when unruptured, these lesions are usually asymptomatic. Large aneurysms may cause mass effect with headache and focal neurological signs. Aneurysms of the posterior communicating artery may cause third nerve palsy. Large aneurysms of the basilar termination may cause brain stem decompression.

Cerebral aneurysms that are at increased risk of rupture (characterized by size and shape) may be treated electively.

Commonly held opinion is that neuraxial blockade may increase the gradient across the aneurysm wall by dropping CSF pressure. However, experience within neurosurgery, where intentional intrathecal lumbar drains are inserted for aneurysm surgery and CSF drainage is actively performed at craniotomy, suggests that this does not increase the risk of rupture.

Literature suggests that normal vaginal delivery with shortened second stage may be preferable, though evidence is lacking. The literature does not exist to give definitive advice regarding uterotonics. Specialist neurosurgical advice should be taken regarding anaesthetic management.

Cerebral arterio-venous malformations (AVM)

Cerebral AVM may increase in size during pregnancy. Up-to-date evaluation of lesions is necessary prior to forming an anaesthetic plan. Providing there is no mass effect, there is no evidence for increased risk of complications with neuraxial anaesthesia.

Cavernomas

Cavernomas can occur in the brain or spinal cord in 1 in 600 persons, of which 50% will be asymptomatic. Exclude lumbar spinal cavernomas prior to performing neuraxial anaesthesia in those known to be affected.

Sub-arachnoid haemorrhage

This is defined as the presence of free blood within the sub-arachnoid space, mixed with CSF. The blood may extend into the brain tissue (intracerebral haemorrhage (ICH)) and into the CSF ventricles (IVH). Risk of aneurysmal SAH is increased during pregnancy, labour and delivery, but is not increased by neuraxial anaesthesia.

Use of recreational drugs, e.g. cocaine, can result in both hypertension and vasculitis, both predisposing to intracranial bleeding. SAH/IVH may be the first presentation of AVM; in the absence of flow-related aneurysms, the risk of rebleeding is much lower than that of aneurysmal SAH.

Presentation (non-traumatic SAH)

Headache is classically accompanied by photophobia and vomiting. Immediate complications can be those of hydrocephalus and seizure. Rebleeding in the acute phase is associated with poor outcome. Alterations in cerebral perfusion may also occur between 2–21 days post primary bleed; these can be severe, causing cerebral ischaemia. Non-cranial complications of SAH include cardiac ischaemia, which may compromise cardiac function. Neurogenic pulmonary oedema may develop.

For differential diagnosis of headache see Chapter 25.

The diagnosis of aneurysmal SAH requires cerebral angiography, performed by CT, MR or formal angiography.

Treatment involves nimodipine orally/IV for 21 days. Prevention of rebleeding can be achieved by endovascular techniques or surgical clipping.

171

Cerebral venous thrombosis (CVT) commonly presents as insidious onset headache though may cause thunderclap headache in approximately 10% of cases. Symptoms may progress to reduced level of consciousness, seizures, lateralizing signs and papilloedema. The venous hypertension results in hypoperfusion and can cause cerebral infarction that commonly undergoes haemorrhagic conversion. Most CVTs (75%) occur post partum, and are linked with low CSF pressure states (e.g. PDPH). Presentation during pregnancy shows an initial peak in the first trimester, possibly due to dehydration resulting from hyperemesis, or related to undiagnosed thrombophilias.

Investigations

CT venogram/MR venogram (gold standard) are diagnostic but be aware, non-contrast CT head *may be negative.*

Treatment requires anticoagulation, though haemorrhagic transformation may impact upon the decision to start this.

Rare vascular conditions of brain and spinal cord, including conditions such as von Hippel–Lindau disease (VHL) and hereditary haemorrhagic telangiectasia (HHT), present the anaesthetist with craniospinal concerns of mass effect and haemorrhage. Such lesions are seldom solitary. Vascular lesions (haemangiomata, haemangioblastomata and arteriovenous malformations) of the cord may result in abnormal venous drainage and increased diameter of the cord within the canal, hence increasing the perceived risk of cord injury, haemorrhagic trauma to the lesion and increased risk of venous bleeding. As vascular lesions may increase in size during pregnancy, a detailed up-to-date evaluation of lumbar spinal anatomy is necessary to evaluate risk of epidural/sub-arachnoid anaesthesia.

Head injury in the obstetric population

Patients with head injury requiring admission have better outcomes (from the head injury) if they are treated in a specific neurosurgical centre, so transfer to a centre with co-located neurosurgery and obstetrics should be considered. It had been thought that the progestogenic and oestrogenic state of pregnancy would afford neuroprotection; however, a large retrospective review suggests that outcome is similar to that of non-pregnant women.

Surgical management of traumatic brain injury may involve insertion of an ICP monitor, EVD, evacuation of haematoma and decompressive craniectomy.

Evidence is lacking to suggest that modification of standard practice is required for management of head injury and neuroanaesthesia in the pregnant patient.

The neuroanaesthetic principles aim to:

- Avoid hypoxia.
- Obtain an optimal cerebral blood volume and perfusion. Patients should be ventilated to a 'normal $PaCO_2$'; this will depend upon the stage of pregnancy.
- Optimize CPP (CPP = MAP (mean arterial pressure) – ICP). Head up position and loose ET ties reduce cerebral venous congestion (the CPP target is 60–70 mmHg).
- Minimize rises in ICP. In the absence of ICP monitoring, an estimate of >20 mmHg should be assumed in the presence of a reduced level of consciousness. Mannitol is widely used in neurosurgical practice; however, evidence on outcome is lacking. Doses of 0.5–2.0 g/kg can acutely reduce ICP by both increasing CPP and also reducing brain water and hence brain volume. Furosemide is also used, and appears safe in pregnancy and breastfeeding.
- Avoid fluctuations in blood pressure. Preanaesthetic blood pressure can guide target postinduction blood pressure. Control excess hypertension using magnesium sulfate infusion rather than cerebral vasodilators, e.g. GTN. Avoid hypotension with its resultant reduced CPP and increased CBV.
- Avoid increasing cerebral metabolic rate (CMR).
- Minimize the risk or duration of seizure activity as this will increase cerebral metabolic rate ($CMRO_2$), particularly post head injury.
- Avoid and treat pyrexia.
- Avoid hypo/hyperglycaemia.

Epilepsy

Epilepsy is a common neurological disorder characterized by recurrent seizures. Women with epilepsy account for 0.3–0.7% of pregnancies in the developed world.

Epilepsy is the commonest cause of seizures during confinement; eclampsia, however, is the most common precipitant for peripartum seizures. (Local anaesthetic toxicity, metabolic derangement, amniotic fluid embolism (AFE) and space-occupying lesions must also be excluded.)

Most pregnancies are uneventful in women with epilepsy. However, there is evidence that parturients taking antiepileptic drugs (AED) are more at risk of developing pre-eclampsia.

Of parturients with epilepsy, 15%–37% will experience an increase in seizure frequency during pregnancy or in the early puerperium. This increase in seizure frequency can perhaps be attributed to poor treatment compliance, altered AED pharmacokinetics or sleep deprivation.

Of parturients with active epilepsy, 1–2% will have a tonic-clonic seizure during labour, and a further 1–2% within 24 hours post partum. A more profound hypoxia is observed in generalized tonic-clonic seizures during pregnancy as a result of the increased oxygen demand; this can adversely impact on the fetus.

There is no evidence that simple focal, complex focal, absence and myoclonic seizures adversely affect the pregnancy or developing fetus.

When managing AED during pregnancy, the risk of maternal and fetal harm from seizures needs to be balanced against the risk of harm from AED. NICE 2012 guidelines recommend aiming for seizure freedom before conception and during pregnancy (particularly for women with generalized tonic-clonic seizures) by using the lowest effective dose of each AED, avoiding polytherapy where possible. AED can cause fetal malformations and possible neurodevelopmental impairments. Studies suggest that valproate is significantly more teratogenic than carbamazepine, and valproate when used in combination (especially with lamotrigine) is particularly teratogenic.

Altered AED pharmacokinetics are observed in pregnancy: an increase in the clearance and a decrease in the concentration of lamotrigine, phenytoin and to a lesser extent carbamazepine is observed; the levels of levetiracetam and the active oxcarbazepine metabolite can also decrease.

Despite this, NICE do not recommend the routine monitoring of AED levels during pregnancy. If seizures increase or are likely to increase, monitoring AED levels (particularly levels of lamotrigine and phenytoin) may be useful when making dose adjustments.

Breastfeeding is encouraged in parturients with epilepsy; however, certain AEDs may be transferred into breast milk in amounts that may be clinically important.

Epidural anaesthesia is a good analgesic option for labour in epileptics, avoiding opiate-induced CNS depression. Slow establishment of the block limits the plasma concentrations of local anaesthetic and reduces the risk of seizures. There are no contraindications to spinal anaesthesia or general anaesthesia.

Migraine

Migraine is a chronic disorder characterized by recurrent moderate to severe headaches, often unilateral and associated with autonomic nervous system symptoms. For diagnostic criteria refer to The International Headache Society.

Approximately one-third of women of childbearing age suffer with migraines. New onset migraines can occur in 1.3–16.5% pregnancies; these are more likely to occur in the first trimester and be accompanied by aura.

Between 50 and 75% of migraineurs experience a reduction in the frequency of migraines or complete cessation of symptoms, normally in their second and third trimesters. This is particularly the case with parturients whose migraines are perimenstrual or pure menstrual. In such cases, as pregnancy progresses, remaining migraines show a reduction in pain intensity.

If a migraineur experiences no reduction in frequency or severity by the end of the first trimester then migraines are likely to continue throughout the peripartum period.

Approximately 8% of migraineurs will experience an increase in frequency and pain intensity of migraines throughout pregnancy. This is more likely in those who suffer with aura. In general, those who suffer with aura are less likely to experience an improvement of symptoms.

Postpartum headache occurs in 30–40% of all parturients. An increased incidence of headache immediately following birth and 3 weeks post partum has been observed. This is postulated to be multifactorial: fatigue, anxiety, hormonal changes and iatrogenic causes at the time of delivery.

Of migraineurs who experience improvement in their symptoms during pregnancy, 50% will have a recurrence of their normal migraine pattern shortly post partum.

Some studies have concluded that whilst breastfeeding, the stable oestrogen levels preventing menstruation also offer some protection against migraine recurrence. Other studies have failed to reproduce these findings. There is no evidence that breastfeeding increases the occurrence of headaches in the postpartum period.

Some studies suggest that parity does not have an effect on migraine symptoms during pregnancy. Other studies show that multiparous patients are more likely to have an increase in migraines at the end of the third trimester and post delivery.

Women with migraine have been shown to have an increased risk of pre-eclampsia and gestational hypertension in pregnancy. They may also have an increased risk of stroke and cerebral vasoconstrictive syndrome.

There are no contraindications to any pharmacological or neuraxial analgesia options for delivery; however, investigation of postpartum headache in migraineurs can be challenging and complications of neuraxial blockade add to the differential diagnosis.

Multiple sclerosis (MS)

MS is an idiopathic inflammatory disease affecting the central nervous system leading to demyelination in the brain and spinal cord. It affects more women compared to men and about 70% of cases present between 20 and 40 years of age. In the UK it is estimated that 20,000 or more women of childbearing age are affected.

MS typically follows a relapsing remitting course that can present with sensory or motor deficit of varying severity. The PRIMS study (a large multicentre study of parturients suffering from MS) demonstrated a significant decrease in the relapse rate during pregnancy with a rebound increase in the first 3 months post partum.

The fetus, having both paternal and maternal antigens, induces a degree of immunosuppression in pregnancy that is necessary for its survival. This is achieved by the upregulation of type 2 helper T cells (Th-2), which encourages a humeral response, while inhibiting type 1 helper T cell (Th-1) response. As MS is an autoimmune disease mediated by activation of Th-1 cells and proinflammatory cytokines, these pregnancy-related changes lead to a decrease in MS disease activity.

A recent survey reported that within a 10-year period, 91% of anaesthetists have encountered <10 cases of MS. Limited case exposure hinders data collection regarding optimal management.

Key anaesthetic issues based on recent available evidence include:

- All patients should be reviewed in an antenatal anaesthetic clinic. Disease severity and extent of pre-existing neurological deficit should be documented. Analgesic and anaesthetic options for labour and operative intervention should be discussed.
- Use of 0.1% bupivacaine with 2 µg/mL fentanyl mixture for epidural labour analgesia is deemed safe. Theoretically, epidural anaesthesia would expose the demyelinated nerves to lower concentrations of local anaesthetic, although this effect might be negated by the use of multiple top-ups.
- Epidurals can be topped up with a higher concentration of local anaesthetic for an operative intervention.
- The majority of surveyed UK anaesthetists would offer regional anaesthesia, with spinal anaesthesia being the preferred anaesthetic option, for elective or emergency caesarean section. Combined spinal-epidural may also be considered on an individual case basis. This could reduce the amount of local anaesthetic in the sub-arachnoid space.
- Due to the upregulation of acetylcholine receptors, it is advisable to avoid succinylcholine, as this can lead to hyperkalaemia and cardiac arrest.
- Dosage of non-depolarizing blocking agents should be guided by neuromuscular function monitoring. Maintenance of normothermia is also important.

Key points

When caring for parturients with co-existing neurosurgical pathology remember:

- A multidisciplinary approach involving obstetricians, neurosurgeons and anaesthetists is necessary. Neurology and endocrinology input may also be required. Timely antenatal assessment and risk/benefit discussions are essential for ongoing care during pregnancy, delivery and post partum.
- Conditions can progress during pregnancy and decisions regarding care must be made upon up-to-date evaluation and imaging.
- 'Non-obstetric causes' of headache or neurological deterioration must *always* be considered.
- Acute neurological deterioration requires urgent attention and involvement of specialists.
- Transfer of care to a centre with co-located neurosurgery and obstetric facilities may be appropriate.

Further reading

Drake, E., Drake, M., Bird, J. and Russell, R. (2006). Obstetric regional blocks for women with multiple sclerosis: a survey of UK experience. *Int. J. Obstet. Anaesth.*, **15**(2), 115–123.

Griffiths, S. and Durbridge, J. A. (2011). Anaesthetic implications of neurological disease in pregnancy. *Contin. Educ. Anaesth. Crit. Care Pain.*, **11**, 157.

Klein, A. and Loder, E. (2010). Postpartum headache. *Int. J. Obstet. Anaesth.*, **19**, 422–430.

Kvisvik, E. V., Stovner, L. J., Helde, G., Bovim, G. and Linde, M. (2011). Headache and migraine during pregnancy and puerperium: the MIGRA-study. *Headache Pain*, **12**, 443–451.

Lindsay, K. W. and Bone, I. (2004). *Neurology and Neurosurgery, 4th edn.* London: Churchill Livingstone.

Matta, B., Menon, D. and Turner, J. (2000). *Textbook of Neuroanaesthesia and Critical Care.* London: Greenwich Medical Media Ltd.

Nolan, J. and Soar, J. (2012). *Anaesthesia for Emergency Care.* Oxford: Oxford Speciality Handbooks.

Vukusic, S., Hutchinson, M., Hours, M. *et al.* (2004). Pregnancy and multiple sclerosis (the PRIMS study): clinical predictors of post-partum relapse. *Brain*, **127**(6), 1353–1360.

Chapter 23

Immunology, including testing and management of allergy during pregnancy

Gareth Kitchen, Tomaz Garcez and Nigel J. N. Harper

Introduction

This chapter focuses on allergic diseases and their relevance to obstetric anaesthesia, with practical advice on management. Ideally, parturients with suspected allergic disease should be assessed prior to pregnancy, in order to identify relevant allergens and to confirm a management plan. Parturients with a history suggestive of adverse drug reaction require further investigation to identify the cause or to exclude allergy. A previous perioperative or peripartum adverse event necessitates review of those anaesthetic and medical records. If a patient has experienced a serious adverse reaction, their notes should be clearly marked with drug allergy information and a hazard-warning bracelet advised.

Pregnancy presents other immunological challenges to the mother and semiallograft fetus. For the pregnancy to succeed, local and systemic immunological changes are required, including reduction in cytotoxic adaptive immunity and enhancement of regulation. The systemic impact of the immunological changes is not clear, but there is an increased risk of atopic and autoimmune dermatoses in pregnancy. There is no clear evidence to suggest that general atopic diseases are affected.

Autoimmune diseases can have a significant impact on pregnancy, particularly when autoantibodies directed against phospholipids, SS-A or SS-B are present. Antiphospholipid syndrome is associated with increased risk of pregnancy morbidity and loss. The presence of antibodies directed against SS-A and/or SS-B is associated with neonatal lupus and congenital heart block. The effect of pregnancy on the course of autoimmune diseases is more variable, with both improvement and deterioration reported without consistency.

Immunodeficiency syndromes may also present challenges in pregnancy. Patients with antibody deficiency syndromes will have increased requirements of immunoglobulin replacement in the third trimester of pregnancy due to active transplacental transfer of immunoglobulin G. Patients with hereditary angioedema (HAE) may improve, remain stable or deteriorate during pregnancy and should receive prophylactic treatment before any instrumental delivery or surgical procedure. Increased vigilance through pregnancy and during delivery is therefore advised for most patients with pre-existent immunologically mediated diseases.

Allergens relevant to anaesthesia

A perioperative allergic reaction is often attributed to drugs, chlorhexidine or latex exposure.

Taking a clinical history for drug allergy

Type I hypersensitivity (IgE-mediated) is often considered to be true allergy. See Table 23.1.

Many patients report allergy to medications: 10% of hospital inpatients self-report penicillin allergy; 90% of patients self-reporting penicillin allergy are able to tolerate penicillin on challenge without adverse reaction (see Box 23.1 and Figure 23.1). The most significant features are time course from exposure to onset of symptoms and nature of the symptoms. In many cases, patients are unable to recall an accurate history, making further assessment challenging. This approach can be applied to other suspected drug allergies.

Investigations for antibiotic allergy include the use of skin prick (SPT) and intradermal (IDT) tests. If the skin tests are negative, graded challenge is required to exclude allergy. Allergen-specific IgE is available for penicillin allergy, but is not sufficiently sensitive to exclude allergy. If either the skin or blood tests are

Core Topics in Obstetric Anaesthesia, ed. Kirsty MacLennan, Kate O'Brien and W. Ross Mcnab.
Published by Cambridge University Press. © Cambridge University Press 2015.

Table 23.1 Classification of hypersensitivity reactions

Type I – Immediate	Mediated by IgE, mast cells and basophils	Allergic anaphylaxis
Type II – Cytotoxic	IgG and IgM antibody mediated	ABO incompatibility, drug induced haemolysis and haemolytic disease of the newborn
Type III – Immune complex	Immune complex mediated	Rheumatoid arthritis and SLE
Type IV – Delayed	T-cell mediated	Contact sensitivity

BOX 23.1 History details required for a drug allergy history

1. Exact drug and route
2. Exact timing of reaction
    a. From last dose
    b. During course (after which dose)
3. Details of infection/symptoms at the time of exposure (what was the infection)
4. Features of the reaction
    a. Itch
    b. Rash
        i. Flushing
        ii. Urticaria
        iii. Maculopapular
        iv. Morbilliform
        v. Bullous/AGEP
        vi. Erythema multiforme/SJS/TEN
        vii. Desquamation
        viii. Mucosal involvement
        ix. Fixed drug eruption
    c. Angioedema
    d. Wheeze
    e. GI symptoms
    f. Hypotension
    g. Fever
    h. Abnormal LFT
5. Other medications at the time
6. Treatment and response to treatment
7. Details of reactions on prior exposure to same drug(s)
8. Details of any subsequent exposure to same or similar drug(s).

Key:

AGEP = Acute generalized exanthematous pustulosis

EM = erythema multiforme

SJS = Stevens–Johnson syndrome

TEN = toxic epidermal necrolysis

LFT = liver function tests

positive in the context of penicillin allergy, a challenge would not be performed as the tests are considered to have high specificity. The reliability of skin testing for non-β-lactam antibiotics is less well understood, but SPT and IDT are generally carried out prior to challenge tests, which are the gold standard test for drug allergy.

Cross-sensitization within antibiotics

The most reliable data exists for penicillin-based (β-lactam group) antibiotics and local antibiotic guidelines should detail antibiotics that are considered safe in patients with documented penicillin allergy. The risk of cross-reactivity or sensitization within the β-lactam group varies. A positive skin test reaction to penicillin infers a 2% risk of reacting on challenge to a cephalosporin and approximately 1% risk to a carbapenem. The safest approach in confirmed penicillin allergy is to avoid all β-lactam antibiotics, as reactions, although infrequent, can include anaphylaxis.

If patients are selectively allergic to the amoxicillin or ampicillin (aminopenicillins) side chain, rather than the β-lactam ring structure, then cephalosporins with an identical side chain should be avoided, but other β-lactam antibiotics do not need to be avoided. The estimated risk of cross-reactivity between aminopenicillins and cephalosporins with an identical side chain is around 24%, but this is based on limited data from a single country. The safest approach in aminopenicillin allergy is to avoid all β-lactam antibiotics unless assessed in an allergy clinic specifically for cross-reactivity.

Reliable data are not available on cross-reactivity for other antibiotic groups and therefore the safest advice is to avoid all structurally similar antibiotics.

Reactions to neuromuscular blocking drugs

Anaphylaxis to neuromuscular blocking drugs may be allergic or non-allergic: the clinical features may be

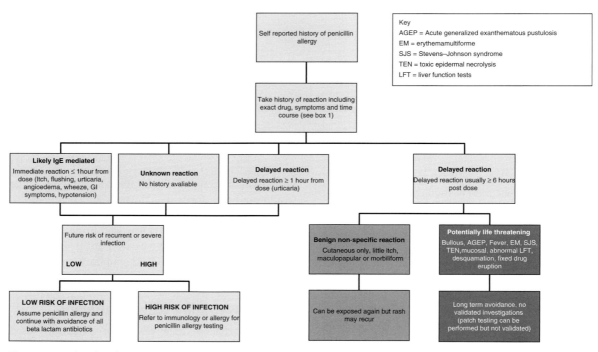

Figure 23.1 Flowchart for management of patients with self-reported penicillin allergy.

indistinguishable. Mivacurium and atracurium commonly cause degranulation of mast cells. Mast-cell degranulation in the skin produces the familiar cutaneous flush, but more widespread degranulation of mast cells and basophils may result in life-threatening bronchospasm, hypotension and angioedema. Cisatracurium, rocuronium and vecuronium are not characterized by non-allergic anaphylaxis. Suxamethonium is the anaesthetic drug most likely to cause an allergic anaphylactic reaction. When a patient reports a previous adverse reaction to suxamethonium, it is often unclear whether the mechanism was anaphylaxis, a plasma cholinesterase deficiency causing 'suxamethonium apnoea', or even malignant hyperthermia (MH). In addition to obtaining copies of the relevant documentation, it is a relatively easy matter to exclude plasma cholinesterase deficiency with the appropriate blood test. The majority of MH-susceptible families, in the UK, are known to the MH Unit at St James' Hospital, Leeds. If any uncertainty persists, the avoidance of trigger agents is straightforward, and rocuronium should be used in preference to suxamethonium to facilitate tracheal intubation. Sugammadex should be available in all obstetric units as a rescue drug in a 'can't intubate can't ventilate (CICV) situation'.

Cross-sensitivity between neuromuscular blocking agents (NMBA) is present in a high proportion of patients who are diagnosed with NMBA-induced anaphylaxis. Contrary to common belief, cross-sensitivity is not confined within classes of NMBA: for example, a patient who has experienced allergic anaphylaxis to atracurium may be co-allergic to rocuronium or suxamethonium. Consequently, a patient with known or suspected allergy to a specific muscle-relaxant drug must not be exposed to any NMBA unless skin testing has confirmed a suitable alternative to which the patient is unlikely to be allergic. In practice this necessitates skin prick testing (SPT) followed, if negative, by intradermal testing (IDT). The sensitivity of IDT for NMBA is high. SPT is performed initially because, although the sensitivity of the test may be less than IDT, SPT is less likely to induce a significant reaction if the patient is allergic to the drug. There are no reliable blood tests for NMBA allergy. The sensitivity of the blood test for specific antibodies to suxamethonium is relatively poor and this test should not be used to exclude allergy because the consequences of a false-negative result could be catastrophic. It must be emphasized that skin testing must be performed only in expert centres with considerable experience of interpreting the results. Pregnancy is not an absolute contraindication to skin testing, but the decision should be left to the expert centre. The decision whether to perform skin testing will depend on the suspected allergen, the prior probability of allergy, the sensitivity and specificity of the test, and the likelihood of a serious reaction occurring if the patient becomes exposed to the allergen. Intubation of the trachea without muscle relaxants has not been investigated in the pregnant patient, but avoiding NMBA is associated with a 52% higher likelihood of difficult intubation in the non-parturient.

Reactions to analgesics

Reported allergy to opioid analgesia is common, which raises the question about management of pain in labour. A careful, unhurried history of events is important. Nausea and vomiting alone is highly unlikely to represent allergy. A localized itchy rash after the administration of IV morphine is characteristic of harmless non-specific histamine release and is not suggestive of allergy. A sensation of being acutely unwell after taking codeine is likely to be the consequence of ultra-fast metabolism to morphine as a result of CYP2D6 gene duplication, seen in 1%–7% of the population. Allergy to fentanyl, alfentanil and remifentanil is vanishingly uncommon. There are recent reports of serious adverse reactions to remifentanil during labour, but these are highly unlikely to be the result of allergy. Skin tests are not useful for investigating suspected allergy to morphine, diamorphine, pethidine or codeine because these drugs cause non-specific degranulation of mast cells in the skin. In contrast, fentanyl, alfentanil and remifentanil are not associated with false-positive skin tests. A blood test for specific-IgE to morphine is marketed, but its reliability is uncertain and it is not widely available in UK immunology laboratories.

Gastrointestinal intolerance to NSAIDs is extremely common. They may also be responsible in some individuals for non-IgE-mediated swelling, rash or bronchospasm. Skin testing is not useful in making the diagnosis, but avoidance is not problematical. A graded challenge test may be the only way to confirm the diagnosis, but should be delayed until after delivery.

Local anaesthetic (LA) allergy

Allergy to LA is a real entity, but is extremely uncommon. The issue of supposed LA allergy usually arises because a patient has experienced unpleasant symptoms during dental treatment. Because LA drugs are the mainstay of obstetric anaesthesia and analgesia, it is important to investigate these suspected reactions to reassure the parturient. Exclusion of allergy on history alone is usually possible; the sensation of palpitations, headache and a feeling of impending catastrophe is characteristic of the systemic effects of vasoconstrictor agents used in dental surgery. Delayed swelling after dental treatment often results from tissue oedema, but occasionally represents stress-induced angioedema. The differential diagnosis includes latex allergy (see below). If allergy to LA cannot be excluded by taking a careful history, the parturient should be referred to a specialist centre for skin testing. The investigation pathway comprises SPT, IDT and sub-cutaneous challenge. Delayed hypersensitivity to prilocaine is sometimes seen after local anaesthetic cream is used to reduce the discomfort of venepuncture. This is not life-threatening and does not preclude the use of spinal or epidural analgesia with bupivacaine.

Allergy to chlorhexidine

Anaphylaxis to chlorhexidine appears to be increasing. Features of anaphylaxis may be immediate or delayed for up to 30 minutes following exposure. Individuals become sensitized by exposure to chlorhexidine in daily life and subsequent exposure in a healthcare setting may cause a life-threatening anaphylactic reaction. Severe anaphylaxis appears to be more likely when chlorhexidine gains access to the circulation during interventional procedures, such as central venous cannulation, cardiac catheterization, dental surgery and urethral catheterization. The MHRA issued a Medical Devices Alert (MDA) in July 2012 relating to chlorhexidine-coated central venous lines and haemo-dialysis catheters, and a second MDA in October 2012 relating to all medical devices and medicinal products containing chlorhexidine.

Some patients previously experience symptoms suggestive of chlorhexidine allergy that goes unrecognized. Increased awareness among healthcare professionals of chlorhexidine allergy might highlight this possibility and allow the patient to be referred for allergy testing before the occurrence of life-threatening allergy. Avoidance of chlorhexidine is a considerable undertaking, especially if an obstetric patient is admitted as an emergency, and therefore efforts to diagnose chlorhexidine allergy should be made as early as possible in pregnancy so that a management plan can be documented. The currently available blood test for IgE antibodies specific to chlorhexidine has a relatively high sensitivity and this should be the first step in the diagnostic pathway in the pregnant patient. If the specific IgE test is negative, despite a strong clinical history, the patient should be referred to a specialist allergy clinic so that the relative merits of skin testing can be discussed.

Latex allergy

All healthcare environments should have a documented protocol for managing patients who are allergic to natural rubber latex (NRL). Allergy to latex is discussed in detail in the AAGBI guidelines, *Suspected Anaphylactic Reactions Associated with Anaesthesia*, 2009. Anaphylaxis to latex is decreasing, probably because non-latex gloves and other equipment are increasingly used in healthcare. Type 1 latex allergy can usually be identified or excluded on history alone. If a patient can blow-up a party balloon without experiencing itch or swelling, it is highly unlikely that they are allergic to latex. If the history is suspicious of latex allergy, a blood test for latex-specific IgE should be performed, but the sensitivity is less than 85%. If the blood test is positive the prevailing latex-avoidance protocol should be invoked and the parturient should be offered referral to a specialist allergy centre for further investigation post partum. If the history is strongly suggestive of latex allergy and the blood test is negative, the parturient should still be offered referral to a specialist allergy centre to discuss skin testing. Preparation of the delivery room and operating theatre for a patient who is allergic to latex does not need to be an onerous undertaking if common sense is applied. All obstetric units should have a list of equipment that contains latex. It is necessary to remove all latex gloves and other latex-containing equipment from the room and a notice should be posted on the door. It is not necessary to remove items of equipment that do not contain latex. Because modern hospital rooms and operating theatres are equipped with forced ventilation, it is unnecessary to prepare the room earlier than a couple of hours before admitting a latex-allergic patient. Allergy to latex is not transmitted from mother to fetus, but the neonatal paediatric team should avoid using equipment that contains latex if they are present in the same room as the mother.

Allergy to intravenous colloids

Intravenous gelatins are a significant cause of anaphylaxis, although often overlooked. Onset is usually within minutes of starting an infusion. The reaction is usually IgE-mediated, but the sensitivity of the blood test for gelatin-specific IgE is very poor; diagnosis requires skin prick testing or intradermal testing. Intravenous starch solutions are no longer available in the UK.

Allergy to adhesive tape/dressings

Suspected allergy to adhesive dressings results from non-specific irritation of the skin or type 4 delayed hypersensitivity. Patch testing can be performed locally (it does not require special expertise) with a selection of adhesive tapes and dressings. A positive test produces a raised, reddened area.

Presentations that may not be allergy

Non-allergic drug reactions

Only a small proportion of drug reactions are allergic in origin. Type A, augmented, reactions are responsible for the majority of the observed instances of hypotension during anaesthesia (see Table 23.2).

Table 23.2 Non-allergic drug reactions

Type A – *Augmented*. An exaggerated, expected pharmacodynamic response, for example respiratory depression with opioids, or bradycardia with remifentanil. These are frequent, predictable and dose related.	Type B – *Idiosyncratic*. These are unexpected and unrelated to the dose administered. Allergy and anaphylaxis belong to this group.
Type C – *Continuing*. Will occur in most patients if the duration of treatment is long enough.	Type D – *Delayed*. The adverse effect can be seen a significant amount of time after the drug has been stopped, for example carcinogenicity and teratogenicity.

Urticaria: 'hives'

Urticaria is a common medical problem affecting 20% of the population at some point in their lives. Urticaria results from histamine release from mast cells. The majority of urticaria occurs during viral infections in childhood, often leading to a presumptive diagnosis of antibiotic drug allergy as the urticaria arises shortly after starting antibiotics for a viral infection. Only 20% of cases of urticaria are caused by allergy, and in these cases the triggering agent is often obvious to the patient. Many cases of urticaria remain of unknown cause and are termed idiopathic urticaria. A diagnosis of chronic idiopathic urticaria is made if urticaria occurs on most days of the week for a 6-week period. It is thought to be autoimmune in origin, although this theory has not been conclusively confirmed. Of patients with chronic idiopathic urticaria, 40% also experience angioedema with episodes of urticaria. Chronic idiopathic urticaria has a prevalence of around 1% and spontaneously remits in most patients within 2 to 5 years. There are a number of recognized aggravating factors for idiopathic urticaria including physical factors, alcohol, stress and histamine releasing medications. The physical and emotional stresses involved in delivery (including instrumental or operative) will contribute to an increased peripartum risk of an urticarial reaction. The use of various medications including those known to release histamine from mast cells, such as atracurium, mivacurium, opiates, contrast, gelatin-based intravenous fluids and non-steroidal anti-inflammatory drugs can increase the likelihood of an urticarial eruption in susceptible patients. In parturients with a background history of urticaria the risk of an eruption may be reduced by premedication with antihistamines prior to exposure to an aggravating factor.

Angioedema: 'swellings'

Angioedema most commonly occurs with urticaria as part of chronic idiopathic urticaria, but may also occur without urticaria (idiopathic angioedema), as a side effect of angiotensin converting enzyme inhibitors (ACEi) or due to hereditary or acquired angioedema (HAE or AAE). The pathogenesis of idiopathic angioedema is not clear. ACEi-related angioedema occurs due to interference with the kinin system and increased production of bradykinin. Bradykinin is a potent vasodilatory mediator and excess causes localized oedema. The only intervention required for ACEi angioedema is to stop the ACEi. HAE is a genetic condition where there is a deficiency of active complement protein C1 esterase inhibitor, which results in increased levels of bradykinin. The prevalence of HAE is estimated at 1 per 50,000. Patients with HAE should be managed in conjunction with a clinical immunologist during pregnancy as their requirements for treatment including prophylaxis prior to labour will need to be customized based on previous history. In the case of emergency intervention, administration of C1 esterase inhibitor concentrate should be provided as soon as possible. The dose of C1 esterase inhibitor concentrate prior to delivery is 500 to 1000 IU. In low-risk pregnancies, where it has been decided not to provide prophylaxis, C1 esterase inhibitor should be available in the delivery room. AAE is a very rare condition where angioedema presents in the absence of urticaria, but often associated with B-cell malignancies or autoimmune diseases. The prevalence of AAE is unknown but is far less than HAE (1 AAE patient per 12 HAE patients in one large angioedema centre). Angioedema occurs secondary to bradykinin accumulation in AAE, similar to HAE, and the treatment is the same.

Atopic illnesses during pregnancy

Rhinitis

See Chapter 16 for asthma.

Ideally patients with rhinitis should be assessed for allergy prior to pregnancy so appropriate avoidance advice can be provided. Rhinitis severity can improve during pregnancy, however oedema of the nasal mucosa can complicate pregnancy and this can worsen or cause rhinitis symptoms. Rhinitis does not appear to have an adverse impact on the outcomes of pregnancy. Non-pharmacological management of rhinitis includes saline nasal spray or irrigation, physical exercise, mechanical airway dilatation with adhesive strips and elevation of the head end of the bed. Pharmacological measures considered safe in pregnancy include nasal cromoglycate, nasal corticosteroids and antihistamines. Nasal and systemic decongestants should be avoided if possible. Immunotherapy for allergic rhinitis can be continued, but is normally not commenced during pregnancy.

Food allergy is managed as per the non-pregnant population.

Exercise-induced anaphylaxis

Exercise-induced anaphylaxis (EIA) is a rare, but increasingly recognized syndrome of anaphylaxis developing in the context of exercise. In some cases EIA occurs only if food has been consumed within a few hours prior to exercise, and often only following specific food (such as wheat-dependent EIA). The prevalence is largely unknown, but has been estimated at 0.03% in a Japanese adolescent population. Management focuses on avoidance of known triggers, fasting prior to exercise and identification of an exercise regimen that does not precipitate symptoms. Pharmacological therapy includes the use of sodium cromoglycate and antihistamines, but there is limited evidence of significant efficacy. There are reports of labour precipitating episodes of EIA and anecdotal reports of early epidural leading to normal labour in parturients at risk. Measures to reduce stress during labour theoretically should reduce the risk of EIA in susceptible individuals. Emergency facilities should be available.

Testing for allergy in pregnancy

Testing for allergy involves taking a clinical history and performing allergy skin and/or blood tests. If the skin and blood tests are negative a provocation challenge is offered as the gold standard test to exclude allergy. Challenge testing is not required in all cases, but is useful to exclude allergy in cases of suspected antibiotic allergy. Ideally a diagnosis of allergy should be made prior to pregnancy to reduce risks and ensure avoidance advice is in place. Parturients are often worried about the risks of allergy testing. There are no significant risks with allergy blood tests. Skin prick tests are also safe with only very rare reports of systemic reactions. In most cases allergy skin testing can be delayed until after delivery, but the parturient can be reassured that the tests are safe if they are required to exclude latex or drug allergy. Intradermal skin testing and challenge testing potentially carry more risk of inducing a severe reaction during the testing procedure; these forms of testing are not usually undertaken in pregnancy unless there is a specific need, such as to exclude penicillin allergy to enable treatment of syphilis.

Management of atopic presentations in pregnancy

Antihistamines in pregnancy

All drugs should be avoided in the first trimester of pregnancy if possible. Chlorphenamine and hydroxyzine at standard dose have appropriate safety data during pregnancy and should be the preferred first-line agents. If chlorphenamine or hydroxyzine are not tolerated due to adverse effects loratadine or cetirizine are suitable alternatives, without any current evidence of teratogenesis, but should be avoided in the first trimester if possible.

Management of patients undergoing desensitization

Desensitization (immunotherapy) therapy is used to modify the allergic response and is currently offered in the UK for respiratory, venom, food and drug allergy. Food and drug desensitization is not widely offered. Desensitization is not started during pregnancy except for the rare cases of syphilis infection occurring in penicillin-allergic mothers. Patients already established on desensitization when they become pregnant do not appear to be at increased risk of pregnancy-related morbidity, despite continuing desensitization and are therefore advised to continue desensitization unless they are not deriving any benefit or have experienced frequent systemic reactions during therapy.

Clinical features and management of anaphylaxis in pregnancy and parturition

Anaphylaxis in pregnancy is rare but may be associated with disastrous consequences for mother and fetus. The incidence of maternal anaphylaxis in the US appears to be approximately 2.7 per 100,000 deliveries. The most recent CMACE triennial report included a maternal death from anaphylaxis to co-amoxiclav given intravenously for pyrexia in labour. There was no history of penicillin allergy nor was there sub-standard care. The report highlighted the importance of immediate medical response, administration of adrenaline and that anaphylaxis management charts should be immediately available in all clinical areas. The UK Obstetric Surveillance

Table 23.3 Distinguishing features of anaphylaxis and amniotic fluid embolism

Feature (frequency +)	Anaphylaxis	Amniotic Fluid Embolism
Suspected exposure to specific trigger agent	+++	–
Coagulopathy	+	++++
Pulmonary oedema	+	+++
Rash	++	+
Bronchospasm	++	+
Right ventricular end-diastolic volume (echocardiogram)	Low (reduced venous return)	High (right heart failure)
Raised mast cell tryptase	+++	+

Table 23.4 Immediate management of anaphylaxis

- ABC approach
- Remove potential causative agents if possible (e.g. IV colloids, chlorhexidine, latex)
- Call for help, note the time
- Maintain a patent airway, high-flow oxygen, intubate the trachea if necessary
- If appropriate, immediate cardiopulmonary resuscitation according to ALS Guidelines
- IM adrenaline 500 μg (0.5 mL 1:1000), repeated if necessary. IV adrenaline if full vital-signs monitoring available, initial dose 50 μg (0.5 mL 1:10,000) repeated if necessary
- Rapid IV crystalloid infusion
- Displace the gravid uterus to the left (manual displacement or wedge)
- Consider immediate delivery of the baby
- Do not sit up the patient

System (UKOSS) 2012–2014 report should provide further incidence data.

The cardinal clinical features of anaphylaxis in pregnancy are the same as in the non-pregnant individual. However, several additional causes of maternal collapse in the third trimester may complicate diagnosis (Chapter 25). Amniotic fluid embolism (AFE) may mimic anaphylaxis but the pattern of clinical features usually enables the clinician to distinguish between them (Table 23.3).

The management of anaphylaxis is described in the AAGBI Safety Guideline (2009) and the Resuscitation Council Guideline (2008). Management algorithms differ depending on resuscitation setting, with additional considerations in pregnancy. Despite the high success rate of maternal resuscitation, there are several reports of hypoxic neurological damage occurring in the neonate as a result of maternal anaphylaxis.

Adrenaline remains the drug of choice for anaphylaxis treatment with α-adrenergic receptor activity and β-adrenergic mast cell stabilizing effects. Limited data exists concerning alternative vasopressor drugs in anaphylaxis, especially in pregnancy. Phenylephrine is used commonly in UK practice to maintain blood pressure during neuraxial blockade. This drug is a suitable vasopressor in anaphylaxis, but only as a second-line drug if the blood pressure fails to respond to repeated doses of adrenaline. There have been several reports describing the efficacy of vasopressin in intractable anaphylaxis, but there is no experience of this drug during pregnancy.

Factors determining the decision whether to proceed urgently to deliver the baby in maternal collapse are discussed in Chapter 25 and the same general principles apply in maternal anaphylaxis (see Tables 23.4 and 23.5).

Table 23.5 Secondary management of anaphylaxis

- Chlorphenamine 10 mg IV (adult dose)
- Hydrocortisone 200 mg IV (adult dose)
- If the blood pressure does not recover despite an adrenaline infusion, consider IV metaraminol, phenylephrine or noradrenaline
- Treat persistent bronchospasm with a metered-dose inhaler or an IV infusion of salbutamol. Consider IV aminophylline or magnesium sulfate
- If the patient takes β-receptor antagonist drugs, consider glucagon IV 1–5 mg followed by an infusion at 5–15 µg/min
- Blood sample for coagulation profile and blood cross-match
- Blood samples for mast cell tryptase (1 h, 2 h, baseline)
- Arrange transfer of the patient to the obstetric operating theatre or critical care unit

Key points

1. Ideally parturients with suspected allergic disease should be assessed prior to pregnancy.
2. Although 10% of hospital inpatients self-report penicillin allergy, 90% of these patients are able to tolerate penicillin on challenge with no adverse reactions.
3. Pregnancy is not an absolute contraindication to skin prick testing.
4. The decision whether to perform skin prick testing during pregnancy depends on the suspected allergen, probability of allergy, sensitivity and specificity of the test, and the likelihood of a serious reaction if the woman is exposed to the allergen.
5. Non-allergic drug reactions account for most drug reactions.
6. It is rare to commence desensitization therapy during pregnancy, but women already on a programme may continue with no increase in pregnancy-related morbidity.

Further reading

Association of Anaesthetists of Great Britain and Ireland (2009). AAGBI Safety Guideline: Suspected anaphylactic reactions associated with anaesthesia. http://www.aagbi.org/sites/default/files/anaphylaxis_2009.pdf (accessed May 2015).

Bhole, M. V., Manson, A. L., Seneviratne, S. L. and Misbah, S. A. (2012). IgE-mediated allergy to local anaesthetics: separating fact from perception: a UK perspective. *Br. J. Anaesth.* **1**, 108, 903–911.

Chaudhuri, K., Gonzales, J., Jesurun, C. A., Ambat, M. T. and Mandal-Chaudhuri, S. (2008). Anaphylactic shock in pregnancy: a case study and review of the literature. *Int. J. Obstet. Anesth.*, **17**, 350–357.

Gompels, M. M., Lock, R. J., Abinun, M. *et al.* (2005). C1 inhibitor deficiency: consensus document. *Clin. Exp. Immunol.*, **139**(3), 379–394. Erratum: 141: 189–190.

Kar, S., Krishnan, A., Preetha, K. and Mohankar, A. (2012). A review of antihistamines used during pregnancy. *J. Pharmacol. Pharmacother.*, **3**: 105–108.

Lundstrøm, L. H., Møller, A. M., Rosenstock, C. *et al.* and the Danish Anaesthesia Database (2009). Avoidance of neuromuscular blocking agents may increase the risk of difficult tracheal intubation: a cohort study of 103,812 consecutive adult patients recorded in the Danish Anaesthesia Database. *Br. J. Anaesth.*, **103**, 283–290.

Nakonechna, A., Dore, P., Dixon, T. *et al.* (2012). Immediate hypersensitivity to chlorhexidine is increasingly recognised in the United Kingdom. *Allergol. Immunopathol. (Madr.)*, **42**, 44–49.

O'Connor, K. (2010). Labour complicated by a history of exercise induced anaphylaxis. *BJA out of the blue.* http://bja.oxfordjournals.org/forum/topic/brjana_el%3B5485 (accessed May 2015).

Soar, J., Pumphrey, R., Cant, A. *et al.*; Working Group of the Resuscitation Council (UK). (2008). Emergency treatment of anaphylactic reactions-Guidelines for healthcare providers. *Resuscitation.*, **77**(2), 157–169.

Sørensen, M. K., Bretlau, C., Gätke, M. R., Sørensen, A.M. and Rasmussen, L. S. (2012). Rapid sequence induction and intubation with rocuronium-sugammadex compared with succinylcholine: a randomized trial. *Br. J. Anaesth.*, **108**, 682–689.

HIV and infectious disease in pregnancy, including herpes, syphilis and hepatitis

Jacqueline E. A. K. Bamfo, Matthew D. Phillips, M. Kingston, K. Chan and Ian Clegg

HIV

Introduction

Human immunodeficiency virus (HIV) is a retrovirus acquired by direct inoculation of infected bodily fluids. This is most often during sexual intimacy, but may also result from contaminated needles or iatrogenic interventions, such as blood transfusion or surgical procedures with contaminated products. The infection is lifelong and if untreated significant morbidity and mortality arise from HIV-associated infections and malignancies; this is termed the acquired immune deficiency syndrome (AIDS). During infection, HIV enters cells presenting CD4 receptors, the most common being the CD4+ T lymphocyte. Within the hosting cell, HIV replication, virion release and eventual cell death occur. The main measurable and prognostic parameters widely used are quantification of peripheral CD4 cells (the CD4 count), and the level of viraemia (HIV viral load). The likelihood of AIDS-defining illness developing increases with progressive CD4+ cell depletion, which occurs steadily over time from infection and more rapidly in individuals with a higher HIV viral load.

The advent of highly active antiretroviral therapy (HAART) in the late 1990s transformed the management of HIV-positive patients, and the infection is now generally treatable with a good prognosis, particularly when detected early. In addition to this, effective HAART together with appropriate obstetric management, infant antiretroviral prophylaxis and avoidance of breastfeeding has reduced rates of mother-to-child transmission (MTCT) of HIV significantly. Universal screening for HIV in UK antenatal clinics from 1999 onwards, followed by appropriate management of mothers and their babies,

has resulted in MTCT rates falling from between 20–30%, depending on maternal viral load in the mid-1990s to less than 1% in 2010. Worldwide, of the 34 million people living with HIV, 69% reside in sub-Saharan Africa, with other high-prevalence areas including Asia, the Caribbean and Eastern Europe. Many HIV-positive parturients receiving their antenatal care in the UK have acquired HIV whilst residing in one of the pandemic areas. The estimated UK prevalence in 2009 was 2.2 per 1000 women giving birth; most of these live in urban areas, with London having the highest rates.

Effect of HIV on pregnancy

HIV infection itself does not cause sub-fertility, although HIV-positive women may have decreased fertility due to associated conditions such as concurrent infections or illnesses, opiate use and low weight. HAART itself, particularly protease inhibitors, has been associated with preterm delivery in some studies, but not in others. Of all the available antiretroviral medications only zidovudine is licensed for use in pregnancy. Current information from the *Antiretroviral Pregnancy Register* and the *National Study of HIV in Pregnancy and Childhood* indicates that in women taking modern HAART, there is no increased risk of congenital abnormalities. During pregnancy, several risk factors increase the risk of MTCT (Table 24.1).

Effect of pregnancy on HIV

There is no evidence that being pregnant has a deleterious effect on HIV disease or increases the rate of progression. Complications of antiretroviral medications such as for hepatitis can at times be difficult to distinguish from pre-eclampsia and obstetric cholestasis.

Core Topics in Obstetric Anaesthesia, ed. Kirsty MacLennan, Kate O'Brien and W. Ross Mcnab.
Published by Cambridge University Press. © Cambridge University Press 2015.

Table 24.1 Risk factors of mother-to-child transmission of HIV during pregnancy

Antenatal risk factors

- High HIV RNA PCR (viral load)
- Low CD4 lymphocyte count
- Co-infection with sexually transmitted infections
- Substance use (including cigarette smoking)
- Maternal symptomatic HIV disease/AIDS

Intrapartum risk factors

- Duration of membrane rupture
- Mode of delivery
- Obstetric interventions (e.g. fetal scalp monitoring, forceps, vacuum)
- Premature delivery prior to 32 weeks of gestation
- Chorioamnionitis

Postpartum

- Breastfeeding

Pregnant women with HIV are at increased risk of puerperal fever and postpartum complications after caesarean delivery.

Preconception

Couples contemplating a pregnancy where one or both partners are known to be HIV positive should ideally discuss their plans with their HIV team and, if appropriate, obstetrician. This allows optimal medical management of the HIV-positive partner. For the parturient, this would include a medication review to minimize teratogenicity and fetal harm and commencement of prophylaxis required for opportunistic infections.

Management of HIV in pregnancy

Screening and diagnosis

HIV testing should be offered and encouraged in all pregnancies at booking, and pathways should exist to facilitate urgent referral of all women following a positive result to specialist HIV services able to offer information, support and medical treatment. This includes addressing partner notification and testing existing children, as appropriate.

Antenatal management

This should be by a multidisciplinary team (MDT) consisting of a consultant obstetrician, HIV physician, specialist nurses and midwives, a paediatrician and, if needed, psychiatric or perinatal mental health specialists and social services. Women with HIV should undergo the standard routine first trimester screening tests and can have chorionic villus sampling or amniocentesis if clinically indicated (only after HIV test results are known and when HIV viral load is suppressed on HAART) (Table 24.2).

Antenatal management aims to optimize maternal health and to prevent MTCT. ART is required to prevent MTCT. If the parturient is not already taking ART prior to pregnancy then, as per national guidelines, this should be initiated by week 24 gestation at the latest and earlier if the HIV viral load is high. Parturients already established on effective HAART prior to pregnancy should continue treatment with regular monitoring of HIV parameters.

The altered volume of distribution during the third trimester can result in the concentration of protease inhibitors being reduced and a higher dose being required. Therapeutic drug-level monitoring (TDM) may be helpful in determining an effective dose and close monitoring of the HIV viral load is vital. Parturients with a CD4 count of less than 200 require prophylaxis against opportunistic infections, including *Pneumocystis jirovecii* pneumonia. Additional prophylaxis is dependent on the CD4 count and previous exposure to such opportunistic infections. If an antifolate drug such as co-trimoxazole is used, then 5 mg folic acid should be co-administered.

Zidovudine monotherapy initiated between 20 and 28 weeks is an alternative to HAART and may be considered for women who do not require HIV treatment for their own health, have a plasma viral load of less than 10,000 copies/mL and are prepared to be delivered by elective caesarean section.

Delivery planning

An intrapartum management plan should be formulated by the members of the MDT and the parturient, ideally by 36 weeks' gestation. If the HIV viral load is undetectable (<50 copies/L) and there are no obstetric contraindications, a vaginal delivery can be planned. A previous caesarean section is not a contraindication to this. HIV-positive women who are booking late for antenatal care, women with poor adherence and detectable HIV viraemia or women diagnosed later in pregnancy, or even during labour, pose particular challenges to the MDT. By using intensive HAART that produces dramatic falls in HIV viral load, the risk of MTCT can be significantly reduced.

Table 24.2 Antenatal management of the HIV-positive parturient

First trimester

- Standard booking tests

Specific tests for HIV-positive women

- Hepatitis B (if HBV infection, quantitative HBV DNA, hepatitis A virus (HAV), HCV and hepatitis delta virus (HDV), liver function tests)
- Hepatitis C (if HCV infection, quantitative VL and genotype, liver function tests)
- Serology for syphilis, toxoplasmosis, varicella zoster, measles
- HIV resistance testing

Monitoring tests for HIV

- Baseline CD4 cell count at booking
- Frequency of checking CD4 count, plasma viral load and drug levels should be according to recommendations of HIV physician
- Pregnant women on HAART will require a viral load (VL) 2–4 weeks after commencing HAART, at least once every trimester, at 36 weeks and at delivery
- Full blood count, renal, bone and liver profile tests before starting HAART treatment and at each antenatal visit
- Vaccination of HIV-positive women for hepatitis B, pneumococcus and influenza

Second trimester

- Second trimester anomaly scan at 18 + 0 to 20 + 6 weeks' gestation
- Offer quadruple test between 15 + 0 to 20 + 0 weeks' gestation in women that have missed combined screening test
- Offer HIV screening at 28 weeks' gestation if previously declined
- Screen for genital tract infections at 28 weeks' gestation
- HIV disease monitoring with plasma viral load and drug toxicities should be performed according to recommendations of HIV physician

Third trimester

- A decision on mode of delivery should be made by 36 weeks' gestation
- A delivery care plan individualized to the woman should be issued and made available to all healthcare professionals involved in her care. A copy should be carried by the patient
- ECV should be offered to women with a VL <50 copies/mL and breech presentation at >36 weeks' gestation in the absence of obstetric contraindications
- Women with a plasma VL of <50 HIV RNA copies/mL at 36 weeks' gestation and in the absence of obstetric contraindications should be offered a planned vaginal delivery
- Women with a plasma VL of 50–399 HIV RNA copies/mL at 36 weeks' gestation should be offered a prelabour planned elective caesarean section at 38 weeks' gestation
- Delivery by prelabour planned elective caesarean section at 38 weeks' gestation is recommended for women taking zidovudine monotherapy, irrespective of plasma VL at the time of delivery and for women with VL >400 HIV RNA copies/mL regardless of ART
- Delivery by prelabour planned elective caesarean section for obstetric indications or maternal request should be delayed until after 39 weeks' gestation in women with VL <50 HIV RNA copies/mL to reduce the risk of transient tachypnoea of the newborn

Intrapartum management

In parturients with detectable HIV viraemia, MTCT can be further reduced by administering intravenous zidovudine either for 4 hours before beginning the caesarean section until the umbilical cord has been clamped, or for those who elect for a vaginal delivery, during labour. Oral HAART should be continued and can be intensified in certain situations, including premature rupture of membranes or if a peripartum HIV diagnosis is made.

For parturients with an undetectable HIV viral load who plan to have a vaginal delivery, artificial rupture of membrane (ARM) should be avoided unless absolutely necessary. ARM and oxytocin may be considered for labour augmentation. Fetal scalp electrode or fetal blood sampling are contraindicated. If instrumental delivery is needed, the instrument of choice is that which will achieve a safe delivery with minimal maternal and fetal trauma. The most senior obstetrician present should perform the procedure. An episiotomy should be avoided unless clinically indicated. Early recourse to caesarean section should be considered if labour is not progressing satisfactorily.

If presenting with threatened or established preterm labour or prelabour rupture of membranes (PROM), a genital infection screen should be performed and any infection treated. Maternal corticosteroids should be administered to reduce the risk of respiratory distress of the newborn. Multidisciplinary team advice (HIV physicians and paediatricians) is essential, particularly for preterm gestations. In PROM after 34 weeks' gestation, delivery should be expedited. In PROM before 34 weeks' gestation, oral erythromycin should be started and broad-spectrum intravenous antibiotic cover should be considered. The presence of chorioamnionitis and fetal distress necessitate immediate delivery.

Where diagnosis of HIV occurs during labour, urgent advice from HIV physicians is essential to facilitate administration of antiretrovirals that produce rapid HIV suppression and that also cross the placenta and effectively deliver prophylaxis to the fetus. Urgent liaison with neonatal colleagues is required to ensure timely infant prophylaxis. Delivery should be by caesarean section, if appropriate, with intravenous zidovudine, if possible.

Healthcare professionals should exercise universal precautions when caring for parturients with HIV, including double gloving and protective eyewear.

Analgesia and anaesthesia

There may be significant drug interactions between analgesic and anaesthetic agents, notably benzodiazepines, and antiretrovirals. This is particularly important when protease inhibitors are being taken as part of the HAART regime, as ritonavir is almost always used as a pharmacological booster due to its profound inhibiting effect on the CYP P450 liver enzyme system. The University of Liverpool maintains a comprehensive reference website where interactions can be checked against all antiretrovirals (http://www.hiv-druginteractions.org/, accessed May 2015).

The choice of anaesthesia for HIV-infected parturients should be based upon the usual obstetric and anaesthetic considerations. Current evidence suggests that both regional and general anaesthesia can be safely used. Neither has been found to be associated with worsening of maternal immune status.

Regional anaesthesia has not been associated with infectious complications or neurologic changes in the peripartum period. The parturients should be examined for pre-existing neurology prior to performing neuraxial anaesthesia. HIV infection is not a contraindication to performing epidural blood patch.

Post partum

Care of mother

Following delivery, cabergoline 1 mg once only is offered to suppress lactation. Measles, mumps and rubella (MMR) and varicella zoster vaccines should be considered in those susceptible, although in the very immunosuppressed with CD4 counts less than 200 the MMR should be deferred until after immune reconstitution as it is a live vaccine. Appropriate contraception should be discussed by the HIV team, as there are significant drug interactions with hormonal contraception and many antiretrovirals. The mother's ongoing care will be based on her prepregnancy care or baseline HIV parameters if she was diagnosed antenatally. Those women who started HAART solely for prevention of MTCT will have the option to continue on HAART or to cease and continue regular monitoring. Women who were on HAART prior to their pregnancy will continue as before. Patients who had their HAART dosages increased in the third trimester, reduce to standard dosages two weeks after delivery.

Genital herpes

Introduction

Genital herpes infection is caused by herpes simplex virus type 2 (HSV-2). This virus is widely distributed throughout the population and is usually acquired through sexual contact. It causes painful vesicular lesions on the skin or mucous membranes of the genital tract; however, women may also be asymptomatic carriers. The primary infection with HSV-2 often causes a viraemia with symptoms including fever and headache. More serious complications such as encephalitis, meningitis and hepatitis can also occur.

Women with primary herpes, or active lesions, at the time of labour should be delivered by caesarean section as this dramatically lowers the risk of vertical transmission to the baby through vaginal delivery. Neonatal HSV infection may also occur by ascent of the organism after maternal membrane rupture. The incidence of neonatal HSV infection is 1:6600 live births in the UK, the majority being from maternal transmission, with few acquired postnatally. The sequelae of neonatal HSV infection can be severe. It may appear initially as a cutaneous lesion, but visceral infection can ensue, carrying a high mortality.

Anaesthetic management

The primary anaesthetic concern is transmission of the virus to the central nervous system from central neuraxial blockade. Several studies have looked retrospectively at the use of neuraxial anaesthesia in patients with genital herpes. A summary of their findings is illustrated in Table 24.3.

These results, although limited in number, suggest that it is considered safe to initiate neuraxial anaesthesia/analgesia in patients with HSV recrudescence. However, the risk of viral translocation following breech of the dura during a primary infection cannot be quantified. The patient is often viraemic during the initial infection and spontaneous CNS infection, although rare, can occur. We would therefore advise caution in performing neuraxial block in those with primary genital herpes.

Viral hepatitis

Hepatitis viruses A, B, C, D and E can cause viral hepatitis. Serology is required in order to confirm diagnosis. Patients present with fever, nausea, abdominal pain and fatigue akin to 'flu'-like illness and jaundice may also be present. Thorough evaluation to determine the degree of hepatic impairment should be undertaken. Blood tests, including full blood count, electrolytes, liver function tests and prothrombin time should be taken. As with herpes, we would advise caution in performing neuraxial anaesthesia in patients with viraemic symptoms. An additional precaution would be to ensure that coagulation studies are within normal limits.

If general anaesthesia is required then drugs with minimal hepatic metabolism should be used. Isoflurane has been shown to have minimal effect on hepatic circulation and is the agent of choice for maintenance of anaesthesia.

Syphilis

Syphilis, caused by the organism *Treponema pallidum*, has increased in incidence 12-fold between 1997 and 2007. It is spread via both sexual contact and placental transfer, with four stages in the disease process: primary, secondary, latent and tertiary. Antenatal syphilis causes significant risk of fetal infection via placental transfer, which can occur at any time throughout pregnancy. Effects on the fetus include preterm delivery, impaired growth and stillbirth. Anaesthetic management of these patients is largely straightforward, including use of universal precautions, avoiding direct contact with lesions and using techniques with a low potential for needle stick injury. General anaesthesia has no specific considerations, with no additional risk to the syphilis patient. Likewise there is no specific contraindication to regional anaesthesia; however, neurosyphilis may present atypically and so a full neurological examination should be documented prior to regional blockade.

Table 24.3 The use of neuraxial anaesthesia in patients with genital herpes.

Study author	Number of patients (all had neuraxial anaesthesia)	% Active disease	% Primary disease	Neurological complications
Crosby *et al.*	93	65	0	0
Bader *et al.*	164	100	3	Transient postoperative weakness in one patient with primary disease following spinal anaesthesia
Ramanathan *et al.*	43	71	0	0

Key points

1. Antenatal screening for HIV became universal in the UK in 1999.
2. Preconception counselling and specialist antenatal care ensures optimal medical management with medication review to minimize MTCT, teratogenicity and provide opportunistic infection prophylaxis.
3. If HIV viral load is <50 copies/mL, vaginal delivery can be considered.
4. MTCT in parturients with detectable HIV viraemia can be decreased by administering 4 hours of IV zidovudine prior to performing a caesarean section.
5. Both general and regional anaesthesia can be used in women with HIV infection.
6. Breastfeeding is not recommended owing to the risk of MTCT.

Further reading

Brown, Z. A., Wald, A., Morrow, R. A. *et al.* (2003). Effect of serological status and caesarean delivery on transmission rates of herpes simplex virus from mother to infant. *JAMA*, **289**, 203–209.

Fiore, S., Newell, M. L. and Thorne, C. (2004). Higher rates of post-partum complications in HIV-infected than in uninfected women irrespective of mode of delivery. *AIDS*, **18**(6), 933–938.

Gershon, R. Y. and Manning-Williams, D. (1997). Anesthesia and the HIV infected parturient: a retrospective study. *Int. J. Obstet. Anesth.*, **6**(2), 76–81.

Kourtis, A. P., Lee, F. K., Abrams, E. J., Jamieson, D. J. and Bulterys, M. (2006). Mother-to-child transmission of HIV0–1: timing and implications for prevention. *Lancet Infect. Disease.*, **6**(11), 726–732.

Read, J. S. and Newell, M. K. (2005). Efficacy and safety of cesarean delivery for prevention of mother-to-child transmission of HIV-1. *Cochrane Database Syst. Rev.*, **2005**(4):CD005479.

Louzada, R. R., Taleco, T., Ricardo, A.S. *et al.* (2007). HIV and epidural blood patch: the state of the art: 312. *Reg. Anesth. Pain Med.*, **32**(5 Suppl. 1), 85.

Royal College of Obstetricians and Gynaecologists (2010). *Management of HIV in Pregnancy. Green-top Guideline No. 39.* London: RCOG Press.

Taylor, G. P., Clayden, P., Dhar, J. *et al.* (2012). British HIV Association guidelines for the management of HIV infection in pregnant women 2012. *HIV Med.*, **13**(2), 87–157.

Tom, D. J., Gulevich, S. J., Shapiro, H. M., Heaton, R. K. and Grant, I. (1992). Epidural blood patch in the HIV-positive patient. Review of clinical experience. San Diego HIV Neurobehavioral Research Center. *Anesthesiology*, **76**(6), 943–947.

Williams, I., Churchill, D., Anderson, J. *et al.* (2012). British HIV Association guidelines for the treatment of HIV-1-positive adults with antiretroviral therapy 2012. *HIV Med.*, **13**(2), 1–85.

Chapter

25

Maternal collapse, including massive obstetric haemorrhage, amniotic fluid embolism and cardiac arrest

Kate Grady and Tracey Johnston

Definition

Maternal collapse is defined as an acute event involving the cardiorespiratory systems and/or brain, resulting in a reduced or absent conscious level (and potentially death), at any stage in pregnancy and up to 6 weeks after delivery. Although collapse is often unpredicted, early warning scoring systems can help to identify deterioration and prompt initiation of interventions that can prevent collapse.

Incidence

Accurate figures are not available as this data is not routinely collected, but the incidence of maternal collapse is estimated to lie between 0.14 and 6/1000 pregnancies. As this is not a commonly encountered scenario, it is essential that care-givers are skilled in effective initial resuscitation techniques and investigation and diagnosis of the cause of the collapse, thus enabling appropriate, directed continuing management. Due to lack of robust data, accurate survival rates following maternal collapse are not available, but the 'near-miss' to death ratios from two large severe morbidity studies are 56:1 and 79:1.

The team

In addition to the standard members, the arrest team should also include a senior midwife, an obstetrician and an obstetric anaesthetist. This ensures that skilled care-givers (who understand the altered physiology of pregnancy and the impact of this on resuscitation) are able to implement directed, cause-specific treatment and effect delivery if indicated. Units must ensure there is a robust system in place for calling the appropriate team. The consultant obstetrician and consultant obstetric anaesthetist should be alerted and asked to attend. If the collapsed woman is over 22 weeks' gestation, the neonatal team should be alerted and prepared if perimortem delivery is required. In cases where resuscitation is successful, the critical care team should then be involved in the ongoing management. Communication and clear definition of roles are essential during the resuscitation process.

In general, roles are as follows:

- Anaesthetist to manage the airway and breathing
- Two care-givers to perform chest compressions (rotating every two minutes to avoid fatigue)
- Two care-givers for the arms (one each), to insert a wide-bore cannula in each arm. One care-giver takes the appropriate bloods, labels and sends the samples, and communicates with laboratories. The other care-giver manages fluid and drug administration
- Obstetrician or midwife to manage the uterus (tilt or manual displacement, perimortem CS, management of postpartum haemorrhage)
- One care-giver as scribe
- One care-giver as runner to obtain any equipment not immediately available
- Porter to take samples to the laboratories and collect blood products
- Laboratory staff and the haematologist to be involved if haemorrhage persists

If collapse occurs in a location without access to the full team e.g. a stand-alone midwifery unit or the community, basic life support should be implemented and emergency transfer via 999 effected to the nearest appropriate environment.

Core Topics in Obstetric Anaesthesia, ed. Kirsty MacLennan, Kate O'Brien and W. Ross Mcnab.
Published by Cambridge University Press. © Cambridge University Press 2015.

Management of maternal collapse

The physiological changes in pregnancy are covered in Chapter 1. The unique problems encountered by the pregnant woman in a state of cardiorespiratory collapse are secondary to a number of physiological and physical changes. The key to successful maternal resuscitation is early recognition, appropriate skilled help and early recourse to emptying the uterus if CPR is initially unsuccessful. Ongoing success is secondary to identification of the cause of collapse and directed treatment. Cardiopulmonary resuscitation should follow the British Resuscitation Council approach of airway, breathing, circulation, with specific adaptations for pregnancy (see Figure 25.1).

- Tilt
  - After 20 weeks' gestation, compression of the IVC and aorta by the gravid uterus must be relieved immediately if resuscitation is to be successful. As the objective of relieving aortic and IVC compression is to improve the efficacy of chest compressions in terms of cardiac output, it is essential that the method used to achieve this does not compromise chest compressions directly. The thorax must be in contact with a rigid surface to ensure effective chest compression, thus improving cardiac output. This can be achieved either by employing a left lateral tilt of 15–30° on a rigid surface that extends from the shoulders to the pelvis e.g. tilting theatre table or an appropriate wedge, or by manual displacement of the uterus to the left whilst supine. If a cardiac output cannot be achieved after 4 minutes of properly performed CPR, the uterus should be emptied to facilitate maternal resuscitation (see Perimortem Caesarean Section below).
- Airway
  - The pregnant airway is potentially complicated by the following: capillary engorgement of the respiratory tract causing swelling of the oropharynx, larynx and trachea, laryngeal oedema secondary to pre-eclampsia, breast hypertrophy and generalized weight gain during pregnancy hindering access to the airway. Given the potential for difficult intubation, careful preparation of airway equipment and a skilled anaesthetist and assistant are required.
  - Nasopharyngeal airways are not recommended on account of the risk of bleeding.
  - Oesophageal sphincter relaxation secondary to progesterone significantly increases the risk of aspiration, therefore early recourse to cuffed endotracheal intubation using cricoid pressure is recommended. During bag and mask ventilation, the risk of aspiration can be reduced by employing cricoid pressure and by performing gentle hand ventilation to avoid insufflation of the stomach. An oropharyngeal airway can assist in reducing the required inflation pressure.
- Breathing
  - A reduction in functional residual capacity and an increased oxygen consumption (by up to 60% at term) can rapidly result in hypoxia during hypoventilation. Irreversible neurological damage can be sustained within 4–6 minutes of collapse. High-flow oxygen should be administered as soon as possible.
  - Ventilation can be more difficult secondary to diaphragmatic splinting by the gravid uterus and reduced chest wall compliance secondary to breast hypertrophy.
  - During CPR, the ratio of chest compressions to ventilation breaths is 30:2. Once intubated, chest compressions are continuous and ventilation maintained at 10 breaths per minute. In the case of respiratory arrest alone, maintain ventilation at 10 breaths per minute.
- Circulation
  - Chest compressions are to be delivered at a rate of 120 per minute. In a left lateral tilt they are more difficult to perform and the resuscitator will tire more quickly, so it is important to rotate the resuscitator performing chest compressions every two minutes.
  - Otherwise healthy mothers can lose up to 35% of their circulating blood volume before becoming symptomatic. Those with pre-existing anaemia do not tolerate haemorrhage as well, and clotting is less efficient if there is significant anaemia.
  - Mothers may compensate for hypovolaemia by reducing fetoplacental blood flow and therefore maternal signs of hypovolaemia are

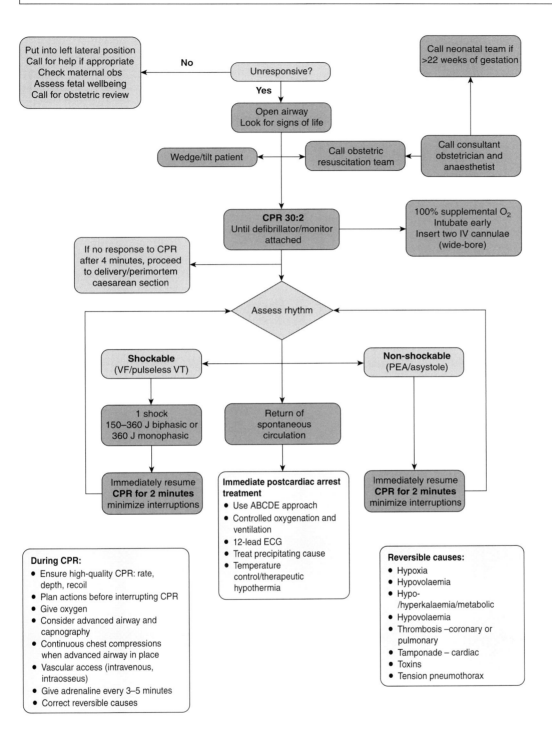

Figure 25.1 Maternal collapse algorithm. (Reproduced from Royal College of Obstetricians and Gynaecologists. *Maternal Collapse in Pregnancy and the Puerperium*. Green-top Guideline No. 56. London: RCOG; 2011, with the permission of the Royal College of Obstetricians and Gynaecologists.) For the colour version, please refer to the plate section.

KEY
ABCDE = airway, breathing, circulation, disability, exposure; CPR = cardiopulmonary resuscitation; RCG = electrocardiogram; PEA = pulseless electrical activity; VF = ventricular fibrillation; VT = ventricular tachycardia

subtle and late. If bleeding is concealed, the significance of tachycardia secondary to hypovolaemia can be overlooked or misinterpreted.

. Maternal blood loss can be rapid and dramatic; large-bore venous access must be secured, haemorrhage controlled and rapid restoration of circulating volume with oxygen transporting red cells is paramount in order to minimize the risk of hypoxic injury. Fluid replacement, in women with pre-eclampsia, needs careful consideration.

- Drugs and defibrillation
  - There should be no alteration in the drugs used during resuscitation, or their dose. Increased doses may be considered in the presence of severe vasodilatation (hypotension) secondary to a dense spinal or epidural block.
  - There is no alteration to the defibrillation energy level. Defibrillator pads should be applied one to the right of the sternum below the clavicle and one in the left mid axillary line, avoiding breast tissue and placing the electrode vertically to maximize efficiency of defibrillation. There is no evidence that shocks from a direct current defibrillator have an adverse effect on the fetus. Fetal and uterine monitoring should be removed prior to defibrillation.

Perimortem caesarean section

As well-performed chest compressions in the non-pregnant situation can achieve only 30% of normal cardiac output and aortocaval compression further reduces this efficiency to an estimated 10%, there should be early recourse to emptying the uterus if CPR is unsuccessful. For this reason, from 20 weeks' gestation, if there has been no response to appropriately performed CPR by 4 minutes, or if resuscitation is continuing beyond this time (e.g. following transfer from the community), the uterus should be emptied to improve the response to CPR. This should be carried out by 5 minutes. This is done purely in maternal interests, whether the baby is alive or dead (do not waste time checking), but a neonatologist should be present in a hospital setting for assessment and resuscitation of the baby after viability (23 weeks onwards). No anaesthetic is required, and it should be performed where resuscitation is taking place. A fixed blade

scalpel should be available on the resuscitation trolley, and the operator should perform the incision they are most comfortable with, although a classical incision is marginally faster. In the absence of circulation, blood loss is minimal, but if circulation is restored, transfer to the theatre environment and anaesthesia should be instigated. Haemorrhage can be controlled in the short term if indicated by compressing the aorta against the spine with a fist just above the bifurcation.

The most robust data available regarding maternal outcome following perimortem caesarean section shows a survival rate of 65% if the cause of collapse is reversible, with survival rates being improved if the procedure is carried out within 5 minutes of collapse. Neonatal survival is influenced by rapid delivery, gestational age and delivery in the delivery suite environment or critical care.

The UK Obstetric Surveillance System (UKOSS) is currently studying outcomes following maternal collapse and will give more current information for the UK.

Postcollapse processes

- Accurate, full documentation is essential detailing events, decisions and interventions.
- Debriefing must be carried out with the woman (if she survives), the family, and with the staff involved, to ensure understanding of events, explain actions taken and to provide support for those in need.
- Incident reporting using the local system allows local data collection of frequency of such events, and should trigger formal event reviews to ensure local and organizational learning, and to enable feedback where care has been optimal.
- All cases of maternal death must be reported to MBRRACE-UK as part of the ongoing confidential enquiries into maternal deaths.

Causes of maternal collapse

Outside pregnancy, the 4Hs and 4Ts aide memoire of reversible causes is useful, and many have modified this for the pregnant patient to 'THE' reversible causes of maternal collapse, with the 4Hs and 4Ts unchanged, and the E added for eclampsia (Chapter 14), including intracranial haemorrhage. Haemorrhage and thromboembolism are the most common causes of collapse. See Figure 25.2 for causes of maternal collapse.

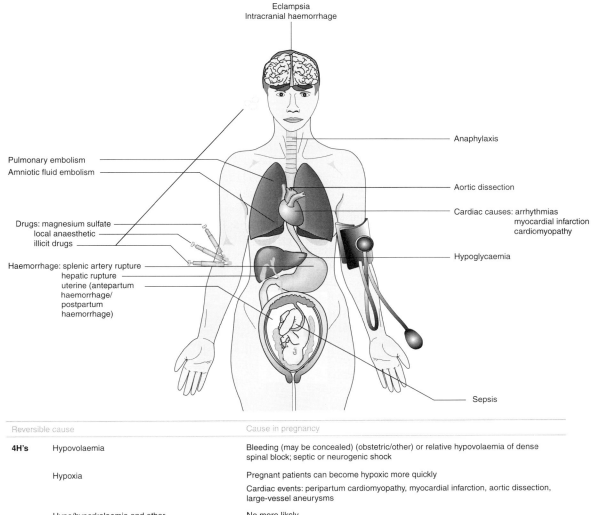

Reversible cause		Cause in pregnancy
4H's	Hypovolaemia	Bleeding (may be concealed) (obstetric/other) or relative hypovolaemia of dense spinal block; septic or neurogenic shock
	Hypoxia	Pregnant patients can become hypoxic more quickly
		Cardiac events: peripartum cardiomyopathy, myocardial infarction, aortic dissection, large-vessel aneurysms
	Hypo/hyperkalaemia and other electrolyte disturbances	No more likely
	Hypothermia	No more likely
4T's	Thromboembolism	Amniotic fluid embolus, pulmonary embolus, air embolus, myocardial infarction
	Toxicity	Local anaesthetic, magnesium, other
	Tension pneumothorax	Following trauma / suicide attempt
	Tamponade (cardiac)	Following trauma / suicide attempt
Eclampsia and pre-eclampsia		Includes intracranial haemorrhage

Figure 25.2 Causes of maternal collapse. (Reproduced from Royal College of Obstetricians and Gynaecologists. *Maternal Collapse in Pregnancy and the Puerperium*. Green-top Guideline No. 56. London: RCOG; 2011, with the permission of the Royal College of Obstetricians and Gynaecologists.) For the colour version, please refer to the plate section.

Another useful mnemonic for causes of maternal collapse by Dr Joel Naftalin (Year 6 Specialist Trainee in Obstetrics and Gynaecology, London Deanery) is 'SHE CAN DIE':

S Sepsis
H Haemorrhage
E Embolism
C Cardiac
A Anaphylaxis
N Non-pregnant causes (4 Hs and 4 Ts)
D Drug toxicity
I Intracranial haemorrhage
E Eclampsia

Amniotic fluid embolism

Amniotic fluid embolism (AFE), also known as the anaphylactoid syndrome of pregnancy, was first described in the 1940s after fetal material was found in the pulmonary circulation of women who had died following maternal collapse in labour. It presents as acute maternal collapse during labour, birth or the first 60 minutes after delivery. The incidence in the UK is around 2/100,000 maternities, and its occurrence, in general, is unpredictable. Survival rates have improved significantly over the last 35 years, and are currently around 80%, but with a significant risk of hypoxic neurological damage in the survivors. If AFE occurs prior to birth, perinatal mortality remains high at 135 per 1000 total births.

Risk factors include induction of labour, caesarean section, abruption, placenta praevia, eclampsia, advanced maternal age and multiple pregnancy. Clinical features of AFE include sudden anxiety and agitation, acute hypotension, dyspnoea, cyanosis, respiratory distress, acute hypoxia, arrhythmias, seizures and cardiac arrest. If it occurs prior to delivery, acute fetal distress is seen. The exact aetiology remains unclear, but it is thought that fetal material enters the maternal circulation and is transported to the lungs. Pulmonary hypertension develops acutely, due to vascular occlusion secondary to vasoconstriction caused by the release of various vasoactive substances, or debris blocking the pulmonary microvasculature, along with acute right ventricular failure leading to a marked reduction in cardiac output and acute hypoxia. This is followed by left ventricular dysfunction or failure. If the mother survives, profound *disseminated intravascular coagulation* (DIC) occurs rapidly, which often results in major postpartum haemorrhage. The pathophysiology of AFE has been likened to anaphylaxis or sepsis,

hence the name anaphylactoid syndrome of pregnancy. The diagnosis is made clinically or at the time of autopsy, but is often a diagnosis of exclusion. Although various other diagnostic tests are being researched, none have been shown to be clinically useful as yet. As the diagnosis is often one of exclusion, other causes of collapse must be investigated and excluded. A useful indicator is a coagulation screen, as if clotting is impaired in the absence of major haemorrhage and replacement therapy, AFE is likely.

Management is supportive and input from senior staff, including an intensivist, is required. Aggressive resuscitation is essential, with rapid oxygenation and early recourse to intubation and ventilation. If AFE occurs antepartum, the baby and placenta should be delivered immediately. Pharmacological support of the cardiovascular system is often required, and central monitoring of cardiac output is useful to avoid fluid overload, as this will increase the risk of pulmonary oedema and acute respiratory distress syndrome (ARDS). Arrhythmias are common, and should be treated as standard. Major postpartum haemorrhage is likely if the mother survives the initial collapse, and is secondary to DIC and uterine atony. Both should be treated aggressively (see below). Following resuscitation, transfer to a critical care setting for ongoing management is indicated, with multidisciplinary support.

Haemorrhage

This is the commonest cause of maternal collapse, and is responsible for up to 50% of the estimated 500,000 maternal deaths that occur worldwide each year, although in the UK deaths from obstetric haemorrhage are uncommon (3.9/1,000,000 maternities). It is also the major cause of severe maternal morbidity in almost all 'near miss' audits, in both developed and developing countries. In many cases, sub-standard care is identified as a contributing factor.

Haemorrhage can occur antepartum, intrapartum or postpartum, and it is well recognized that visual blood loss estimation often underestimates actual losses. Major haemorrhage is defined as a blood loss of greater than 1000 mL. The main causes of major antepartum/intrapartum haemorrhage are placental abruption and placenta praevia.

Placental abruption

This occurs when part of the placenta separates from the uterus prior to delivery of the baby, with resultant haemorrhage, which may be revealed, concealed behind the placenta, or a mixture of both (thus blood loss is often greater than that seen). With large placental abruption, the uterus has a hard wooden consistency. The diagnosis is a clinical one, as ultrasound is not a reliable method to diagnose placental abruption. Significant placental abruption carries an increased risk of DIC, and this should be screened for early. Bleeding can often go unrecognized or underestimated, and it predisposes to postpartum haemorrhage secondary to atony +/− DIC.

Placenta praevia

This occurs when the placenta lies within the lower uterine segment and partially or completely covers the internal cervical os. It is now routine practice to document the placental site on the mid-trimester scan and a quick review of the scan report, if available, will often rule out placenta praevia. In the absence of knowing the placental site, vaginal examination should not be performed until the placental site has been identified by ultrasound, to avoid provoking further, potentially catastrophic haemorrhage in cases of placenta praevia.

The causes of postpartum haemorrhage are easily remembered using the 4 Ts – tone, tissue, trauma and thrombin. Uterine atony accounts for over 70% of cases and can co-exist with the other causes.

Management of major obstetric haemorrhage

- Management should follow the initial resuscitation processes as above, ensuring that all relevant personnel are involved, i.e. in addition to the arrest team, consultant obstetrician and consultant anaesthetist asked to attend, laboratory staff informed specifically of major obstetric haemorrhage, on-call haematologist informed, dedicated porter available to take samples to laboratories and collect blood products, and dedicated scribe to record timings, treatments and events. Maternal blood should be sent for FBC, coagulation screen, urea and electrolytes and cross-match for four units.
- If the fetus is not yet delivered and is still alive, delivery should be effected rapidly to enable control of the bleeding and improve the chances of survival for the baby, but this should not compromise maternal resuscitation.
- If the fetus is dead, delivery should usually be effected vaginally following maternal resuscitation and stabilization, but occasionally caesarean section will be indicated either as part of the resuscitation process or to control and arrest haemorrhage rapidly in maternal interests. This decision should be taken by the consultant obstetrician, in conjunction with the consultant obstetric anaesthetist. In such cases, general anaesthesia would usually be employed due to maternal cardiovascular instability and potential DIC.
- In cases of postpartum haemorrhage secondary to atony, rubbing up a contraction and emptying the bladder can be all that is required. In cases where these measures are ineffective, bimanual compression of the uterus can be lifesaving, while resuscitation is taking place and cause-specific treatment instigated. This is performed by placing a fist in the vagina and acutely anteverting the uterus abdominally with the other hand and compressing the uterus firmly between both hands. This has the dual effect of compressing the open vascular sinuses in the placental bed, and reducing blood flow through the uterine arteries with the acute anteversion.
- Hypothermia should be avoided by actively warming the woman in order to improve the function of endogenous and exogenous coagulation factors.
- Volume replacement and replacement of oxygen-carrying capacity, i.e. red cells, is paramount, whilst simultaneously addressing the underlying cause of bleeding. The objective is to maintain the haemoglobin above 80 g/L, platelets above 75×10^9/L, APTT less than $1.5 \times$ mean control, PTT less than $1.5 \times$ mean control and fibrinogen above 1.0 g/L.

Fluid replacement

- Commence resuscitation with crystalloids. Colloid can be considered.
- Blood, in the form of red cell concentrate, should be rapidly infused. Ideally fully cross-matched blood should be used. In the absence of this, group-specific blood should be given. In an emergency, O Rhesus-negative blood can be used until group-specific or cross-matched blood is available.
- Platelets should be administered if the platelet count falls below 50×10^9/L.
- In cases of major haemorrhage causing collapse, the risk of DIC is high and should be actively prevented if possible. With ongoing haemorrhage,

fresh frozen plasma should be given in a ratio of 1:1 with red cells.

- Cryoprecipitate should be given if the fibrinogen falls below 1 g/dL.

Cause-specific treatment

In cases of antepartum or intrapartum haemorrhage, delivery will often resolve the problem, but the incidence of postpartum haemorrhage is increased and this should be addressed according to cause. The four main causes of postpartum haemorrhage are uterine atony, retained tissue, genital tract trauma and DIC. DIC can result from any of the other three if blood loss is sufficient, and both retained tissue and uterine trauma can lead to atony, so a systematic assessment and exclusion of the four causes is essential. Often atony can be diagnosed by abdominal palpation, and the act of rubbing up a contraction can improve uterine tone. There should be a careful exploration of the genital tract for trauma, which can be difficult if bleeding is heavy and this should be done in theatre. Any retained tissue should be removed and trauma repaired. Rarer traumatic causes of haemorrhage that will not be diagnosed by this approach include broad ligament haematoma, hepatic sub-capsular haemorrhage, ruptured spleen and rupture of splenic artery aneurysm; thus if all other causes of bleeding have been excluded, abdominal ultrasound, paracentesis or laparotomy may be required.

Management of atonic haemorrhage can be divided into first-line pharmacological management and mechanical/surgical methods.

Pharmacological methods

- *Syntocinon* – this is synthetic oxytocin and is the drug of choice for active management of the third stage of labour, and many women with postpartum haemorrhage will already have received up to 10 IU following delivery. It acts within 1–2 minutes via oxytocin receptors in the myometrium to cause myometrial contraction, but has a short half-life so does not provide a sustained contraction. It also has antidiuretic hormone properties and in large doses can cause water intoxication. In the case of uterine atony, 5–10 IU of syntocinon by IV injection (diluted in 10 mL water for injection and given slowly to avoid the risk of profound hypotension) is the first-line management. This can be repeated after 10 minutes.

- *Ergometrine* – this is a potent smooth muscle contractor causing myometrial contraction within approximately 3–5 minutes. It has a longer half-life of up to 30 minutes, resulting in a more sustained contraction of up to three hours. It also causes contraction of vascular smooth muscle and can result in acute hypertension. It is contraindicated in parturients with hypertension, cardiac disease, Raynaud's disease, AV shunts and peripheral vascular disease. Another common side effect is vomiting. The dose is 0.5 mg either IM or by slow IV injection.

- *Syntometrine* – this is a premixed combination of 5 IU syntocinon for immediate effect and 0.5 mg of ergometrine for sustained action.

- *40/40 syntocinon* – a continuous infusion of syntocinon 40 IU in 36 mL of 0.9% normal saline infused over 4 hours (10 mL/h) provides prolonged uterine contraction, without the risk of fluid overload secondary to the antidiuretic effect of the syntocinon.

- *Carboprost (Hemabate)* – this is a synthetic prostaglandin F2α analogue which is an effective uterotonic agent. The dose is 250 μg given by IM injection, and repeated every 15 minutes to a maximum of eight doses. It also acts on the bronchial smooth muscle and is contraindicated in asthma. It must never be given IV, but can be given directly into the myometrium, ensuring that it is not injected intravascularly, although it is not licensed for this route of administration. In cases of hypotension and reduced peripheral perfusion, this method may be more effective compared to peripheral IM injection (although be aware it may cause localized myometrial contraction and ischaemia).

- *Misoprostol* – this is frequently used in the management of atonic haemorrhage, although the evidence shows carboprost to be more effective, and systematic reviews have demonstrated that the optimal route of administration or dose is not known. It can be given rectally in a dose of 800–1000 μg. As it has not been demonstrated to have benefits over other more effective uterotonics, its place in the developed world is limited, but as it is inexpensive, heat stable and light stable, and does not require injection or infusion, it has been shown to be of benefit in under-resourced countries.

- *Recombinant factor VII* – this is licensed for use in haemophiliacs and has proven to be an effective haemostatic agent when used in the right conditions. It replaces a missing factor and actively initiates and promotes coagulation. It binds to tissue factor and activates platelets, activating factor II to thrombin and X to Xa, providing a local fibrin burst at the site of tissue damage. Effects occur within around 30 minutes, providing the patient is not hypothermic or acidotic at the time of administration. Successful effect is also dependent upon adequate concentration and function of other clotting factors. The platelet count must be above 20×10^9/L and fibrinogen above 1 g/L before its use is considered. A recent Cochrane review (2012) of 29 RCTs reported that the effectiveness of rFVIIa as a more general haemostatic drug, either prophylactically or therapeutically, remains unproven. The results indicate increased risk of arterial events in patients receiving rFVIIa. The use of rFVIIa outside its current licensed indications should be restricted to clinical trials. For all these reasons a consultant haematologist should be involved in the decision to use this agent.

- *Tranexamic acid* – 1 g oral or IV can be given three times daily to minimize bleeding. There are trials currently underway looking at its role in major haemorrhage in both obstetrics and trauma.

Mechanical/surgical methods

- *Balloon tamponade* – this is an established and effective, relatively non-invasive mechanical method for controlling uterine haemorrhage. Different balloons have been used, the commonest being Rusch or Bakri balloons. The balloon is inserted into the uterine cavity and inflated with water – on average about 300 mL. In cases where the cervix has been dilated, a vaginal pack is often required to stop the balloon being expelled. This method has been shown to be effective in almost 80% of cases, avoiding the need for hysterectomy. The balloon should be left in for a minimum of 6 hours, and should be removed during the day when facilities and staff are available should further bleeding occur.
- *Brace sutures* – If bimanual compression controls bleeding secondary to atony, then the insertion of compression sutures to vertically compress the body of the uterus is often successful.

- *Stepwise uterine devascularization* – if bleeding continues, then stepwise devascularization of the uterus can be considered, starting with bilateral uterine artery ligation, bilateral ovarian artery ligation and ultimately bilateral internal iliac ligation. Uterine artery ligation is more successful for controlling haemorrhage from the upper rather than the lower segment. Ligation of the internal iliac arteries can be technically challenging. It must be remembered that these techniques will preclude the option of arterial embolization.
- *Arterial embolization* – selective arterial occlusion or embolization by interventional radiology can prevent major blood loss, obviating the need for blood transfusion and hysterectomy.
- *Hysterectomy* – in some cases, the only way to control life-threatening haemorrhage is to perform hysterectomy. This should not be done too early, as it is associated with a significant risk of increased transfusion, other organ damage, ITU admission and return to theatre, nor should it be left too late. It is good practice to involve another consultant in the decision to perform hysterectomy. Studies show that there is little difference in morbidity between total and subtotal hysterectomy.

Cardiac disease

Cardiac disease was the most common overall cause of maternal death in the last CEMACH report, being responsible for 48 maternal deaths. The majority of deaths secondary to cardiac causes occur in women with no previous history. The main cardiac causes of death are myocardial infarction, aortic dissection and cardiomyopathy. The incidence of primary cardiac arrest in pregnancy is much rarer at around 1 in 30,000 maternities, and most cardiac events have preceding signs and symptoms. Aortic root dissection can present in otherwise healthy women, and signs and symptoms such as central chest or interscapular pain, a wide pulse pressure, mainly secondary to systolic hypertension, and a new cardiac murmur must prompt referral to a cardiologist and appropriate imaging. The incidence of congenital and rheumatic heart disease in pregnancy is increasing secondary to increased survival rates owing to improved management of congenital heart disease, and increased immigration. These cases should be managed by an appropriately skilled and experienced multidisciplinary team, usually in regional centres. Other cardiac causes include dissection of the coronary artery, acute left ventricular failure, infective endocarditis and pulmonary oedema. With the increasing incidence of obesity, diabetes and advanced maternal age, acute myocardial infarction is also becoming more prevalent.

Training

There is good evidence that training in obstetric emergencies improves outcomes. All team members should undergo specific training in the adaptations and complexities of maternal cardiac arrest and resuscitation, and nationally based courses are available. Local policies should be in place for annual training for all staff, and it would appear that integrating clinical teaching with teamwork training in small groups, with all members of the team training together is the best way. It must, however, be remembered that delivery of teaching and training does not necessarily equate to learning and acquisition of skills.

Key points

1. Altered physiology of pregnancy complicates resuscitation in the case of maternal collapse.
2. Senior anaesthetists and obstetricians should be present to guide management.
3. Relieving compression of the IVC and aorta in the supine position is essential for successful resuscitation.
4. Maternal haemorrhage can be rapid. Maternal compensation for haemorrhage can give a falsely reassuring blood pressure measurement that can

delay diagnosis and management of hypovolaemia.
5. Consideration of the neonate is required. Ensure a neonatal resuscitation team is present and, where appropriate, consider early delivery of the neonate to aid both maternal and neonatal resuscitation.
6. Teams caring for parturients should be trained in the adaptations and complexities of maternal resuscitation.

Further reading

Centre for Maternal and Child Enquiries (CMACE). (2011). Saving mothers' lives: reviewing maternal deaths to make motherhood safer: 2006–08. The Eighth Report on Confidential Enquiries into Maternal Deaths in the United Kingdom. *Br. J. Obstet. Gynaecol.*, **118** (1), 1–203.

Knight, M. (2007). Peripartum hysterectomy in the UK; management and outcomes of the associated haemorrhage. *BJOG*, 114(11), 1380–1387.

Knight, M., Tuffnell, D., Brocklehurst, P. *et al.* (2010). Incidence and risk factors for amniotic fluid embolism. *Obstet. Gynecol.*, **115**(5), 910–917.

Royal College of Obstetricians and Gynaecologists (2011). *Antepartum Haemorrhage*. Green Top Guideline No. 63. London: RCOG Press.

Royal College of Obstetricians and Gynaecologists (2011). *Maternal Collapse in Pregnancy and the Puerperium*. Green Top Guideline No. 56. London: RCOG Press.

Royal College of Obstetricians and Gynaecologists (2011). *Prevention and Management of Postpartum Haemorrhage*. Green Top Guideline No. 52. London: RCOG Press.

Chapter 26

Postpartum complications, follow-up and maternal satisfaction

Richard Wadsworth and Kailash Bhatia

Introduction

Over the last three decades, the use of regional anaesthesia has led to a significant decrease in maternal morbidity and mortality. However, obstetric anaesthesia remains one of the leading causes of litigation in anaesthesia in the UK. All anaesthetic techniques carry a risk of complication and potential patient harm. Although complications cannot be entirely eliminated, risks can be reduced with a combination of:

- Appropriate training and supervision
- Meticulous technique
- Reliable follow-up with vigilance for complications
- Sound multidisciplinary communication
- Regular audit.

Post dural puncture headache (PDPH)

PDPH is one of the most common complications encountered following neuraxial anaesthesia in obstetrics. A tear in the dura leads to leakage of cerebrospinal fluid (CSF), which results in reduction in intracranial pressure and a downward traction on pain-sensitive intracranial structures, including meninges, veins and cranial nerves. Following CSF loss, compensatory vasodilatation occurs, which further exacerbates symptoms.

In parturients receiving epidural anaesthesia, the incidence of accidental dural puncture (ADP) is between 0 and 2.6%. The incidence of PDPH varies: up to 80% of women will have a headache after an ADP following a labour epidural with a 16G Tuohy needle, 0–5% following spinal anaesthesia with a 25G Whitacre needle, whilst a tertiary unit reported an incidence of 0.5% following 16,000 combined spinal epidurals (CSE).

In addition to the size and type of needle, the incidence of ADP is inversely proportional to the experience of the person performing the procedure and directly proportional to the number of attempts at needle insertion. In almost 30% of patients, ADP is not recognized at the time of epidural needle placement, suggesting that the epidural catheter is responsible.

PDPH is classically described as an occipitofrontal headache, often radiating to the neck and shoulders with postural features (exacerbated by sitting, standing, coughing and straining, and alleviated by lying flat). A majority (90%) of patients will report symptoms within 72 hours post puncture, although both immediate and later presentations have been described. Other features of PDPH include: nausea, vomiting, neck stiffness, tinnitus and visual disturbances. Rarely, cranial nerve palsies, convulsions or subdural haematomas have been reported as a result of PDPH. Criteria for PDPH have been described by The International Classification of Headache Disorders (ICHD) and are summarized in Table 26.1.

The parturient should be reassured, a full explanation given for the signs and symptoms experienced, and a management plan should be agreed upon.

Initial management includes adequate hydration, simple analgesics including paracetamol and non-steroidal anti-inflammatory drugs. The pharmacological management of PDPH has recently been subjected to a Cochrane review, which concluded that caffeine (150–300 mg 6–8 hourly) may provide symptomatic relief and possibly reduce the need for further interventions. Gabapentin, sumatriptan, ACTH and steroids have been suggested, but the evidence base for their use is weak.

Therapeutic epidural blood patch (EBP) forms the mainstay of management of PDPH. There is limited evidence to support the use of prophylactic (before

Core Topics in Obstetric Anaesthesia, ed. Kirsty MacLennan, Kate O'Brien and W. Ross Mcnab.
Published by Cambridge University Press. © Cambridge University Press 2015.

Table 26.1 Diagnostic criteria for PDPH as per ICHD

A	Headache that worsens within 15 min after sitting or standing, and improves within 15 min after lying, with at least one of the following, and fulfilling criteria C and D: • Neck stiffness • Tinnitus • Hyperacusia • Photophobia • Nausea
B	Dural puncture has been performed
C	Headache develops within 5 days after dural puncture
D	Headache resolves spontaneously either: • Spontaneously within 1 week • Within 48 hours after effective treatment of CSF leak (usually by epidural blood patch)

Table 26.2 Differential diagnosis of postpartum headache:

- Hypertensive disorders of pregnancy
- Migraine
- Tension-type headache
- Stroke
- Subdural haematoma
- Subarachnoid haemorrhage
- Venous sinus thrombosis
- Posterior reversible encephalopathy syndrome
- Benign intracranial hypertension
- Space-occupying lesion
- Others – sinusitis, dehydration, drugs

the development of headache) EBP. The procedure involves injection of autologous blood into the epidural space in a theatre environment. Contraindications include sepsis, coagulopathy and patient refusal. The risks of EBP include all the risks associated with epidural, back pain, neck pain, fever, cranial nerve palsy and possible worsening of headache. The timing of EBP is controversial, but good results have been obtained when it is performed over 24–48 hours after the development of symptoms.

To perform an EBP, a senior anaesthetist locates the epidural space using a loss of resistance technique, while another anaesthetist takes 20 mL of blood from the patient. This is then slowly injected into the epidural space.

Strict asepsis is mandatory. The interspace at or below the original puncture is recommended, as injected blood has been shown to track upwards on MRI scans. The optimal blood volume for injection is unknown, but general recommendations are 15–20 mL. If the patient reports pain during injection of blood then the procedure should be stopped.

The blood not only seals the dural leak site, but also increases the CSF pressure, leading to an immediate relief of headache in up to 65% of cases. Parturients in whom the first EBP has failed may be offered a repeat procedure, which has a 90–95% success rate. Maintenance of a supine position for 2–4 hours post procedure is recommended. Further follow-up initially via the telephone and later at the anaesthesia clinic is recommended to confirm resolution of symptoms.

Failure of headache resolution 48 hours after blood patch should raise suspicion of acute subdural bleeding and haematoma (ASDH), or other causes of postpartum headache (see Table 26.2).

Remain vigilant for any of the following:

1. Focal neurological symptoms
2. Change in mental status
3. Headache of unilateral nature not responding to normal pain killers
4. Sudden uncontrollable vomiting
5. Above symptoms with co-existing medical issues (e.g. bleeding disorder or immunocompromise).

Presence of any of these signs necessitates neurological referral and consideration of further investigation, including a computerized tomography (CT) scan/ magnetic resonance imaging (MRI). An obstetric patient with ASDH is best treated in a facility providing both neurosurgery and obstetric care. ASDH may be treated conservatively; however, the presence of localizing signs or neurological deterioration will require neurosurgical intervention.

Itching

The use of intrathecal opioids during neuraxial anaesthesia makes itching one of the most common side effects observed at follow-up. Itching is more pronounced when opioid is administered intrathecally compared with systemically. The incidence varies from 30–100% with neuraxial anaesthesia. The incidence is highest for intrathecal morphine and lowest with lipophilic drugs such as fentanyl and sufentanil. The exact causal mechanism for itching is not absolutely clear but one theory postulates the existence of an 'itch centre' in the lower medulla, including the trigeminal nucleus. Neuraxial opioids (μ receptor and serotonin receptor mediated) seem to remove the inhibitory effects of pruritis pathways leading to itching, especially along the face and upper thorax.

Less than 1% of patients request treatment for severe itching. Various regimes have been tried. Propofol in sub-hypnotic doses, droperidol, ondansetron, nalbuphine and naloxone are some of the common ones. The best results have been obtained with naloxone given sub-cutaneously (50–150 μg) or via a low-dose infusion (0.4–0.6 mg/h), and by using nalbuphine and naltrexone, though higher doses of these opioid antagonists result in a diminishing quality of analgesia.

Postoperative nausea and vomiting (PONV)

PONV is common in pregnancy; other factors during the peripartum period increase the risk. These incude the use of neuraxial opioids, intraoperative hypotension associated with sympathetic blockade, supplementation with systemic opioids, use of ergometrine, exteriorization of uterus (visceral pain), and pain postoperatively are the chief factors responsible for this side effect. The incidence is higher during caesarean delivery after spinal anaesthesia (20–30%) as compared to general anaesthesia (10%) with the incidence falling somewhere in between for epidurals. Intrathecal morphine has the highest incidence of around 50–60% compared to the more lipophilic agents like diamorphine (10–30%) and fentanyl (<10%). The incidence of PONV is higher when the dose of intrathecal opioid is increased.

Several pharmacological and non-pharmacological strategies (oxygen, acupressure at P6 point, intravenous fluids) have been investigated to prevent this side effect, with variable success. Prophylactic 5-HT3 antagonists, cyclizine, scopolamine, droperidol, and dexamethasone or a combination of them have been used and have the best evidence of reducing PONV. A review emphasized the need to optimize intraoperative care by reducing hypotension with vasopressors, aiming for adequate block height, giving appropriate doses of neuraxial opioids, minimizing surgical stimuli and by judicious use of uterotonics. Prophylactic antiemetics should be reserved for high-risk patients. A Cochrane review 2012 on the interventions for reducing nausea and vomiting during caesarean section concluded that there was insufficient data to demonstrate any class of intervention (5HT antagonist, dopamine antagonist, sedative) was superior to another. There were no significant differences observed in the comparison of combined vs. single interventions.

Awareness

This refers to a state where patients can recall intraoperative events and is caused as a result of inadequate general anaesthesia. This complication is known to cause significant dissatisfaction, anxiety, sleep and behavioural disturbances, including post-traumatic stress disorder (PTSD) in a parturient. The incidence in obstetrics is estimated at 1:200–1:350. Factors contributing to this include: the use of rapid sequence induction, use of thiopentone in inappropriately low doses, use of muscle relaxants, the concern of exposing the fetus to anaesthetic agents, increased risk of difficult intubation, obesity, short 'obstetric gap' i.e. time from induction to start of surgery, the effect of volatile agents on uterine tone, junior staff managing surgery out of hours. The results of the 5th National Audit Project, 'Accidental Awareness during General Anaesthesia in UK and Ireland 2014', made a number of recommendations for obstetric anaesthesia. Anaesthetists should be aware of the increased risk of awareness in obstetric patients, particularly when undergoing caesarean section. Appropriate doses of induction agents, nitrous oxide, volatile agents and opioids should be used. If airway management proves difficult, plans should be in place regarding additional IV anaesthesia or plans to allow return of consciousness. Failed regional anaesthesia progressing to general anaesthesia in obstetric surgery is an additional risk factor for awareness.

It has been suggested that parturients having general anaesthesia be warned about this risk. A minimum alveolar concentration (MAC) of at least 0.7–1 of volatile agent (monitored with a volatile agent monitor) has been suggested as the minimum during GA for lower segment caesarean section (LSCS). Assessing depth of anaesthesia during LSCS is difficult and none of the available monitors have shown to be superior to monitoring simple vital signs like pulse blood pressure, sweating and tears (PRST).

A senior anaesthetist should review any patient complaining of awareness. The events surrounding the event, including the anaesthetic chart, should be reviewed. The patient should be offered an apology and appropriate counselling and all the conversation and assessments documented for future reference in case of legal action.

Respiratory depression (RD)

The use of neuraxial opioids in the obstetric anaesthesia setting makes this one of the most feared complications after an operative intervention. The true incidence is not known though figures ranging from 0.01–7% have been quoted in the literature. This large variation is due to the fact that there is lack of agreement on the definition of the term 'respiratory depression'. The risk is higher with neuraxial morphine, which exhibits a biphasic response – initially RD is caused by intravascular absorption (30–90 min) whilst late RD is caused by rostral spread in cerebrospinal fluid and slow penetration into the brainstem. RD caused by lipophilic opioids (fentanyl, sufentanil (0.02% or less) and diamorphine) is rare, though early onset RD has been reported in the literature. Risk factors in obstetrics include morbid obesity, pre-eclamptics on magnesium sulfate and patients receiving concomitant doses of opioids via other routes.

It is important that nursing staff monitor the respiratory rate, sedation score and oxygen saturation, following neuraxial opioid administration for at least 10–12 hours if diamorphine has been used and to at least 24 hours if morphine is used to provide analgesia. Local protocols should exist in each delivery unit to ensure a swift response to respiratory events noted by staff. These include administration of naloxone as a bolus and/or an infusion, and if necessary by securing the airway to prevent hypoxia and aspiration.

Neurological complications

Neurological complications during the peripartum period could be intrinsic to the process of labour and delivery or could result from an extrinsic intervention such as a neuraxial anaesthetic. Those resulting from regional anaesthesia are fortunately rare, though it is difficult to ascertain their exact incidence. Studies from Sweden (over 250,000 obstetric neuraxial blocks) quote an incidence of 1:25,000 and from France quote an incidence of neuropathy of 1:1000–1:3000 for spinal and 1:5000–1:10,000 for epidural anaesthesia.

A meta-analysis (15 studies, 987,218 patients) reported a calculated rate of transient neurologic (< 1 y) injury of 2.57/10,000. In the UK, a national audit project (NAP3 January 2009) by the Royal College of Anaesthetists (RCOA) described an incidence of permanent nerve damage of between 0.2 (optimistically) and 1.2 (pessimistically) in 100,000 of the obstetric population, based on a study of 320,000 regional blocks. One study, looking for postpartum neurological symptoms from anaesthesia and obstetric factors combined, found the incidence to be much higher – almost 1 in 150 patients.

Intrinsic nerve damage

Intrinsic nerve damage (1% incidence) mainly presents as peripheral nerve lesions and is caused as a result of obstetric and fetal reasons. Rarely the fetal head can compress blood vessels supplying the trunk, conus medullaris or cauda equina.

Almost all major peripheral nerves of the lower limb can be damaged, with factors ranging from exaggerated lumbar lordosis, maternal obesity, diabetes, fetal macrosomia, use of forceps, use of retractors during LSCS and lithotomy position. For the anaesthetist, it is important to know the functional anatomy to delineate the possible nerves implicated in injury. Lateral cutaneous nerve of thigh or meralgia paraesthetica, femoral nerve palsy (affecting sensation on the anterior thigh, hip flexion and knee reflex), obturator nerve palsy (affecting medial thigh and hip adduction) and the common peroneal or the lumbosacral trunk injury (presenting as foot drop) are the most common lesions. Fortunately most are neuropraxial in nature and will recover within a few months. Nerve conduction studies will help in diagnosis and determine whether the lesion is central or peripheral.

Extrinsic nerve damage

This can be caused by a number of factors: traumatic, chemical, ischaemic, infective and others (caused by CSF leakage and unknown factors):

- *Nerve root damage* – this is most likely caused by the needle/catheter whilst establishing a neuraxial block in the parturient. Pain and/or paraesthesia are often experienced at the time of instrumentation. The occurrence and site of pain whilst performing the block must always be documented on the anaesthetic chart. It usually

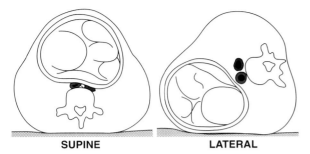

Figure 1.1 The relationship between the gravid uterus and the IVC in the supine and lateral positions. A black and white version of this figure will appear in some formats.

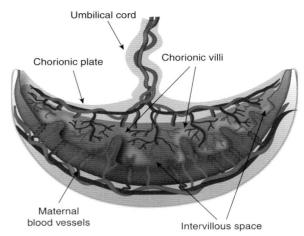

Figure 2.2 Structure of the placenta. A black and white version of this figure will appear in some formats.

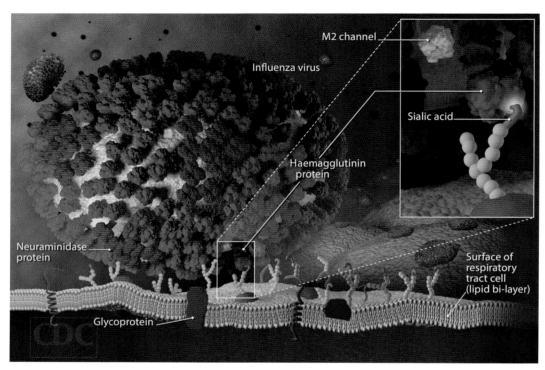

Figure 15.1 Structure of influenza virus (http://www.cdc.gov/flu/images/influenza-virus-fulltext.jpg (accessed 25/2/2013). A black and white version of this figure will appear in some formats.

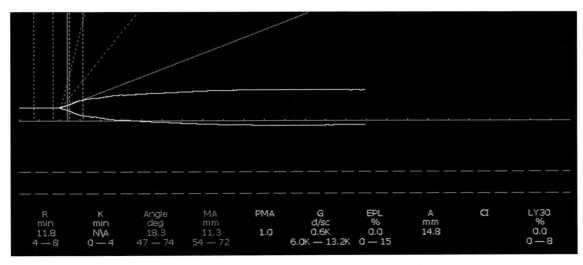

R	K	Angle	MA	PMA	G	EPL	A	CI	LY30
min	min	deg	mm		d/sc	%	mm		%
11.8	N\A	18.3	11.3	1.0	0.6K	0.0	14.8		0.0
4 — 8	0 — 4	47 — 74	54 — 72		6.0K — 13.2K	0 — 15			0 — 8

Figure 21.2 TEG at presentation. A black and white version of this figure will appear in some formats.

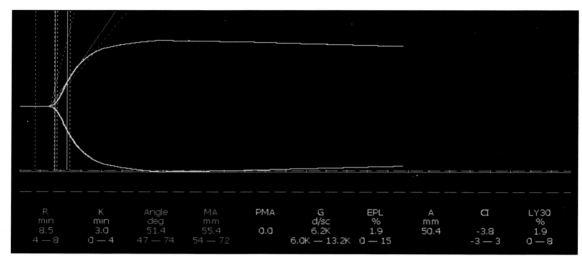

R min 8.5 4 — 8	K min 3.0 0 — 4	Angle deg 51.4 47 — 74	MA mm 55.4 54 — 72	PMA 0.0	G d/sc 6.2K 6.0K — 13.2K	EPL % 1.9 0 — 15	A mm 50.4	CI -3.8 -3 — 3	LY30 % 1.9 0 — 8

Figure 21.3 TEG after correction with blood products. A black and white version of this figure will appear in some formats.

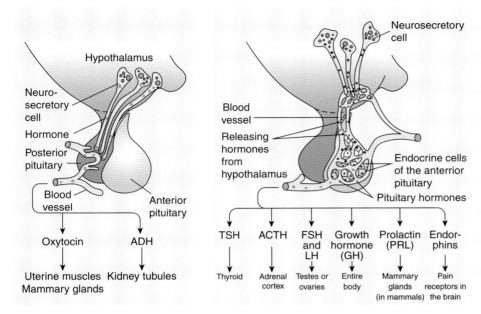

Figure 22.1 The pituitary. A black and white version of this figure will appear in some formats.

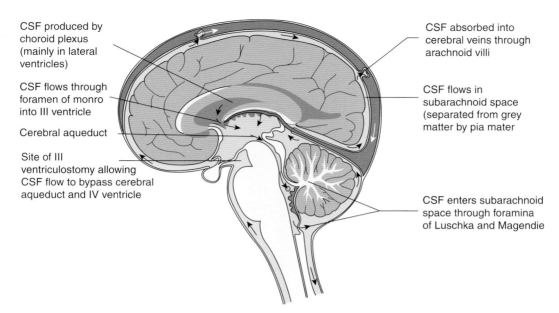

Figure 22.2 Cerebrospinal fluid production and flow. A black and white version of this figure will appear in some formats.

The labels on the figure read:

CSF produced by choroid plexus (mainly in lateral ventricles)

CSF flows through foramen of monro into III ventricle

Cerebral aqueduct

Site of III ventriculostomy allowing CSF flow to bypass cerebral aqueduct and IV ventricle

CSF absorbed into cerebral veins through arachnoid villi

CSF flows in subarachnoid space (separated from grey matter by pia mater

CSF enters subarachnoid space through foramina of Luschka and Magendie

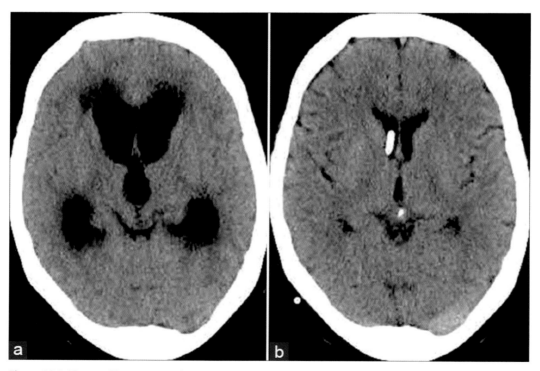

Figure 22.3 The two CT scan images demonstrate (a) dilated lateral venticles with a teardrop-shaped third ventricle and periventricular oedema. (b) An image of treated hydrocephalus with a ventricular drain *in situ* (this may be an EVD or ventriculo- shunt. A black and white version of this figure will appear in some formats.

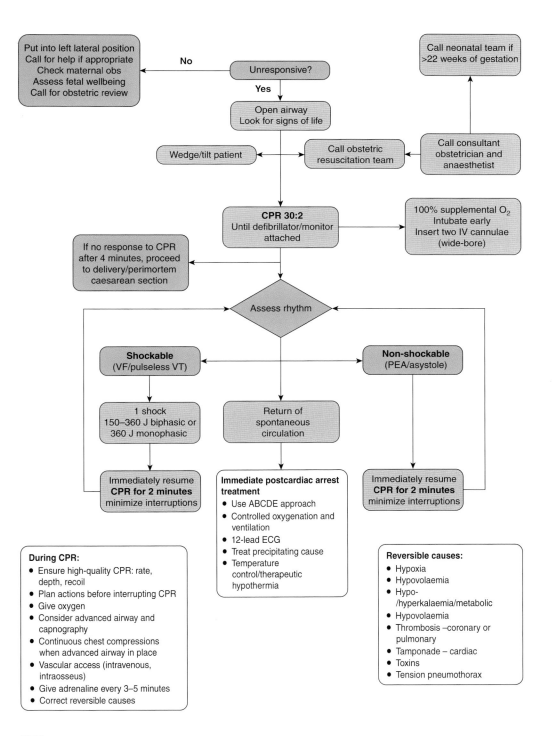

Figure 25.1 Maternal collapse algorithm. (Reproduced from Royal College of Obstetricians and Gynaecologists. *Maternal Collapse in Pregnancy and the Puerperium*. Green-top Guideline No. 56. London: RCOG; 2011, with the permission of the Royal College of Obstetricians and Gynaecologists.) A black and white version of this figure will appear in some formats.

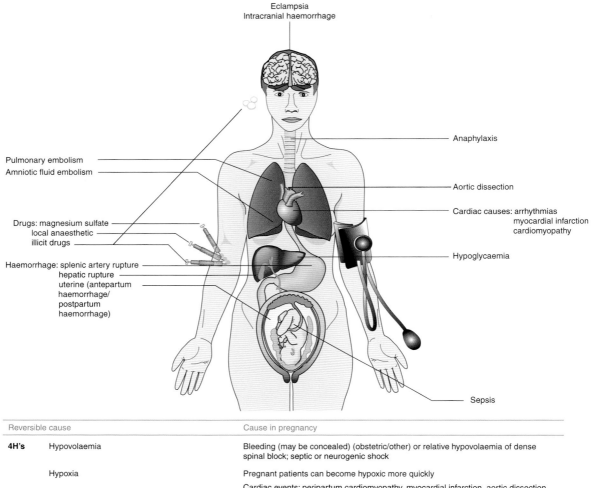

Eclampsia
Intracranial haemorrhage

Anaphylaxis

Pulmonary embolism
Amniotic fluid embolism

Aortic dissection

Cardiac causes: arrhythmias
myocardial infarction
cardiomyopathy

Drugs: magnesium sulfate
local anaesthetic
illicit drugs

Hypoglycaemia

Haemorrhage: splenic artery rupture
hepatic rupture
uterine (antepartum
haemorrhage/
postpartum
haemorrhage)

Sepsis

Reversible cause		Cause in pregnancy
4H's	Hypovolaemia	Bleeding (may be concealed) (obstetric/other) or relative hypovolaemia of dense spinal block; septic or neurogenic shock
	Hypoxia	Pregnant patients can become hypoxic more quickly
		Cardiac events: peripartum cardiomyopathy, myocardial infarction, aortic dissection, large-vessel aneurysms
	Hypo/hyperkalaemia and other electrolyte disturbances	No more likely
	Hypothermia	No more likely
4T's	Thromboembolism	Amniotic fluid embolus, pulmonary embolus, air embolus, myocardial infarction
	Toxicity	Local anaesthetic, magnesium, other
	Tension pneumothorax	Following trauma / suicide attempt
	Tamponade (cardiac)	Following trauma / suicide attempt
Eclampsia and pre-eclampsia		Includes intracranial haemorrhage

Figure 25.2 Causes of maternal collapse. (Reproduced from Royal College of Obstetricians and Gynaecologists. *Maternal Collapse in Pregnancy and the Puerperium*. Green-top Guideline No. 56. London: RCOG; 2011, with the permission of the Royal College of Obstetricians and Gynaecologists.) A black and white version of this figure will appear in some formats.

presents as hypoaesthesia or paraesthesia along the relevant dermatome and very rarely with muscular weakness. Most recover within a few weeks. The patient should be reassured and if symptoms persist or lead to mobility issues, a neurological opinion should be sought. Damage to the conus medullaris has been described following spinal and epidural anaesthesia, and could be caused by a block placed at a relatively high level in the neuraxis or by abnormally low-lying conus. A lumbar disc prolapse may cause nerve root damage, and this usually presents as back pain and sciatica (see Chapter 17).

- *Chemical* – this can lead to aseptic meningitis or chronic adhesive arachnoiditis (CAA). Previously, detergents, contaminants in epidurals, contrast agents and more recently 2% chlorhexidine have been implicated in CAA, where incidence is not known. Rice *et al.* have defined CAA after neuraxial block as: back pain, increasing with activity, leg pain, which may be bilateral, neurological abnormality on examination, most commonly hyporeflexia and MRI changes consistent with CAA (Table 26.3). Leg weakness, sphincter disturbances, paraplegia and hydrocephalus have been described in case reports of CAA. Rarely, aseptic meningitis has been described following neuraxial blockade, where patients present with signs and symptoms of meningism, but no organism is isolated from CSF. Fortunately, it has a self-limiting benign course.

- *Infective* – meningitis (*Streptococcus viridans*) and epidural abscess (*Staphylococcus aureus*) have been described following neuraxial anaesthesia, but are fortunately rare in obstetrics. The NAP3 audit revealed an incidence of epidural abscess of 1 in 300,000. The source of infection could arise from the skin flora, vaginal flora or the airway of the anaesthetist. Strict asepsis is mandatory for all procedures. Cases of suspected CNS infection

necessitate a senior anaesthetic review. MRI spine should be performed urgently to confirm epidural abscess, antibiotics commenced and neurosurgical referral for emergency decompressive laminectomy if necessary.

- *Ischaemic* – anterior spinal artery syndrome has been reported as a result of hypotension and hypoperfusion of the spinal cord. Spinal/epidural haematoma has been reported in coagulopathic patients and has a low incidence of 1 in 200,000. In the NAP3 audit no vertebral canal haematomas were reported.

- *Others* – abducens and facial nerve palsy associated with intracranial hypotension have been reported following ADP and EBP. Transient neurological symptoms (TNS), a benign self-limiting condition, presents with moderate to severe lower limb pain with no neurological deficit. It is most commonly attributed to spinal hyperbaric 5% lignocaine. Cauda equina syndrome as a result of damage to sacral nerve roots (S2–4) either by needle trauma or due to the use of spinal microcatheters using 5% lignocaine have been reported. This leads to a bowel/bladder dysfunction with saddle anaesthesia and varying degrees of lower limb weakness. Urgent MRI spine to exclude a haematoma or an abscess is mandatory, along with neurological referral.

Pre-existing neurology should be documented prior to neuraxial anaesthesia. Document any intraprocedural paraesthesia. Neurological issues raised during follow-up should prompt a full clinical examination and senior input. Patients presenting with red flags (Table 26.4) should have appropriate imaging and neurological/neurosurgical referral. Figure 26.1 is an example of a diagnostic algorithm used in our institute.

Table 26.3 Magnetic resonance imaging criteria for diagnosis of adhesive arachnoiditis

1. Conglomerations of adherent nerve roots residing centrally within the thecal sac
2. Nerve roots adherent peripherally giving the impression of an 'empty sac'
3. Soft tissue mass replacing the sub-arachnoid space

Table 26.4 Red flags on postpartum neurological examination

1. Persistent or progressive neurological deficit
2. Signs and symptoms of meningism
3. Bladder, bowel dysfunction
4. Saddle anaesthesia
5. Any bilateral signs
6. Back pain associated with fever
7. Any back pain in an immunocompromised patient

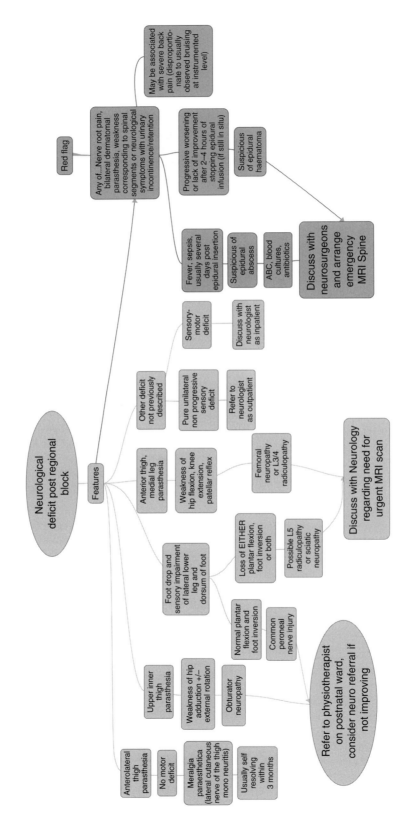

Figure 26.1 Neuropraxia algorithm. (Courtesy of Adam Zermansky, Kirsty MacLennan, Peter Sandbach and Rachel Stoeter.)

Follow-up

Anaesthetic contact with the parturient may occur at any time during the antenatal or peripartum period. Quality of care delivered at each point of contact is important. Patient safety, clinical effectiveness and patient experience have been highlighted as some of the key attributes of quality. Without appropriate follow-up of patients postoperatively, the quality of service provided cannot be evaluated.

The Association of Anaesthetists of Great Britain and Ireland (AAGBI) and The Obstetric Anaesthesia Association (OAA) in the UK recommend that all women who have received regional analgesia, anaesthesia or general anaesthesia be reviewed following delivery. The review provides feedback for the anaesthetic team. This helps to improve the service and maternal satisfaction based on real patient feedback.

The main aims of follow up are to:

- Identify issues regarding anaesthetic management
- Determine any side effects of the anaesthetic intervention
- Determine the quality of the postoperative care rendered to the parturient
- Gauge maternal satisfaction.

Most UK hospitals use a postanaesthetic intervention follow-up questionnaire. An example is highlighted in Figure 26.2. Follow up should focus on the quality of analgesia provided, any relevant side effects and whether those could affect the patient's daily routine (e.g. PDPH, sensory or motor symptoms). A recent study by Nguyen *et al.* highlighted open questions about follow-up (e.g. how are you feeling?) and specific questioning (do you have any pain at the moment?) might be necessary to identify pain after surgical intervention. All women should feel able to offer constructive criticism about the care they received as this can help guide service improvement. Concerns identified warrant swift senior attention. Clear lines of communication should exist between anaesthetists, obstetricians, midwifery staff, other specialities, e.g. neurology, and the parturient.

Most inpatient follow-ups occur 24–36 hours after delivery. Telephonic follow-up may be possible in those discharged early. Community midwives and general practitioners provide support once the parturient has been discharged.

Parturients experiencing the anaesthetic complications in Table 26.5 should be seen in clinic 6–8 weeks following delivery. This enables explanation of events, time for questions and can lead to a discussion about how care could be improved. This may help reduce litigation and improve service delivery.

Maternal experience

Childbirth is one of the most significant events in a woman's life. Maternity services strive to ensure a positive overall experience irrespective of the mode of delivery.

Most developed nations now publish a survey about women's experience of all aspects of childbirth, including postnatal care. Examples include, *What Mothers Say, Delivered with Care* and *Listening to Mothers* from Canada, UK and USA. These surveys cover a wide range of information pertaining to:

- Socio-economic and demographic status
- Social habits
- Antenatal care
- Antenatal and peripartum parturient information
- Medical interventions
- Postpartum health and care including length of stay in hospital
- Partner involvement
- Infant feeding
- Community midwife involvement.

By analysis of regional variations, statistics of perinatal care and review of real-life experiences, these surveys are able to make recommendations to improve education, quality of care and maternal satisfaction.

Maternal experience has been assessed as overall maternal satisfaction after birth, which serves as a marker of quality of care provided by the 'child birthing team'. Salmon *et al.* introduced the concept of birth experience as a multidimensional phenomenon defining emotional distress, physical discomfort and fulfilment in the form of a 20-item, validated questionnaire using a Likert scale. Studies looking into maternal experience and satisfaction using Salmon's questionnaire have found that women planning caesarean reported a more favourable birth experience than women planning vaginal birth, due in part to low satisfaction associated with unplanned caesarean. The studies concluded that maternal satisfaction with childbirth could be improved by efforts to reduce unplanned caesarean, but also by support for maternal-choice caesarean, a theme that has recently

Follow-up Proforma (Please tick all that apply)

1) **Anaesthetic Interventions**

Single Shot Spinal   Epidural   CSE
Intrathecal Catheter   Remifentanil Patient-Controlled Analgesia (PCA) for Labour
General Anaesthesia   Transversus Abdominal Plane Block

2) **Mode of Delivery**

Vaginal   Vaginal Instrumental
LSCS   Grade of LSCS: 1 2 3 4

3) **Quality of Pain Relief in Labour**

In Labour   Good Moderate Poor
During Delivery   Good Moderate Poor
Problems Identified
1) Unilateral Block   2) Missed Segments   3) Re-sited

4) **Intraoperative Discomfort**

None   Mild   Moderate   Severe

5) **Postoperative Pain Relief Prescription**

Paracetamol   NSAIDS   Oral Opioids (specify)   PCA (specify)

6) **Postoperative Pain**

None   Mild   Moderate   Severe

7) **Side Effects**

None   Sore Throat   Nausea   Vomiting   Itching

Headache

1) Post Dural Puncture Headache
2) Other

Neurological Issues

1) Sensory Symptoms
2) Motor Symptoms
3) Urinary Catheter > 24 hours

Others (e.g.: Myalgia/ Untoward Dreams etc.)

8) **Critical Care Admission Required**: Yes/No

9) **Is anaesthetic follow-up in the clinic required**: Yes /No (If yes please discuss with consultant)

10) **Maternal Satisfaction**

Very satisfied   Satisfied   Dissatisfied

Figure 26.2 Suggested questionnaire for follow-up of patients

been supported by the National Institute of Clinical Excellence (NICE) in the UK.

Measuring satisfaction with respect to childbirth is complex as it is influenced by many factors. A poor maternal or neonatal outcome can result in a negative experience, irrespective of standard of care. Key factors identified in systematic reviews of maternal satisfaction with childbirth experience included: personal expectations, sense of control, support from caregivers, quality of care-giver–patient relationship and involvement in decision-making. All other factors, including woman's demographics, childbirth preparation, pain and continuity of care seemed to be less important.

Most anaesthetists use visual analogue or numerical rating scales to measure maternal satisfaction. Although simple, they are not very objective. Further, we still await a reasonable tool to measure labour pain experience. Can anaesthetists influence maternal experience and satisfaction during childbirth, despite the findings

Table 26.5 Patients to follow up in clinic 6–8 weeks post-delivery

- Pain during LSCS (the most common reason for litigation in the UK)
- Traumatic delivery because of failed regional anaesthesia
- PDPH ± EBP
- Persistent neurological symptoms
- Awareness or unpleasant dreams experienced by the patient
- Any critical incident such as wrong drug/wrong route error

in most studies that absence of pain during childbirth does not equate to satisfaction? The answer is a resounding 'Yes!' Anaesthetists play a major role in many aspects of maternal care in the peripartum period, including: maternal medicine, managing parturients with morbid obesity, operative interventions (25% CS rate in UK), maternal high-dependency care on delivery suite and responding to early warning scores in sick parturients.

For some women, analgesia and anaesthesia can have an enormous impact on maternal satisfaction. Studies have shown that maternal experience is enhanced if adequate information is provided about the anaesthetic options and if participation in decision-making is encouraged. For labour analgesia, using low-dose local anaesthetic/opioid mixtures and mobile epidurals, which decrease motor block and promote vaginal delivery, enhance a woman's feeling of control in labour and are perceived to encourage satisfaction.

Some of the main factors decreasing parturient satisfaction are:

- Poor satisfaction with the anaesthetic procedure (commonly pain or nausea)
- Delay in analgesia
- Perceived poor co-ordination within healthcare teams
- Maternal or neonatal complications.

Negative maternal experience should be explored to identify any deficiencies in care and guide service improvements.

Key points

1. The risk of developing a PDPH is related to the experience of the operator, the number of attempts, and the size and type of needle used.

2. When treating a PDPH, 65% of patients will experience immediate relief of headache after a first EPB, 90–95% after a second EBP.

3. Although itching is common following intrathecal opiates, <1% of patients require treatment.

4. Peripartum neurological complication can be caused by intrinsic nerve damage (most common, due to obstetric causes) or extrinsic nerve damage (less common, including central neuraxial blocks).

5. Postanaesthetic follow-up allows teams to evaluate and further develop their service.

Further reading

Balki, M. and Carvalho, J. C. (2005). Intraoperative nausea and vomiting during cesarean section under regional anesthesia. *Int. J. Obstet. Anesth.*, **14**, 230–241.

Carvalho, B. (2008). Respiratory depression after neuraxial opioids in the obstetric setting. *Anesth. Analg.*, **107**(3), 956–961.

Cook, T. M., Counsell, D. and Wildsmith, J. A. W. (2009). Major complications of central neuraxial block: report on the Third National Audit of The Royal College of Anaesthetists. *Br. J. Anaesth.*, **102**(2), 179–190.

Klein, A. M. and Loder, E. (2010). Postpartum headache. *Int. J. Obstet. Anesth.*, **19**, 422–430.

Paech, M. J., Scott, K. L., Clavisi, O., Chua, S. and McDonnell, N.; ANZCA Trials Group (2008). A prospective study of awareness and recall associated with general anaesthesia for caesarean section. *Int. J. Obstet. Anesth.*, **17**, 298–303.

Robins, K. and Lyons, G. (2009). Intraoperative awareness during general anesthesia for caesarean delivery. *Anesth. Analg.*, **109**, 886–890.

Royal College of Anaesthetists and Association of Anaesthetists of Great Britain and Ireland (2014). *Accidental Awareness During General Anaesthesia in UK and Ireland*, 5th National Audit Project. London: RCOA.

Szarvas, S., Harmon, D. and Murphy, D. (2003). Neuraxial opioid-induced pruritus: a review. *J. Clin. Anesth.*, **15**(3), 234–239.

Turnbull, D. K. and Shepherd, D. B. (2003). Post-dural puncture headache: pathogenesis, prevention and treatment. *Br. J. Anaesth.*, **91**(5), 718–729.

Van de Velde, M., Schepers, R., Berends, N., Vandermeersch, E. and De Buck, F. (2008). 10 years of experience with accidental dural puncture and post dural puncture headache in a tertiary obstetric anaesthesia department. *Int. J. Obstet. Anesth.*, **17**, 329–335.

Chapter

27

Multidisciplinary teaching and training on the delivery unit

Catherine Robinson and Cathy Armstrong

Introduction

In addition to the central role of training anaesthetic trainees in obstetric anaesthesia, working on the delivery unit presents many opportunities for the anaesthetist to become involved in education of the multidisciplinary team. Areas of education particularly pertinent to the skills and expertise of anaesthetists are:

- Training midwives and junior doctors in delivering critical care on the delivery unit and recognition and management of the sick parturient
- Skills/drills or simulation team training for emergencies on the delivery unit
- 'Pain relief for childbirth' education for midwives, including regional analgesia/anaesthesia.

One of the main challenges in education provision on the delivery unit is the ability to allocate adequate time for staff, away from clinical duties, to attend training. It is known that when units are busy and understaffed, staff are unable to take up scheduled teaching sessions. Anaesthetists should help champion education needs at management level and also consider strategies to deliver education in novel ways that can be accessed more flexibly, for example, with e-learning packages or video podcasts of lectures.

Education on the sick parturient

Care of the sick parturient on the obstetric unit has been closely examined in recent years. Recurrent themes in the triennial reports from the Centre for Maternal and Child Enquiries (CMACE) have included:

- Late recognition by midwifery and medical staff of the seriously unwell woman

- Inadequate and infrequent performance of basic observations
- Inappropriate or no action taken in women found to have abnormal observations.

Obstetric anaesthetists should be prominent in the education of midwives and junior doctors in the recognition and management of the critically ill obstetric patient.

Midwives must be able to accurately measure and record observations, recognize when they are abnormal and alert the appropriate staff. Many midwives now qualify after a direct-entry degree course and often have had no prior general nursing exposure. While skilled in many areas of parturient management, they often lack the experience of caring for sick medical or surgical patients, and may have an incomplete understanding of the relevance of abnormal physiological observations. The current undergraduate midwifery courses focus mainly on well women, with less emphasis on sick patients or those with pre-existing medical conditions. Future curriculum development within undergraduate midwifery training should aim to address this.

With the 2011 document: 'Providing equity of critical and maternity care for the critically ill pregnant or recently pregnant woman' (see Further reading), we now have national guidance on the competencies required for midwifery and medical staff caring for critically ill obstetric patients. Critically ill parturients should have the same standard of care, whether in a general critical care unit or a maternity unit. Midwives and medical staff on the delivery unit must have the competencies outlined in the Department of Health document 'Competencies for Recognising and Responding to Acutely Ill Patients in Hospital'.

Core Topics in Obstetric Anaesthesia, ed. Kirsty MacLennan, Kate O'Brien and W. Ross Mcnab.
Published by Cambridge University Press. © Cambridge University Press 2015.

Table 27.1 Suggested minimum acute care practical skill competencies to be undertaken by midwives (those in italics could be taught to a subgroup of 'maternal critical care trained midwives')

System	Practical skill
Cardiovascular	Can set up 3-lead ECG monitoring Can perform a 12-lead ECG *Successfully completed* <u>*arterial line competencies*</u> *including: assisting with insertion, checking components of arterial line system, checking for complications, common causes of inaccuracy Taking out arterial lines* *Successfully completed* <u>*central venous line competencies*</u> *including: assisting with insertion, checking components of CVP line system, checking for complications, common causes of inaccuracy. Taking out CVP lines*
Respiratory	Can set up and administer oxygen via: non-rebreathing mask, MC mask, nasal cannulae Can set up and administer nebulized medication Can set up, check and use suction equipment including portable suction Can perform peak flow monitoring (PEFR) and act on abnormality *Can set up, check and use equipment for administering humidified oxygen*
Renal	Can accurately complete fluid balance chart
Neurological	Can complete basic neurological observations, including pupillary responses and conscious level (AVPU or GCS), recognize and act on abnormality
Haematological	Completed local blood administration competencies
Communication	Gives structured handover of acutely unwell patient, including clear communication of management plan

These competencies are wide-ranging and require significant educational input. Courses on acute illness recognition and management have been developed, which can help units achieve some of these staff competencies, but to cover all of them requires a co-ordinated educational strategy. These acute care competencies are not specific to obstetrics, so training on specific obstetric problems and management of medical illness during pregnancy needs to be incorporated into the training provided. There are also practical skills outlined in the document which may be best taught and assessed by in-house hospital training (Table 27.1).

The training required for midwifery and medical staff caring for the acutely unwell parturient can be provided with a combination of the following:

- Courses on acute illness recognition and management
- Maternal early warning score training
- Life support training
- Specific obstetric critical care training courses: formal courses available, some with postgraduate qualification or in-house formal obstetric critical care training

- Communication training
- Obstetric emergencies training: skills/drills training, simulation training
- Practical skills teaching (see Table 27.1).

All midwifery and junior medical staff need to be competent in the recognition and management of the acutely unwell parturient, management of obstetric emergencies and life support in the pregnant woman. A subset of midwives should be given further formal training in care of the critically ill woman on the delivery unit, including competence in caring for women with invasive monitoring.

A designated group of clinicians (obstetric, anaesthetic, midwifery and critical care) need to take on the role of facilitating this training and ensuring that the competencies are met. Ongoing audit is essential to identify how many staff have achieved these competencies. The Department of Health document states that there should be a board-level sponsor for the implementation of these competencies. Support at senior management level is essential to facilitate the provision of time and resources for the competencies to be achieved.

Obstetric early warning scores

A top 10 recommendation in the 2003–2005 CMACE report was to introduce a specific early warning score system for obstetric patients, in order to aid detection of the patient who is becoming unwell, and trigger the appropriate response.

Early warning scores (EWS) were introduced over 10 years ago in the non-obstetric setting. It is known that physiological abnormalities are a marker for clinical deterioration. A 'track and trigger' early warning score system consists of periodic recording of a set of physiological variables, such as heart rate, respiratory rate, blood pressure, temperature (*track*) with pre-defined criteria then *triggering* an appropriate response, i.e. the right personnel attending within an agreed time frame.

Non-obstetric EWS are not appropriate for the obstetric population as the normal physiological changes of pregnancy would result in inappropriate triggering. Scores must also be altered to detect pathology specific to the parturient, such as pre-eclampsia.

There is potential for any woman to be at risk of physiological deterioration in the peripartum period, this cannot always be predicted. 'Equity in Critical Care' recommends that all women have physiological observations done on admission. Following labour and delivery, observations should be done a minimum of 12-hourly.

Over the last few years, many obstetric units across the UK have independently introduced modified early warning scores for obstetric patients (MEOWS). This has unfortunately resulted in a wide variety of charts being used throughout the country – some using a colour-coded scheme and others producing a numerical aggregate score that determines the response triggered. The physiological variables included also vary: most systems track heart rate, respiratory rate, blood pressure and temperature. Some also include urine output, oxygen saturations, pain score and conscious level.

This lack of consistency in early warning systems between hospitals can cause confusion and is a potential patient safety issue. Movement of staff between hospitals necessitates further education on the new track and trigger system. This same problem occurred in the non-obstetric setting and resulted in the development of a National Early Warning Score (NEWS), launched in 2012 (see Further reading). This means training can be standardized and national education

training tools set up – the NEWS e-learning package can be accessed for free.

Most obstetric early warning scores have not yet been validated, but Singh *et al.* have studied the validity of the obstetric early warning score system recommended by CEMACH and found that the system had good sensitivity and reasonable specificity for predicting morbidity in obstetric patients.

Agreement on a national obstetric early warning score would be welcomed. A standardized training program similar to the NEWS on-line training package would equip staff with transferable skills and avoid duplication of training if a healthcare professional moves hospital.

MEOWS training for midwives and medical staff needs to include:

- How to accurately measure and document observations
- Clinical relevance of abnormal physiological observations
- How to calculate overall MEOWS score
- Ability to trigger an appropriate response, including correct personnel contacted to review in an appropriate time frame and changes to the frequency of observations if indicated
- What to do if MEWS reassuring, but staff member still concerned about patient.

When teaching staff about the track and trigger system it must be emphasized that a full set of observations must be completed to produce an accurate score and that once the patient has triggered then a response *must* be activated.

Early warning scores may help in the early recognition of the sick obstetric patient, but we must teach the midwives and junior medical staff not to be totally reliant on them. Early warning scores shouldn't replace thinking about the whole clinical picture. Most pregnant women initially compensate well physiologically so may have a falsely reassuring early warning score. Women with any concerning symptoms or signs need full assessment, even if their early warning score is normal.

Multidisciplinary team training in maternity

Organization and delivery of multidisciplinary team training is an important part of curriculum design when identifying and planning the training needs of a maternity service.

Obstetric emergencies require complex management in a time-constrained, often life-threatening situation. There is significant pressure on the assembled team, necessitating effective clinical management and efficient teamwork. The team can be large, consisting of midwives, obstetricians, anaesthetists, paediatricians, theatre staff and support workers, all with an important role to play.

Traditional healthcare teaching occurs within individual disciplines. For example, obstetricians attend training programmes separately from anaesthetists and midwives attend training programmes away from doctors. In an urgent clinical situation all of these disciplines are expected to work together, often performing multiple complex tasks. While intradisciplinary training is important to allow individuals to develop expertise within their own field, it is widely agreed that a group of individual experts does not automatically constitute an expert team.

Multidisciplinary training is nationally recognized as a risk management strategy. In the UK, evidence of provision of multidisciplinary emergency skills drills is a criterion laid out in the Clinical Negligence Scheme for Trusts (CNST) document for maternity services. The required scenario topics are listed in Figure 27.1. Compliance with these standards will impact on the level of indemnity cover offered to the Trust by the NHS Litigation Authority.

There are various recognized formats for multidisciplinary team training within maternity. These include:

- Workplace-based emergency skills drills on delivery suite
- Formal simulation programmes – either 'in-house' or within a simulation centre setting.

Whatever the format, simulated multidisciplinary training provides an environment where learners can make, detect and correct errors without adverse consequences.

Workplace-based emergency skills drills

Workplace-based emergency skills drills involve the organization of an emergency simulation scenario within the delivery suite or maternity theatre setting. While the organizers, management and selected clinical staff are informed prior to the exercise, other front-line staff should be unaware that this is a simulated emergency until they attend.

This form of multidisciplinary team training has many advantages. In particular it can highlight local logistical issues and potentially identify unexpected training needs. For example, it may highlight that the defibrillator trolley is located too far from a particular delivery room, or that staff were not aware of its location.

One major disadvantage, however, is that while these drills may test the logistics and protocols of the organization as a whole it may not always be tailored towards the individual learner. The simulation is often run while other clinical activities are taking place, and participants may feel that their attention is being deflected from actual patient care, thereby devaluing the educational impact for those learners. The organizers should therefore guarantee patient safety and optimize educational impact by ensuring that these simulations are not run when the labour ward is busy. Conducting comprehensive debrief sessions for participants and increasing familiarity by regular simulations will also help to enhance the learner experience.

Formal multidisciplinary team training simulation programmes

Formal multidisciplinary simulation programmes are those run either 'in house' within the hospital or in a simulation centre that are not run alongside actual clinical work. They necessitate staff to be released from their clinical duties for protected study time.

They require a faculty of trainers to run a pre-planned set of scenarios with clearly defined learning objectives. These should include a mixture of clinical knowledge/skills and communication/team behaviours. Time should be taken to ensure adequate introduction to the intended learning objectives and course format. The main body of the course will comprise a selection of structured simulation scenario cycles (see Figure 27.2 for suggested format). Some programmes will include elements of didactic teaching to consolidate knowledge further. A wrap-up session to highlight lessons learned is deemed to be useful.

The main advantage of this formal format over the workplace-based emergency skills drills is the time taken to consolidate learning for the individual. There

- Cord prolapse
- Shoulder dystocia
- Vaginal breech
- Antepartum and postpartum haemorrhage
- Eclampsia

Figure 27.1 Clinical scenarios for emergency skills stipulated in CNST criteria

Briefing

- Roles are allocated (as much as possible, participants should perform in their normal roles, to aid fidelity and relevance)
- Facilitator gives some clinical details and 'sets scene' for upcoming scenario
- Any procedural queries are answered by facilitator

Scenario

- Simulated scenario is commenced
- One or more faculty members form part of the multidisciplinary team to ensure smooth running of the scenario and allow some direction if necessary
- Another faculty member operates the mannequin (it is useful to have a communication link between the mannequin operator and any faculty members participating)
- A separate faculty member observes and then facilitates the debrief (use of performance assessment checklists/tools can be helpful)
- Any candidates not participating may observe via cameras/one-way screen from a viewing room or directly *in situ*

Debrief

- Arguably the most important element which aims to complete the experiential learning cycle
- Faculty members facilitate inclusive debrief discussion encouraging comments from participants and observers. Aim to identify learning points and desirable/undesirable behaviours
- Use of video debriefing can be a particularly effective demonstration tool.

Figure 27.2 Suggested format of simulation scenario cycle

are no conflicting workload pressures and several simulation cycles will be completed allowing repetition and consolidation of many of the learning points.

An obvious disadvantage is the significant resources required, including expert faculty, equipment and time away from the workplace.

Components required for successful simulation team training in obstetrics

Planning and implementation of any type of training programme within a healthcare institution is challenging. Some of the components thought to be required for the success of an obstetric simulation programme include the following.

Institutional backing

A simulation programme requires significant resources, not just in terms of money for equipment, but also time. Organizers of emergency drills will require planning time and formal programmes will require both faculty and participants to be given time away from their clinical duties to attend. It is vital, therefore, to have enthusiastic support for the programme at both a departmental and Trust level.

Strong leadership

An enthusiastic leader of the program is vital to maintain momentum and keep the programme continuously updated and relevant. Ideally, obstetric team training should be an ongoing process rather than a once-only event.

Curriculum design

Outcome-based curriculum design is crucial and it is important to conduct a needs assessment within your own organization to ensure the course is specifically tailored and fit for purpose. A close relationship between the faculty and the clinical risk team can allow development of scenarios based on actual problems experienced in the department and their subsequent solutions to produce highly relevant local learning.

Setting: 'in-house' versus simulation centre

An 'in-house' programme does offer some obvious advantages in terms of cost, accessible location for attendance by staff and perhaps more importantly, the ability to tailor the course to local needs. The 'in-house' course will utilize the equipment, protocols and general set-up that the participants will be exposed to within their normal working environment, therefore bearing more relevance for those attending.

The simulation centre setting offers different advantages, including expert simulator facilitators, often better equipment and debriefing facilities (i.e. video feedback). The learning environment is away from the workplace, so the staff are far less likely to be affected by workload pressures on the delivery suite.

Many large healthcare institutions now have their own simulation centres on site.

Equipment

When considering communication/behavioural team training there is no educational benefit in the use of complex high-fidelity mannequins over low-tech simple mannequins, so a successful team training programme can be developed without necessarily needing to buy expensive equipment. The key is to create psychologically realistic 'high fidelity' scenarios. Patient actors and role-play can have an excellent effect on the fidelity of the scenario. Fidelity can be further increased by the use of a delivery room with all equipment set out in a familiar way.

High-fidelity mannequins do have a recognized role for some procedural skills within obstetric simulation. For example, specialized mannequins can allow measurement of pressures applied during delivery and can aid with training of shoulder dystocia and vaginal breech delivery techniques.

The key is to identify the main aims and objectives of the course during curriculum design, therefore allowing planning of the equipment required.

Performance assessment tools

Development of tools to assess both clinical and teamwork performance within the scenario is important, not necessarily just to provide standardized evaluation of performance, but also to facilitate the feedback discussion in the debrief session and ensure that the intended outcomes are discussed. These tools often comprise a checklist of desired actions and behaviours that can be used by faculty members or course participants observing the scenario. Designing performance assessment tools that are fit for purpose is a challenging task. Skills-based markers can be relatively easy to highlight within scenario design (e.g. timely administration of magnesium in eclampsia). Desirable team behaviours are harder to outline. Some suggestions are listed below:

- Stating the emergency in specific terms
- Management of critical tasks using closed-loop communication
- Use of an SBAR style of communication
- Reduced number of exits from the room
- A leader with high global situational awareness.

It is widely agreed that simulation is a useful educational tool; however, in the literature there is little robust evidence demonstrating the cost effectiveness and patient safety impact of multidisciplinary simulation training in obstetrics. It is clear, however, that obstetric emergencies require a skilled and functional multidisciplinary team. Provision of a controlled environment where team members can make, detect and correct errors without adverse consequences remains very attractive. The popularity and development of simulation team training initiatives in obstetrics is likely to continue whilst awaiting quality research to guide content and design.

Education on 'pain relief for childbirth' for midwives

Anaesthetists have traditionally been key in providing epidural training for midwives, but are also ideally placed to provide education for all methods of pain relief for labour. Anaesthetic involvement in this teaching is essential, as new techniques or drugs are introduced onto the labour ward that are unfamiliar to non-anaesthetists, such as remifentanil patient-controlled analgesia (PCA).

The undergraduate midwifery syllabus does not specify how much time should be given to learning about analgesia in labour and the time given to this important area of learning can vary widely between university courses. By getting involved as anaesthetists in providing education for midwives at the undergraduate level, we can introduce clinically important issues, such as recognition and management of complications of opioids, epidurals and spinals, which will equip them well when they qualify and start work on the delivery unit (see Table 27.2).

Midwife training on regional analgesia and anaesthesia

Management of epidural analgesia is a significant part of the modern midwife's workload. When the midwife board agreed in 1970 that midwives could give epidural top-ups independently, it was under the condition that they were properly instructed in the procedure. As anaesthetists we are ultimately responsible for all women with ongoing regional anaesthesia in labour. It is vital, therefore, that we provide robust training for our midwives on the management of women with epidurals or spinals.

Table 27.2 Core topics for 'pain in childbirth' education for midwives

Physiology of pain in labour

Non-pharmacological methods of analgesia including TENS – transcutaneous electrical nerve stimulation

Entonox

Opioid analgesia – routes of administration: oral, intramuscular, intravenous (PCA systems – including remifentanil), intrathecal, epidural. Monitoring required. Side effects and their management

Pain management after caesarean section

Regional analgesia (see Table 27.3)

Table 27.3 Recommended topics for midwife teaching on regional analgesia/anaesthesia

Anatomy of the epidural space, dura and intrathecal space

Basic pharmacology of local anaesthetics and opioids

Physiology of pain in labour – nerve roots involved in labour pain

Differences between epidurals, spinals and combined spinal-epidurals

Beneficial effects of epidurals

Contraindications to epidurals

Side effects of epidurals

Major complications with epidurals: recognition and management

How to assist anaesthetist for epidural insertion: positioning, equipment

Monitoring the woman with an epidural, including assessment of epidural sensory level and degree of motor block

How to give a bolus epidural top-up

Practical 'epidural pump competencies' if using continuous epidural infusions/patient-controlled epidural analgesia

Simple 'troubleshooting' of epidural problems

Documentation

National guidance on education for practitioners caring for patients with epidurals has come from the National Patient Safety Agency (NPSA) Epidural Safety Alert (2007) and the OAA/AAGBI (Obstetric Anaesthetists' Association and the Association of Anaesthetists of Great Britain and Ireland) Guidelines for Obstetric Anaesthetic Services (2013)(see Further reading). The NPSA recommend that training for new staff should include theoretical and competency-based assessment; there should also be a programme of continuing education, including regular updates. Both documents emphasize the need for specific training on potential epidural complications. Although serious complications with epidurals are rare, they are potentially life-threatening and demand prompt recognition and effective early management.

In summary, the documents recommend:

- Midwives must undergo formal training to an agreed standard in regional analgesia
- Training should be competency-based

- Anaesthetists need to be involved in midwife education on regional analgesia/anaesthesia
- Midwives must be aware of potential epidural complications and their management
- Midwives must be able to assess and document sensory block height
- Midwives must undergo regular refresher training.

Also, the NPSA specifically recommends that if epidural bolus top-ups are being used, 'a second practitioner independently confirms that the correct product and line connection have been selected and prepared…' to reduce the risk of wrong route errors. We should ensure that our anaesthetic trainees are also aware of this, as well as our midwives.

Key points

1. One of the main challenges facing education provision on delivery suite is the allocation of adequate time for staff training.
2. Obstetric anaesthetists should be prominent in the education of midwives and junior doctors in the recognition and management of the critically ill obstetric patient.
3. National guidance is available detailing competencies required for midwifery and medical staff caring for critically ill obstetric patients.
4. Midwifery and medical staff should be trained in interpretation of MEOWS.
5. Multidisciplinary team training is nationally recognized as a risk-management strategy.
6. Anaesthetic involvement in analgesia and anaesthesia training for midwives is essential.

Further reading

Ayres-de-Campos, D., Deering, S. and Siassakos, D. (2011). Sustaining simulation training programmes – experience from maternity care. *BJOG*, **118**, Suppl. 3: 22–26.

Centre for Maternal and Child Enquiries (CMACE) (2011). Saving Mothers' Lives: reviewing maternal deaths to make motherhood safer: 2006–2008. The Eighth Report on Confidential Enquiries into Maternal Deaths in the United Kingdom. *BJOG*, **118**, Suppl. 1: 1–203.

Department of Health (2008). Competencies for Recognising and Responding to Acutely Ill Patients in Hospital. http://webarchive.nationalarchives.gov.uk/+/www.dh.gov.uk/en/Consultations/Closedconsultations/DH_083630 (accessed May 2015).

Eppich, W., Howard, V., Vozenilek, J. and Curran, I. (2011). Simulation-based team training in healthcare. *Simul. Healthcare*, **6**, Suppl. S14–S19.

Maternal Critical Care Working Group (2011). Providing equity of critical and maternity care for the critically ill pregnant or recently pregnant woman. http://www.rcoa.ac.uk/document-store/providing-equity-of-critical-and-maternity-care-the-critically-ill-pregnant-or (accessed May 2015).

Merien, A. E. R., van de Ven, J., Mol, B. W., Houterman, S. and Oei, S. G. (2010). Multidisciplinary team training in a simulation setting for acute obstetric emergencies: a systematic review. *Obstet. Gynecol.*, **115**(5), 1021–1031.

National Patient Safety Agency (2007). Safety Alert 21: 'Safe practice with epidural injections and infusions. http://www.nrls.npsa.nhs.uk/resources/?entryid45=59807 (accessed May 2015).

Obstetric Anaesthetists' Association and the Association of Anaesthetists of Great Britain and Ireland (2005). *Guidelines for Obstetric Anaesthetic Services.* London: OAA/AAGBI.

Royal College of Physicians (2012). *National Early Warning Score (NEWS): Standardising the assessment of acute illness severity in the NHS. Report of a working party.* London: Royal College of Physicians.

Singh, S., McGlennan, A. and England, A. (2012). A validation study of the CEMACH recommended modified early obstetric warning system (MEOWS). *Anaesthesia*, **67**(1), 12–18.

Strachan, B. and Crofts, J. F. (2008). *The SaFE study – Simulation and Fire-drill Evaluation: Proof of principle study of the effect of the individual and team drill on the ability of labour ward staff to manage acute obstetric emergencies – Study Report.* London: Department of Health.

Chapter 28

Clinical governance and patient safety

Kate O'Brien

Introduction: how clinical governance originated

The NHS was established in 1948 and there was no agenda for quality of care. In the early years of the NHS most doctors rarely looked at their clinical practice or results. In the late 1960s hospital activity analysis was introduced to provide better patient-based information.

In 1969 the Ely Hospital report was published; this was the first of the modern inquiries into failure of care: this included cruelty to patients, threatening behaviour, indifference to complaints and lack of care by the physician superintendent. Subsequently there have been more than 30 reports highlighting the exact same failings.

The NHS had become a victim of its own success and it had to acknowledge that there had to be clear financial bounds. The Griffiths report (1983), commissioned by the government, described a lack of accountability for quality of care at the local level. This led to:

- Appointment of managers to lead healthcare units
- Medical staff involvement in the management teams
- More flexibility in team structures
- Introduction of clinical responsibility for quality of the service.

The first government white paper was published in 1997. 'The New NHS, Modern, Dependable' was the first document to directly address the issues of quality and effectiveness of clinical care and the introduction of a national framework to drive improvements in NHS performance.

On the back of this paper two new organizations were commissioned:

- National Institute for Clinical Excellence (NICE)
    - To assess treatments using up to date evidence
    - To provide high-quality national guidelines

- The Commission for Health Improvement (CHI)
    - This body was set up to ensure that high standards of quality and safety for patients and staff were established and maintained.

In 1998 a white paper was published 'A First Class Service: Quality in the New NHS'. This was the first paper to mention the concept of clinical governance. The rationale was to have a framework, which would ensure that high standards of care are achieved. The paper also stated that:

- Staff must undertake lifelong learning
- Staff must maintain professional standards
- The NHS needs to be more open and accountable to the public.

Scally and Donaldson (1998) commented on the fact that quality of care issues had become secondary to fiscal and activity targets, subsequent to the Griffiths report. The white paper outlined, for the first time in the NHS:

- 'all health organizations will have a statutory duty to seek quality improvement through clinical governance'.

Clinical governance will provide:

- 'a framework through which NHS organizations are accountable for continually improving the quality of their services and safeguarding high standards of care by creating an environment in which excellence in clinical care will flourish'.

'Clinical governance in the New NHS' (1999) provided guidance on how to implement clinical governance.

The 'Darzi Report' (2009) aimed for high-quality care for all patients, with the emphasis on moving from centrally set targets to local services focused on quality. This encompassed:

Core Topics in Obstetric Anaesthesia, ed. Kirsty MacLennan, Kate O'Brien and W. Ross Mcnab.
Published by Cambridge University Press. © Cambridge University Press 2015.

- Improved information on clinical performance e.g. Dr Foster
- Greater choice and control for patients
- Strengthened incentives for providers
- New assessment processes to focus on quality of care, patient safety and patient experience.

Background: why good clinical governance processes are necessary

In the 30 years before 'The New NHS' paper there had been a number of inquiries into the appalling treatment by staff of patients in certain institutions.

The biggest reforms, however, were as a result of two inquiries; these have resulted in significant changes to professional regulation and the clinical governance process.

1. The Royal Liverpool Children's Inquiry (1999)
2. The Bristol Royal Infirmary Inquiry (2001).

The lessons from all these inquiries were strikingly similar:

- Inadequate leadership
- Systems and process failures
- Poor communication
- Disempowerment of staff and service users
- Organizational or geographic isolation
- Lack of internal and external transparency regarding the problems that exist
- Ineffective complaints systems.

The 'Bristol Inquiry' (1997) was one of the major catalysts for the introduction of clinical governance:

An independent expert review (1995), looking at the excess deaths in under one-year-old infants undergoing complex open-heart surgery, showed that one surgeon had mortality figures fourfold those of his colleagues performing the same operation. There had been concerns raised by an anaesthetist about the high death rates as early as 1991. Despite sharing his concerns with colleagues, a senior medical officer at the hospital and the Department of Health, no action was taken by the Bristol Healthcare Trust until April 1995.

With the changes implemented in the child cardiac surgery service in Bristol, following the review in 1995, the mortality had fallen from:

- 29% (April 1991–March 1995)
- 3% (April 1999–March 2002).

The Mid Staffordshire NHS Foundation Trust Public Inquiry final report (2013) was published, and the root causes were almost identical to all the previous inquiries; however, the report emphasized poor clinical governance structures as one of the main factors.

Clinical governance in obstetric anaesthesia

The NHS Clinical Governance Support Team was established to support the implementation of clinical governance.

Clinical effectiveness

This is the efficacy of an intervention and/or treatment provided to a population. The most reliable evidence comes from large randomized control trials and systematic reviews.

NICE and national service frameworks were put in place to standardize healthcare provision. For any treatment or intervention the recommendations will also include clinical and cost effectiveness and efficacy.

Clinical guidelines should contain the best available evidence for the management of a particular condition. Guidelines reduce variation in management, improve quality of care and are used to set standards. In anaesthesia we have several professional bodies that provide guidance and standards of care.

Clinical audit is central to effective clinical governance. The process consists of:

- Identifying the problem
- Setting criteria and standards, e.g. adherence to a guideline
- Data collection
- Comparing the performance against the criteria and standards
- Implementing change to address deficiencies.

The GMC document 'Good Medical Practice' is explicit in stating that all doctors have a duty to participate in clinical audit.

An integrated care pathway (ICP) is multidisciplinary, locally agreed practice for a specific patient group. Documentation is standardized and in one place, this assists team working and communication.

One example is an ICP for enhanced recovery for elective caesarean section. The pathway starts at the preoperative visit and finishes at discharge home. All the key stages in the process of an elective caesarean section are explicitly stated in the multidisciplinary document. There may be variances from the pathway and these must be documented.

It is essential that ICPs are evaluated and reviewed on a regular basis. This ensures the pathway is based on the best evidence and is an easy tool to use. Often it is not until the ICP is used clinically that the problems become apparent. Audit of the ICP should include the process, the content, agreed targets and outcomes, and non-adherence (variance) to the pathway.

Risk management

Effective risk management is fundamental to governance in any organization. The risks may be at the patient level or at an organizational level. Healthcare is a vast and complex organization, which will never be free from error. Risk management is a way of assessing risk awareness, identification, assessment, controls and assurance.

Risk awareness

This is the recognition of the likelihood of risks, hazards and situations that may result in patient harm. Being risk aware can modify hazards by putting contingencies in place to mitigate the risk.

A successful patient safety culture is when there is a high awareness of safety issues at all levels of the organization. There are barriers to developing this culture, and this is seen in the majority of the national inquiries:

- A blame culture
- Failure to understand human factors:

  . Bystander apathy – people are less likely to take responsibility if they assume that someone else will do it
  . Fixation – errors occur because the person is convinced that their first interpretation was correct
  . Groupthink – usually large groups, fixate on doing things one way; no other options are explored, often to avoid confrontation and conflict.

Improving risk awareness should be part of the curriculum for all healthcare professionals, this involves:

- Types of patient safety incidents
- Human error and human factors
- How to report risks and incidents

- Mechanisms for learning from error, e.g. root cause analysis
- Safety briefings, e.g. WHO Safe Surgery Checklist.

Risk identification

This follows risk awareness in the risk management process. The definition of a patient safety incident is 'Any incident which could have or did cause harm, loss or damage to a patient receiving care in the NHS'.

Clinical risks may be identified by many sources:

1. Incident reporting

   a. System for submission of reports
   b. Need clear indications on what to report; a list of triggers may be available
   c. Ease of reporting
   d. Confidential reporting
   e. Centralized reporting with links to other services, e.g. complaints and claims
   f. Needs to be a factual and objective account
   g. Needs to be regarded as a positive action

Where there is a culture of incident reporting it helps to identify risk promptly and facilitates the introduction of preventative measures.

Root cause analysis is a method of looking at the reasons why an incident happened. A multidisciplinary team is tasked with investigating the incident and then produces an action plan to put preventative strategies in place. Communicating the lessons learned is an essential part of the action plan process.

2. Claims and complaints

This is an important source of feedback from our patients. Often with the complaints investigation there are failings in:

- Systems of care delivery
- Patient pathways
- Facilities
- Individual practice

There is a specific timeframe for complaints and it is important that feedback to the patient is prompt.

3. Clinical audit
4. Morbidity and mortality meetings
5. Executive safety walk-rounds
6. Proactive risk assessment, e.g. high-risk injectable medicines
7. National reports and surveys, e.g. confidential enquiries into maternal deaths
8. Patient safety alerts, e.g. MHRA.

Risk assessment

This is the tool that is used to stratify any particular risk; this estimates the likelihood and the consequence of the risk being realized (Table 28.1).

Table 28.1 Risk assessment tool

Consequence	Likelihood				
	1	**2**	**3**	**4**	**5**
	Rare	*Unlikely*	*Possible*	*Likely*	*Almost certain*
5 Catastrophic	5	10	15	20	25
4 Major	4	8	12	16	20
3 Moderate	3	6	9	12	15
2 Minor	2	4	6	8	10
1 Negligible	1	2	3	4	5

1–3	Low risk
4–6	Moderate risk
8–12	High risk
15–25	Extreme risk

The process:

- Proactive assessment
  - Undertaken to prevent a patient safety incident
  - For example, increasing numbers of deliveries in the unit. Rate of significant postpartum haemorrhage 1%. The fluid warming devices available were old and inadequate to manage the potential risk, put on the risk register (Consequence 5 × Likelihood 3 = 15). Two rapid infusors purchased within 6 weeks.
- Reactive assessment (Table 28.2)
  - In response to an incident

Table 28.2 Reactive assessment

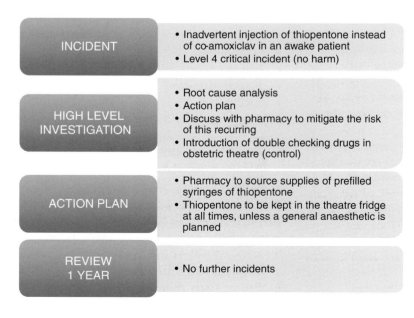

INCIDENT	• Inadvertent injection of thiopentone instead of co-amoxiclav in an awake patient • Level 4 critical incident (no harm)
HIGH LEVEL INVESTIGATION	• Root cause analysis • Action plan • Discuss with pharmacy to mitigate the risk of this recurring • Introduction of double checking drugs in obstetric theatre (control)
ACTION PLAN	• Pharmacy to source supplies of prefilled syringes of thiopentone • Thiopentone to be kept in the theatre fridge at all times, unless a general anaesthetic is planned
REVIEW 1 YEAR	• No further incidents

Risk control options

The main aim of risk management is to ensure effective controls are in place to mitigate established risks. As stated before, risks are inevitable in any healthcare system and it is important to understand that risks cannot be eliminated completely.

The controls put in place target both the elements of the risk and reduce the consequence to the patient and organization. Measures used to implement controls include: policies, guidelines, procedures, checks and human factors that are used by the organization. The residual risk must be regularly monitored and reviewed.

Complaints

Approximately 140,000 are made to the NHS annually. Any complaint about an aspect of treatment or care can be submitted by the patient or by someone else affected. This has to be within 12 months of the clinical episode. The patient advice and liaison service (PALS) will often resolve the issue at the time, if not then they will provide the information to make a formal complaint.

As a clinician, the best way to deal with dissatisfaction is to be honest and open about the patient's concerns. The vast majority of complaints involve poor communication.

Written complaints must be acknowledged within 3 working days, together with an offer to discuss the matter. A response should be made within 6 months. Complaints should be part of the agenda at each clinical governance meeting.

Clinical negligence claims

The NHS Litigation Authority (NHSLA) was established in 1995: its purpose was to manage clinical negligence claims on behalf of the NHS in England.

The Clinical Negligence Scheme for Trusts (CNST) is administered by the NHSLA. The remit of the organization was to provide indemnity to member trusts and their employees with respect to clinical negligence claims.

The NHSLA provided a framework of risk management standards to reduce the likelihood of patient safety incidents. The Maternity CNST standards were related to all aspects of obstetric care. The assessment relied predominantly on guidelines and audit for each domain. The benefit of the assessment, if passed, was a reduction in the Trust indemnity payment to the

NHSLA. The NHSLA website stated that assessments provided organizational information, but did not reflect quality of care or patient outcomes.

From 1st April 2014, there will be no more assessments and no further updates to the standards from the NHSLA. The standards will be devolved to clinical teams. The agenda will be focused on patient care, quality and patient safety improvements to reduce harm and provide meaningful outcome data.

Other aspects of clinical governance

Dashboards

Dashboards can be very useful to monitor changes over time, usually the data per month is collated and added to the existing data.

The main datasets are:

- Bookings, including date of first contact with a midwife
- Delivery numbers and types of delivery
- Where was the delivery
- Caesarean section rate
- Staffing levels: sickness is often a surrogate marker of a stressful working environment
- Training and education attendance
- Maternal morbidity, e.g. postpartum haemorrhage, eclampsia
- Risk management: number of SUIs level 4 and 5
- Neonatal transfers
- Complaints
- Infection: MRSA, *Clostridium difficile*
- Teaching and training (Chapter 26)
- Research effectiveness.

Patient safety

'The protection of patients against harm that results from the efforts or lack of efforts of the healthcare system.'

Patient safety is central to clinical governance. About 10% of inpatients in NHS hospitals have an adverse event, which impacts on their outcome, and 50% of these are preventable.

The Patient Safety First Campaign (2008):

- Patient safety to be the highest priority

- Make all avoidable death and harm unacceptable
- Trust board leadership. The aim was to have executive accountability for certain strategic priorities with regards to harm and deliver a patient safety culture.

The campaign was effective in that the patient safety agenda had a much higher profile.

Key points

1. Clinical governance and patient safety is the key to providing a sound basis for quality improvement in all aspects of care.
2. Assessment of risk is a powerful tool to ensure patient safety. The Royal College of Anaesthetists and Association of Anaesthetists publish evidence-based standards, which should be used as evidence if there are resource shortfalls.

Further reading

Department of Health. (1997). *The New NHS: Modern, Dependable*. London: The Stationery Office.

Department of Health. (1998). *A First Class Service – Quality in the New NHS*. Consultation Document.

Department of Health (2008). *High Quality Care for All: NHS Next Stage Review Final Report*: (Cm7432). London: The Stationery Office.

Francis Inquiry Report (2013). www.midstaffspublicin quiry.com/report

Haynes, A. B., Weiser, T. G., Berry, W. R. *et al.* (2009). A surgical safety checklist to reduce morbidity and mortality in a global population. *N. Engl. J. Med.*, **360**, 491–499.

Higgins, J. (2001). The listening blank. *Health Serv. J.*, **111** (5772), 22–25.

NHS Litigation Authority www.nhsla.com

The Report of the Public Inquiry into Children's Heart Surgery at Bristol Royal Infirmary 1984–1995: (Cm 5207) (2001). London: The Stationery Office.

Chapter 29

Ethics, consent and the law

Andrew Heck and Ross Clark

Introduction

Obstetric anaesthesia poses a convergence of all the ethical and consensual dilemmas only encountered infrequently in other areas of anaesthetic practice. The patient population typically ranges from teenagers upwards, with varying degrees of capacity to consent, a varying level of understanding and information provision, but a universally high degree of expectation. Patients can present in a time-critical manner and the treatment of the mother or the baby may cause risk to one to save the other. The anaesthetist, however, is well placed to provide a unifying voice of reason in this difficult arena. Therefore it is incumbent on us to have a good grasp of all the pertinent issues. This chapter will cover the issues of consent in the obstetric population, the legal background which underpins our current situation, and finally the ethical controversy that surrounds pregnancy testing in the under-16s.

Consent

We perform consent for a number of reasons: ethical, legal and regulatory body requirements.

Ethical considerations

Ethically there are a couple of underlying principles which govern our actions in this area. The Select Committee of Medical Ethics ruled in their report in 1994 that:

> Alongside the principle that human life is of special value, the principle is widely held that an individual should have some measure of autonomy to make choices about his or her life … As the law stands medical treatment may be given to competent adult patients only with their informed consent, except in an emergency.

Making your own decisions, whether this involves consenting or withholding consent, of itself promotes welfare. Seeking consent helps to establish trust between the doctor and patient, and actively involves the patient in their own care. The requirement of consent therefore promotes individual autonomy and encourages rational decision-making. These derive from the basic principle of the right to self-determination, complemented by the principle of respect for persons.

Legal considerations

The Department of Health has released the Reference Guide to Consent for Examination or Treatment (2009), which provides a guide to the legal framework that all health professionals need to take account of in obtaining valid consent for any examination, treatment or care that they propose to undertake. It stems from the case law that exists within English law and from Court of Appeal judgements, as well as the European Court of Human Rights.

The classic legal statement comes from an American case (*Schloendroff v Society of New York Hospital*, 1914) where the presiding Judge stated:

> Every human being of adult years and sound mind has a right to determine what shall be done with his own body; and a surgeon who performs an operation without the patient's consent commits an assault.

In English law the concept of 'informed consent' exists in a very limited form in *Chatterton v Gerson* (1981) where it was deemed the patient need only be informed in broad terms of the nature of the procedure. As ethically and legally acceptable consent must always be 'informed' it has been argued that this phrase represents a tautology, and that 'valid consent' is more appropriate. Valid

---

Core Topics in Obstetric Anaesthesia, ed. Kirsty MacLennan, Kate O'Brien and W. Ross Mcnab.
Published by Cambridge University Press. © Cambridge University Press 2015.

consent comprises three main aspects: the voluntary nature of consent, information provision and time for deliberation, and that the patient must be competent and autonomous. The requirements for valid consent in UK law were set out in the case highlighted below:

> **Re. C (Adult: refusal of treatment) [1994] 1 WLR 290, Fam Div**. An inpatient at Broadmoor Hospital for over 30 years due to schizophrenia had developed advanced gangrene of the foot. He was given an 80% chance of dying despite treatment, but he refused surgical treatment. The judge acknowledged that although his general capacity was impaired, he understood the nature, purpose and effect of the proposed treatment; he retained relevant treatment information and had arrived at a clear choice. This case confirmed the three-stage test that is now required for valid consent and also that mental disorder per se does not preclude someone from making a legally competent medical decision.

The three-stage approach to establish capacity to consent

1. Can the patient comprehend and retain the necessary information?
2. Does the patient believe the information?
3. Has the patient weighed the information, balanced the risks and benefits, arrived at a choice and communicated it?

With the concept of a legal requirement for valid consent in law, to proceed to administer treatment without consent carries the risks of criminal trespass, any of which could affect the medical practitioner depending on the circumstances:

- *Battery*. This is non-consensual touching – i.e. any act on another person without consent. In law there is no need for the plaintiff to establish loss and all direct damages are recoverable.
- *Assault*. This is criminal assault and battery and is an offense against the Persons Act and has a maximum fine of £5000 and/or up to 6 months imprisonment.
- *Actual bodily harm*. This is any hurt or injury calculated to interfere with health or comfort – so anything from a bruise upwards – and carries up to 5 years imprisonment.

- *Medical negligence*. The plaintiff needs to establish that the negligence of touching without consent has led to the injury for which damages are being claimed. There is therefore a need to establish factual causation in negligence and only foreseeable damages can be recovered.
- *Gross negligence manslaughter*. This charge is attributable when a lawful act is carried out in a reckless manner leading to the death of a patient.
- *Murder*. Where the death of the patient is intended.

With the legal precedent for valid consent established and the litigious consequences outlined, it remains to consider what information provision is considered adequate for valid consent. In the United Kingdom the 'professional practice standard' has been the norm since the *Chatterton v Gerson* case mentioned earlier, where the doctor decides what information the patient should be told. Two contrasting, more recent cases are worth mentioning – *Sidaway v Board of the Bethlem Royal hospital and the Maudsley hospital* [1985] and *Chester v Afshar* [2004].

> **Sidaway v Board of Governors of the Bethlem Royal hospital and the Maudsley hospital AC 871; [1985] 1 All ER 1018, HL**. A patient was consented for spinal surgery, but the surgeon did not disclose a 1–2% risk of cord damage. The patient suffered a spinal cord injury, but the action for negligence failed. The judgement stated that the physician had the right of therapeutic privilege to withhold information from the patient if they thought that passing on the information could harm the patient.

> **Chester v Afshar [2004] UKHL 41**. Again a patient was consented for spinal surgery and the risk of cord damage was not disclosed. The patient suffered a spinal cord injury, but in this instance the surgeon was found guilty of negligence. The judge concluded that the necessary causal connection between the negligence and the injury had been established on the basis that C, if duly warned, would not have undergone surgery as soon as she had, but would have wished to discuss matters further and explore other options.

Clearly the mandate now is to provide information that the individual in front of you needs to know to make a decision. This requires two-way communication and may be the most time-consuming method; nevertheless it is the standard to which we now aspire.

There are situations where the normal consent process may be suspended:

- Where the patient is deemed to have incompetent capacity judged by the three-stage rule. This is covered by the Mental Capacity Act (2005) and Mental Health Act (2007) mentioned below.
- Children <16 years old who are not 'Gillick competent' (see below).
- 16–17 years of age is normally considered competent, but they may not necessarily refuse treatment under certain circumstances – where the illness is very grave or a threat to life and parents consent to treatment, or where the courts over-rule a parental decision.
- Treatment under public health legislation.
- The unconscious patient requiring life-saving surgery under the doctrine of necessity. In these circumstances two requirements must apply: that it is impossible to communicate with the patient and that what is done is what was necessary to save the person's life.

Under 16 years old

This population group are encountered with reasonable frequency in a busy obstetric unit and have a number of ethical and legal concerns:

- What is the extent of their capacity to consent to treatment? It should not be assumed that consent to intercourse equates to capacity for competence.
- Where under-age sexual intercourse has taken place there may be safeguarding concerns, especially if the partner is significantly older or where there is any suspicion of coercion or abuse. The validity of capacity to consent is nearly always questionable in these cases and should almost always involve the close participation of the safeguarding team. These cases must be considered on a case by case basis.

Fraser competence or Gillick competence

- To be 'Gillick' competent, a child must have sufficient maturity to understand the nature, risks and purpose of the proposed treatment.
- 'Gillick' competence is a sliding scale: the level of competence required to consent to having a BP

check is obviously different to consenting to a bone marrow transplant.

- If competent, the child can consent to treatment without parental involvement.
- The child may not refuse treatment when consent has been given by a parent or a court.

Patients without capacity

These patients are provided for within law in England and Wales by the Mental Capacity Act (2005) and the 2007 revision of the Mental Health Act (1983). In Scotland this is provided by Adults with Incapacity (Scotland) Act 2000.

The Mental Capacity Act 2005

- This defined a lack of capacity: ' … a person lacks capacity in relation to a matter if at the material time he is unable to make a decision for himself in relation to the matter because of an impairment of, or a disturbance in the functioning of, the mind or brain'.
- A person lacks capacity if they cannot pass the three-stage assessment.
- The Act also sought to promote capacity by ensuring that clinicians:
  - Provide relevant information, including alternatives
  - Are aware of specific communication and cognitive problems and communicate in an appropriate way
  - Use technology/alternate methods of communication
  - Are aware of factors undermining capacity and alleviate where possible
  - Give sufficient time for discussion
- New provisions were made for:
  - The Lasting Power of Attorney (replaced the Enduring Power of Attorney and allowed those so nominated to make decisions regarding an incapacitated patient, including withholding life-saving treatments).
  - Advance directives, which now have a statutory basis. These have direct applicability to the obstetric situation where blood products may be refused by virtue of an advance directive. To be valid these must have been made by someone over the age of 18, it must specify the treatment(s) to be refused, it must not have been modified verbally or in writing

since it has been made; with refusal of life-sustaining treatment it must include the statement that the decision should stand 'even if life is at risk', that this is in writing and has been signed and witnessed. The validity of an advance directive may be questioned if the patient's behaviour is clearly inconsistent with the decision, if the current situation could not have been anticipated by the patient or if the patient is being treated under the Mental Health Act.

- The Court of Protection, which has the power to make decisions on behalf of individuals that lack capacity, usually in a 'one-off' situation.
- Independent mental capacity advocates. An NHS Trust is now obliged to appoint an independent advocate for decision-making in serious illness where a patient lacks capacity and cannot be represented by other means.

Mental Health Act 1983

This legislation is designed to provide legal stature for the detention, assessment and treatment of the mentally disordered. The umbrella term of what is acceptable medical treatment has been broadened to include such treatments as caesarean section, provided they can be demonstrated to be therapeutic in treating the underlying mental illness. One such case within the arena of obstetrics is published and this will be examined in detail later. It is anticipated that the provisions now made in the Mental Capacity Act provide a more appropriate tool to guide treatment in those that are mentally incompetent.

Where patients are deemed to lack capacity then physicians may proceed in a manner consistent with the patient's best interests within the confines of the Bolam principle (that what is done is considered appropriate by a like-minded body of responsible peers) or under the direction of the courts, Mental Health Capacity Advocate or Lasting Power of Attorney.

Adults with Incapacity (Scotland) Act 2000

This Act aims to safeguard those without capacity over the age of 16 through mental disorder or some inability to communicate. It also lays down guidelines in how others may act on their behalf.

Table 29.1 Factors affecting competence in the obstetric patient

Pain	Influence of others
Fear	Unrealistic expectations
Drugs	Age
Exhaustion	Mental incapacity

Regulatory body requirements

The General Medical Council has laid down guidance in the revised 2008 document 'Consent: patients and doctors making decisions together'. In summary it reinforces that patient consent should be patient-centred with the delivery of accurate, appropriate and timely information with valid alternative therapies and a balanced approach to risk discussion. It also highlights how this should be documented and under what circumstances it may be considered appropriate to withhold information. It is worthwhile to note that the GMC requirements exceed the minimum legal requirements in the United Kingdom.

The obstetric patient

With the underlying principles and stature that guide consent now outlined, it is time to consider how this translates into the obstetric setting. The capacity to consent may be impaired in the obstetric setting for a number of reasons. This incorporates patients who have long-term mental impairment, as well as those in whom capacity to consent would be considered intact in normal circumstances. These factors are outlined in Table 29.1.

There are five obstetric cases represented in case law which highlight how these factors have been dealt with.

Re. S (Adult: refusal of treatment) [1992] A11 ER 671. A 30-year-old women presented in established labour for her third child, but with a transverse lie with the elbow protruding through the cervix. The obstetric team recommended a caesarean section for the health of the mother and fetus as 'a life and death situation', but the woman refused on the basis of religious grounds. The court declared to proceed with caesarean section following an 18-minute hearing.

Tameside and Glossop Acute Services Trust v CH [1996] 1 FLR 762. A 41-year-old patient was detained under s.3 of the MHA due to paranoid schizophrenia. A caesarean section was permitted under s.63 of the 1983 Act as ' achievement of a successful pregnancy was a necessary part of the treatment of her psychiatric condition'. In addition 'the doctor was entitled, if he considered it clinically necessary, to use restraint to the extent reasonably required to achieve the birth of a healthy baby'.

Rochdale NHS Trust v C [1997] 1 FCR 274. The patient arrived at hospital in arrested labour with clinical suspicion of a rupturing uterus due to a previous caesarean section. The obstetrician recommended a life-saving caesarean, but the patient refused. An urgent psychiatric opinion was sought, but unavailable immediately and the obstetrician was of the opinion the woman had full capacity. After a 2-minute hearing the judge was of the opinion she lacked capacity: 'the patient being in the throes of labour with all that involved and who could speak in terms which accepted the inevitability of her own death and that of the child, was not a patient who was able to properly weigh-up the considerations that arose so as to make any valid decision.'

Norfolk and Norwich Trust v W [1997] 2 FLR 613. A patient arrived in arrested labour in the emergency department, but denied she was pregnant. She had a previous history of mental illness with three previous pregnancies all terminated by caesarean section. A psychiatric review judged there was no mental disorder, but were unable to say whether she had capacity. The judge ruled she did not have capacity: although not suffering from a mental disorder she lacked mental competence to make a decision about the treatment as she was incapable of weighing up the considerations involved.

This string of cases led to the Court of Appeal (Butler-Sloss, Saville and Ward, L.JJ.) providing guidance for future caesarean section refusal cases. This guidance is summarized below:

- A mentally competent patient has an absolute right to refuse treatment even if this might lead to her death.

Re. MB (Adult: Medical Treatment) [1997] 2 FLR 426, CA. A caesarean section was recommended for a term breech delivery to which the patient consented. On numerous attempts the patient refused at the point of anaesthesia due to needle phobia. The court applied for a compulsory order for section, which was granted on the grounds that at the point of having her desired treatment her phobia was causing an impairment of her mental functioning, and she was temporarily incompetent. She appealed the decision but the Court of Appeal upheld the decision. The following morning she consented to section voluntarily.

- The only situation in which it is lawful to proceed is if the adult patient did not have the capacity to decide, the treatment was necessary and what was done was no more than was in the best interests of the patient.
- Panic, indecisiveness and irrationality do not necessarily amount to incompetence. However they may indicate incompetence and the gravity of the consequences of the decision are commensurate with the level of competence required to make the decision.
- A person could lack the capacity to make a decision by impairment of mental function due to shock, pain, fatigue, drugs or confusion, but only if the ability to clearly decide is absent as a result.
- Panic induced by fear could influence capacity when extreme, as in the case of *Re. MB*, but fear can also be a rational response to surgery, so every case requires careful scrutiny.
- The interests of the unborn fetus (i.e. *the sanctity of life*) do not take precedence over its mother (i.e. *the principle of autonomy* and *self-determination*) unless she is incapable of making a reasoned choice because of an impairment of mental functioning.
- The unborn fetus does not have a legal status until it is born.

It remains to provide some handy tips on what this means on a day to day obstetric unit. This is summarized in Table 29.2.

The ethics of pregnancy testing in the under-sixteens

Based on National Statistics from 2010 on the rate of conception in under 16-year-olds and the total number

Table 29.2 Putting it into practice

Know GMC and Department of Health guidance

Identify potential competency problems early

Provide evidence-based information early

Minimize factors that erode capacity – pain, fear, panic

Ensure 24-hour access to translation services

Make use of acute pain protocols

See patients early in labour

Clear documentation of the information provided

When in doubt seek expert opinion

of procedures performed on females aged 12–15, some 200 to 300 young women present for surgery each year with a wanted pregnancy. The National Institute for Health and Clinical Excellence and the Health Protection Agency require that the pregnancy status of all reproductive females should be established prior to any procedure that may harm the mother or fetus. There remain, however, some ethical and clinical concerns around mandatory pregnancy tests for this age group:

- Compulsory testing is increasingly being viewed as unethical and, as a certain number of these females would be deemed to be 'Gillick' competent, it has the potential to be discriminatory by not seeking valid consent.
- Preprocedure these young persons are frequently seen in the company of parents or guardians where a sexual history may be embarrassing, and likely uninformative.
- Physical examination to establish pregnancy is unreliable and the menstrual history is often erratic in this age group, making them poor discriminators.
- There is concern that not testing for pregnancy may expose a mother and fetus to harm and may lead to litigious repercussions.
- Capacity to consent can be difficult within this age group.
- Revelation of active sexual history under the legal age of consent may have implications for safeguarding, especially where there is coercion, abuse or where the partner is over the age of 18.
- Given the extremely low rate of positive pregnancies in the under-15 group, enquiring may cause undue distress.

Recent guidance has been issued from an expert working group convened by the Royal College of Paediatrics and Child Health to assist clinicians and institutions in developing local procedures that strike a balance between minimizing harm and complying with national guidelines. A summary of some of their key recommendations is presented below:

1. Preadmission information is invaluable in reducing anxiety and allaying fears concerning questions about sexual activity.
2. The incidence of pregnancy in the under-13 age group is so negligible that this group may be considered exempt.
3. A key component to establishing trust and complying with guidance is an assessment of capacity.
4. Privacy and confidentiality is essential to this process.
5. When a sample is positive it should be repeated, together with serum confirmation. A senior member of the team should be involved and appropriate advice given regarding the risks of proceeding. Where there is suspicion of coercion, abuse or a partner over the age of 18 then local safeguarding procedures should be followed.
6. Any positive pregnancy test under the age of 13 should prompt concerns of safeguarding issues.
7. In the case of clinical emergencies where a sexual history cannot be obtained or competency cannot be assessed then a balance of risk approach must be taken and documented accordingly.

Key points

1. Obstetric patients may have compromised capacity due to many reasons – age, pain, fear, fatigue, drugs and pre-existing mental illness.
2. Department of Health and GMC guidance on consent exist and should be adhered to.
3. All attempts to minimize the erosion of capacity should be made.
4. The provision of information and the assessment of capacity must be carefully documented.
5. Expert opinion should be sought early where there is doubt.
6. Recent guidelines exist on how to approach the issue of pregnancy testing in the under-16 age group.

Further reading

General Medical Council. Consent: Patients and Doctors making Decisions Together (online). http://www.gmc-u

k.org/guidance/ethical_guidance/consent_guidance_index.asp (accessed May 2015).

Montgomery, J. (2002). *Health Care Law, 2nd edn*. Oxford: Oxford University Press.

Royal College of Paediatrics and Child Health (2012). Pre-procedure Pregnancy Checking in Under 16s: Guidance for Clinicians (online). Available: http://www.rcpch.ac.uk/system/files/protected/page/pregnancy%20checking%20guidance%20final.pdf (accessed May 2015).

Stauch, M., Wheat, K. and Tingle, J (2002). *Sourcebook on Medical Law, 2nd edn*. London: Routledge Cavendish Publishing Ltd.

Index